Fat-Soluble Vitamins: Biochemistry and Clinical Applications

Fat-Soluble Vitamins: Biochemistry and Clinical Applications

Editor: Lucy Taylor

AMERICAN
MEDICAL PUBLISHERS
www.americanmedicalpublishers.com

AMERICAN
MEDICAL PUBLISHERS
www.americanmedicalpublishers.com

Cataloging-in-Publication Data

Fat-soluble vitamins : biochemistry and clinical applications / edited by Lucy Taylor.
p. cm.
Includes bibliographical references and index.
ISBN 978-1-63927-670-7
1. Vitamins, Fat-soluble. 2. Vitamins, Fat-soluble--Therapeutic use. 3. Biochemistry.
4. Clinical biochemistry. 5. Vitamin therapy. 6. Therapeutics, Physiological. 7. Vitamins.
I. Taylor, Lucy.
QP772.F37 F383 2023
612.399--dc23

American Medical Publishers,
41 Flatbush Avenue,
1st Floor, New York,
NY 11217, USA

ISBN 978-1-63927-670-7 (Hardback)

Contents

Preface

Vitamins are organic molecules and essential micronutrients that are required by organisms in small quantities for appropriate functioning of their metabolism. Essential nutrients are usually not synthesized or if at all, are synthesized in insufficient quantities in the body of organisms. Therefore, organisms must obtain vitamins through proper diet. The majority of vitamins contain groups of related molecules known as vitamers. For instance, vitamin E has eight vitamers comprising four tocotrienols and four tocopherols. In humans, 13 vitamins are found. They are vitamins A, E, C, K, D, B1, B5, B9, B2, B12, B3, B7, and B9. The vitamins are classified as being either fat-soluble or water-soluble based on their solubility. Vitamins A, D, E, and K are fat-soluble vitamins whereas all others are water-soluble. The fat soluble vitamins are absorbed by the body along with the fats. They are stored within the liver and the fatty tissue. This book explores the biochemistry and clinical applications of vitamins. Those in search of information to further their knowledge on fat soluble vitamins will be greatly assisted by it.

This book unites the global concepts and researches in an organized manner for a comprehensive understanding of the subject. It is a ripe text for all researchers, students, scientists or anyone else who is interested in acquiring a better knowledge of this dynamic field.

I extend my sincere thanks to the contributors for such eloquent research chapters. Finally, I thank my family for being a source of support and help.

Editor

1

Multiple Modes of Vitamin K Actions in Aging-Related Musculoskeletal Disorders

Kotaro Azuma [1] and Satoshi Inoue [1,2,*]

[1] Department of Systems Aging Science and Medicine, Tokyo Metropolitan Institute of Gerontology, 35-2 Sakae-cho, Itabashi-ku, Tokyo 173-0015, Japan; azumak@tmig.or.jp

[2] Division of Gene Regulation and Signal Transduction, Research Center for Genomic Medicine, Saitama Medical University, 1397-1 Yamane, Hidaka-shi, Saitama 350-1241, Japan

* Correspondence: sinoue@tmig.or.jp

Abstract: Vitamin K is a fat-soluble vitamin that was originally found as an essential factor for blood coagulation. With the discovery of its role as a co-factor for γ-glutamyl carboxylase (GGCX), its function for blood coagulation was understood as the activation of several blood coagulation factors by their γ-carboxylation. Over the last two decades, other modes of vitamin K actions have been discovered, such as the regulation of transcription by activating the steroid and xenobiotic receptor (SXR), physical association to 17β-Hydroxysteroid dehydrogenase type 4 (17β-HSD4), covalent modification of Bcl-2 antagonist killer 1 (Bak), and the modulation of protein kinase A (PKA) activity. In addition, several epidemiological studies have revealed that vitamin K status is associated with some aging-related diseases including osteoporosis, osteoarthritis, and sarcopenia. Clinical studies on single nucleotide polymorphisms of GGCX suggested an association between higher GGCX activity and bone protective effect, while recent findings using conditional knockout mice implied that a contribution in protective effect for bone loss by GGCX in osteoblastic lineage was unclear. GGCX in other cell lineages or in other tissues might play a protective role for osteoporosis. Meanwhile, animal experiments by our groups among others revealed that SXR, a putative receptor for vitamin K, could be important in the bone metabolism. In terms of the cartilage protective effect of vitamin K, both GGCX- and SXR-dependent mechanisms have been suggested. In clinical studies on osteoarthritis, the γ-carboxylation of matrix Gla protein (MGP) and gla-rich protein (GRP) may have a protective role for the disease. It is also suggested that SXR signaling has protective role for cartilage by inducing family with sequence similarity 20a (*Fam20a*) expression in chondrocytes. In the case of sarcopenia, a high vitamin K status in plasma was associated with muscle strength, large muscle mass, and high physical performance in some observational studies. However, the basic studies explaining the effects of vitamin K on muscular tissue are limited. Further research on vitamin K will clarify new biological mechanisms which contribute to human longevity and health through the prevention and treatment of aging-related musculoskeletal disorders.

Keywords: γ-glutamyl carboxylase (GGCX); steroid and xenobiotic receptor (SXR); pregnane X receptor (PXR); osteoporosis; osteoarthritis; sarcopenia; osteocalcin; matrix Gla protein (MGP); Gla-rich protein (GRP)

---

1. Introduction

Vitamin K is a fat-soluble vitamin that is classified into three forms, namely vitamin K1 (phylloquinone), K2 (menaquinone), and K3 (menadione) (Figure 1). Among them, vitamin K1 and K2 are natural compounds, whereas vitamin K3 is an artificial one. Vitamin K1 is abundant in vegetables [1] and vitamin K2 is contained in fermented foods [2,3]. For example, Japanese fermented soybeans (called "natto") contain high concentrations of vitamin K2 [2]. Vitamin K2 is referred as "MK-n" depending on the number of isoprene units in its side chain. For example, vitamin K2 abundant in "natto" is MK-7 [2], whereas MK-9, -10, and -11 are major forms of vitamin K2 in dairy food [3]. Although mammals do not have the ability to synthesize vitamin K2 de novo, they are able to convert vitamin K1 into MK-4 form of vitamin K2 by UbiA prenyltransferase domain containing protein 1 (UBIAD1) [4]. The *Ubiad1* knockout mice were embryonic lethal [5], suggesting essential physiological roles of vitamin K2, although the contribution of other substrates of UBIAD1 cannot be excluded. Vitamin K3 is widely used as a source of vitamin K in animal food. However, it is actually toxic in that it generates reactive oxygen species and has been banned from human consumption by the U.S. Food and Drug Administration since 1963.

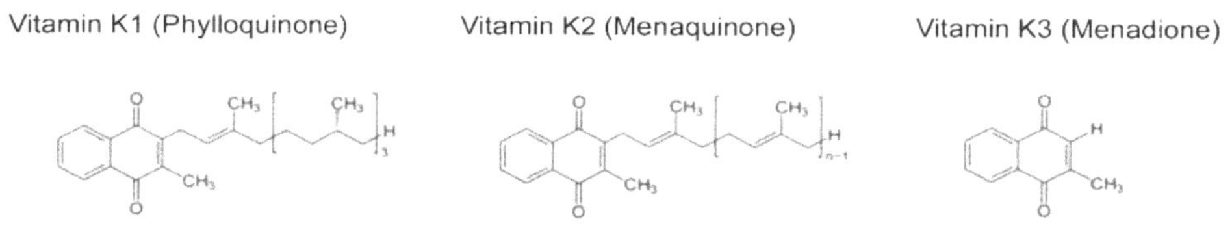

Figure 1. Molecular structures of the three forms of vitamin K. Vitamin K1, K2, and K3 share naphthoquinone ring, but differ in their side chains. Vitamin K1 has a phytyl side chain. Vitamin K2 has a side chain with varying number of isoprene units and called "MK-n" depending on the number of isoprene units. Vitamin K3 is a synthetic vitamin K without a side chain.

Vitamin K was discovered by Danish biochemist Dr. Henrik Dam in 1929 as a fat-soluble diet substance necessary for blood coagulation [6]. The substance was named after the German word 'Koagulationsvitamin' by adopting the first letter of this word. Dr. Henrik Dam was awarded the Nobel Prize in Physiology or Medicine in 1943 with an American biochemist, Dr. Edward A, doisy, who determined the structure of both vitamin K1 and K2 [7]. It was not until the 1970s that part of the mechanism of vitamin K functions began to be clarified. Vitamin K was found to be a necessary factor for γ-carboxylation of some coagulation factors which is catalyzed by an enzyme called γ-glutamyl carboxylase (GGCX) [8,9].

Now, vitamin K is known to be involved in many biological processes other than blood coagulation. In addition, other modes of vitamin K action have been elucidated by studies from independent laboratories, including ours. In this review, we will introduce the mechanisms of vitamin K functions, including novel modes of action other than classical vitamin K action mediated by GGCX. Then, we discuss the functions of vitamin K in three aging-related musculoskeletal disorders; osteoporosis, osteoarthritis, and sarcopenia.

2. Vitamin K Function Mediated by γ-Carboxylation of Proteins

The earliest discovery of vitamin K function was its essential role in GGCX activity [8,9]. GGCX adds a carboxyl group to the gamma-position carbon of glutamate residues in the substrate proteins (Figure 2). The modified glutamate residue is called "Gla" residue. This reaction requires oxidization of vitamin K hydroquinone to vitamin K epoxide (Figure 2). This function of vitamin K was blocked with warfarin by inhibiting an enzyme called vitamin K epoxide reductase (VKOR) [10] which is necessary for cyclic use of vitamin K [11]. Coagulation factors II [8,9], VII [12], IX [13], and X [13] are well known substrates for GGCX. Activities of coagulation factors II, VII, IX and X are shown to be regulated by the γ-carboxylation of these glutamate residues, explaining the anti-coagulative function of warfarin [10].

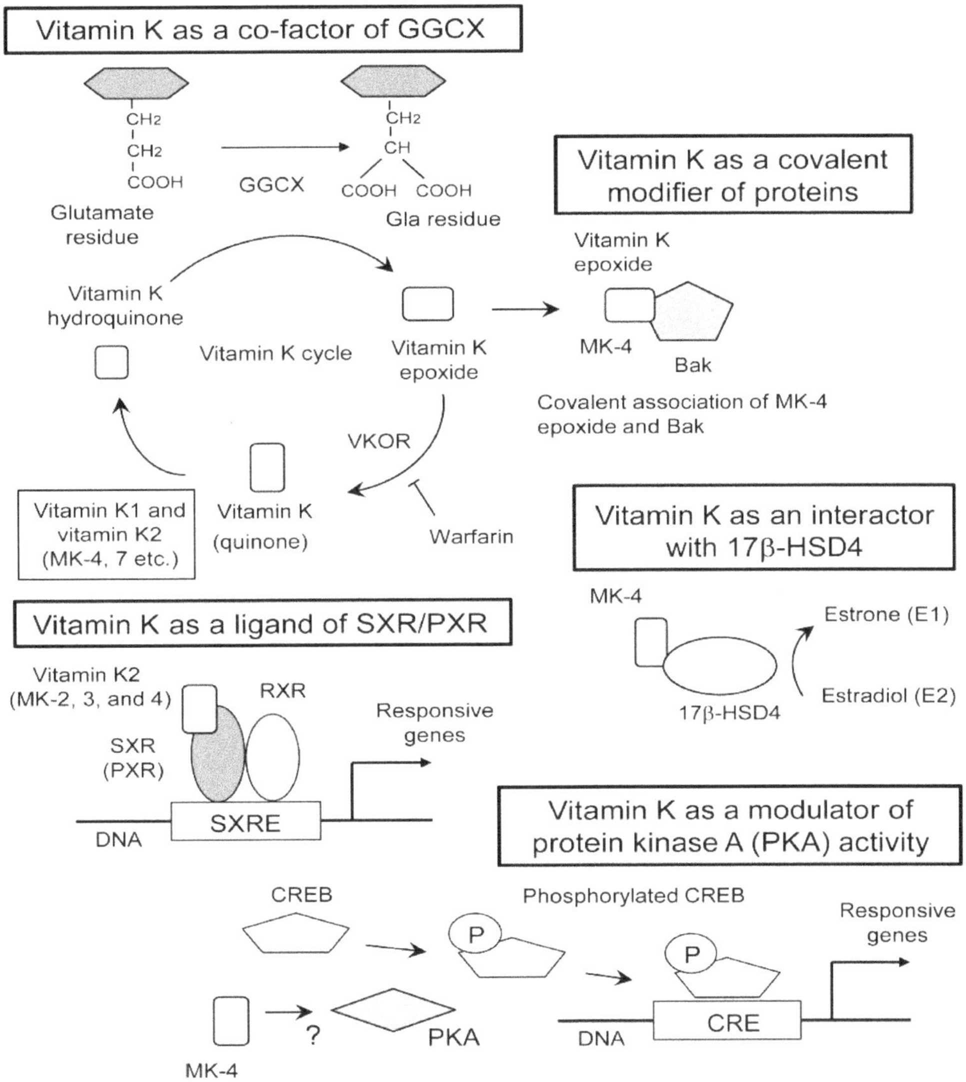

Figure 2. Multiple modes of vitamin K actions. The classical mechanism of vitamin K action is a co-factor for γ-glutamyl carboxylase (GGCX) [8–11]. This reaction requires cyclic use of vitamin K. Both vitamin K1 and K2 work in this mode of action. Vitamin K epoxide reductase (VKOR) is required for recycling vitamin K which is oxidized during γ-glutamyl carboxylation. Warfarin inhibits VKOR and vitamin K recycling, thereby suppressing GGCX activity. Vitamin K also functions as a ligand of steroid and xenobiotic receptor (SXR) and its murine homolog, pregnane X receptor (PXR) [14]. Some forms of vitamin K2 (MK-2, 3, and 4) are reported to have the ability to activate SXR [15], while vitamin K1 is not capable of activating SXR [16]. On vitamin K binding, SXR/PXR form heterodimers with 9-cis-retinoid acid receptor (RXR), and this complex binds to SXR-responsive elements (SXRE) within the regulatory regions of target genes. Covalent binding of vitamin K epoxide and a target protein, Bcl-2 antagonist killer 1 (Bak), is also proposed as a novel mode of vitamin K action [17]. This function is reported only in MK-4. Association of vitamin K with 17β-Hydroxysteroid dehydrogenase type 4 (17β-HSD4) can be different mode of vitamin K action [18], although mechanism of binding and regulation of enzymatic activity is unknown. Only MK-4 was used in this study. Finally, MK-4 activates protein kinase A (PKA) with unknown mechanism [19]. Typical substrate of PKA is CREB (cyclic AMP responsive element binding protein) and it binds to CRE (cyclic AMP responsive element) within the promoter or enhancer regions of target genes when CREB is phosphorylated. The arrows indicate conversion, association, or induction. The T bar indicates inhibition.

GGCX resides in the membrane of the endoplasmic reticulum [20]. Typical substrates of GGCX have pro-peptides on their N-terminus and the substrates bind GGCX with carboxylase recognition site, a conserved motif within the pro-peptide [21]. Many of the substrates of GGCX have Gla domain next to the pro-peptide, where γ-carboxylation of multiple glutamate residues occurs in processive manner [22] (Figure 3). After the substrates are carboxylated, they become a mature protein by the dissection of pro-peptides.

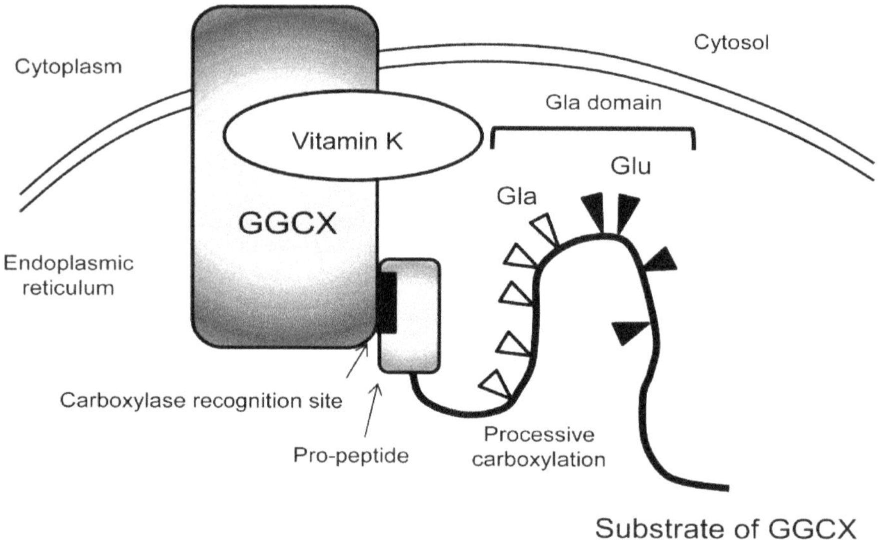

Figure 3. Processive γ-carboxylation of typical GGCX substrates. In the endoplasmic reticulum, typical substrates of GGCX bind with GGCX with the carboxylase recognition site in the pro-peptide at their N-termini (indicated by arrows). Then, multiple glutamate residues (Glu, black triangles) in the Gla domain are converted into Gla residues (white triangles) in processive manner.

As far as we know, 20 human proteins are found to be γ-carboxylated so far (Table 1). Among the γ-carboxylated proteins, we introduce 9 proteins which are shown to be related with musculoskeletal diseases, or potentially related to them.

Table 1. Musculoskeletal disease-related γ-carboxylated proteins. Among 20 kinds of proteins known to be γ-carboxylated, 9 proteins are related or possibly related to musculoskeletal diseases.

Proteins	Expression	Function	References
Osteocalcin (Bone Gla protein, BGP)	Osteoblast	Regulation of bone calcification, Regulation of glucose metabolism? Enhancing male fertility?	[23–30]
Matrix Gla protein (MGP)	Chondrocyte, vascular smooth muscle cell, etc.	Regulation of calcification	[31–34]
Growth arrest specific-6 (GAS6)	Lung, heart, kidney, intestine, endothelium, vascular smooth muscle cell, bone marrow, osteoblast, osteoclast, monocyte, etc.	Thrombus formation; Inflammation; Cell proliferation; Enhancing osteoclast activity	[35–38]
Protein S	Liver, endothelium, monocyte, etc.	Anti-coagulation; Enhancing osteoclast activity	[37,39–41]
Periostin	Periosteum, periodontal ligament, heart valve, adrenal gland, lung, thyroid, intestine, ovary, testis, prostate	Maintenance of periodontal ligament; Bone development and maintenance	[42,43]
TGFβ induced (TGFBI)	Bone, joint, skin, cornea, kidney.	Bone development; Maintenance of cornea	[42,44,45]
Gla-rich protein (GRP)/Upper zone of growth plate and cartilage matrix associated protein (Ucma)	Chondrocyte, osteoblast, osteocyte, vascular smooth muscle cell, skin	Suppression of inflammation; Suppression of calcification in blood vessels and articular cartilages	[46–48]
Androgen receptor	Testis, prostate, muscle, brain, prostate cancer	Induction of male sexual characteristics; Promotion of prostate cancer; Bone protection; Enhancing skeletal muscle mass	[49–53]
γ-glutamyl carboxylase (GGCX)	Systemic (High expression in liver)	γ-carboxylation of proteins	[54]

Osteocalcin (also called bone Gla protein) [23,24] and matrix Gla protein (MGP) [31], which regulate the calcification of bone and cartilage, are substrates of GGCX. Their roles in osteoporosis or osteoarthritis will be disscussed later.

Growth arrest specific 6 (GAS6), which has multiple functions such as thrombus formation, inflammation, and cell proliferation, is also known as a substrate of GGCX [35]. GAS6 is shown to be a ligand for receptor tyrosine kinases such as Axl, Tyro3, and Mer. The γ-carboxylation of GAS6 is necessary for the activation of these receptors [36]. In relationship with the bone metabolism, GAS6 is shown to increase bone resorbing activity of osteoclast by binding Tyro3 expressed in osteoclast [37]. Another γ-carboxylated protein, protein S, was originally discovered as a protein involved in the fibrinolysis cascade [39]. Protein S, which is highly homologous to GAS6 [40], is also a ligand for Tyro3 [41], and activates osteoclasts [37]. In terms of cartilage metabolism, GAS6 is reported to have suppressive effect on chondrogenic differentiation [38].

In 2008, periostin and TGFβ induced (TGFBI) was reported to be members of γ-carboxylated proteins [42]. Periostin is involved in the maintenance of ligaments and bone development [43]. TGFBI is a protein homologous to periostin and has been shown to be involved in the maintenance of cornea and bone development [44,45]. In either periostin or TGFBI the significance of γ-carboxylation is not clarified. In fact, there is a study suggesting that the γ-carboxylation of periostin and TGFBI is doubtful [55].

In 2008, Gla-rich protein (GRP) which is also known as Upper zone of growth plate and cartilage matrix-associated protein (Ucma) was discovered from sturgeon cartilage and human fetal growth plate [46,47]. GRP is supposed to prevent the aberrant calcification of cartilage, which will be mentioned later.

Androgen receptor (AR) is a member of nuclear receptors. It mediates transcriptional regulation when the cells are stimulated with androgen. In 2017, it was shown that glutamate residue 2 of AR can be γ-carboxylated [49]. When the activity of VKOR was suppressed with warfarin or siRNAs, the transcriptional activity of AR was also suppressed. On the other hand, suppression of GGCX with siRNAs did not affect the transcriptional activity of AR [49], which makes it difficult to understand the biological significance of γ-carboxylation. In terms of bone metabolism, AR deficient mice display bone loss with enhanced bone resorption [50]. The suppressive effect of androgen on bone resorption was shown also in humans by a clinical study [51]. In the relationship between androgen and muscular tissue, the administration of testosterone is shown to increase skeletal muscle mass and strength in normal men [52]. In the animal model, AR deficient male mice displayed decreased skeletal muscle mass [53].

The final human protein carboxylated by GGCX is GGCX itself. In 1998, it was reported that three Gla residues in a GGCX molecule were carboxylated [54]. It was speculated that γ-carboxylation of GGCX may facilitate the release of GGCX substrates and suppressively regulate the processive γ-carboxylation of its substrates.

3. Vitamin K Function as a Ligand of SXR/PXR

In 2003, we discovered a completely different mechanism of vitamin K2 action mediated by transcriptional regulation. We showed that MK-4 form of vitamin K2 is one of the ligands for the nuclear receptor, steroid and xenobiotic receptor (SXR) and its murine ortholog, pregnane X receptor (PXR) [14,56] (Figure 2). This receptor is also known as NR1I2, according to standardized nomenclature designated by the nuclear receptor committee. Blumberg et al. cloned SXR/PXR as a novel nuclear receptor that is mainly expressed in the liver and intestine [57].

SXR/PXR is a ligand-dependent transcription factor and is activated by various drugs and xenobiotic compounds [58]. At the time of cloning, endogenous ligands of SXR/PXR had not been discovered. For that reason, SXR/PXR was originally classified as an orphan receptor. Now, secondary bile acids are known to be endogenous ligands for this receptor [59,60]. When SXR/PXR is activated by a ligand, it forms a heterodimer with 9-cis retinoid acid receptor (RXR). Then, this heterodimer is shown to bind with SXR-responsive elements (SXRE) in the regulatory regions of typical SXR/PXR-responsive genes [57] (Figure 2). Typical SXR/PXR-responsive genes include the drug metabolizing enzyme, *CYP3A4*, and the ABC family transporter, *MDR1*, which are involved in detoxification and drug excretion [61]. These responsive genes indicate that one of the roles of SXR/PXR function is a xenobiotic sensor. The expression of SXR/PXR has also been detected in the kidney, lung [62], and peripheral mononuclear cells [63].

Because of the difference of ligand-binding domain, the ligand specificity of SXR/PXR is known to be different among mammalian species. For example, rifampicin, an antibiotic drug, is an effective activator of human and rabbit SXR, while it has little activity on mouse SXR (PXR) or rat SXR. On the other hand, pregnane 16α-carbonitrile (PCN) activates mouse SXR (PXR) and rat SXR efficiently, while it does not activate human or rabbit SXR [15]. We reported that SXR is expressed in human osteoblastic cell lines and is activated by both rifampicin and MK-4 [14]. We also demonstrated that MK-4 can be a ligand for mouse SXR (PXR) by using osteoblastic cells derived from PXR-deficient mice [14]. Therefore, despite the difference of ligand specificity among mammalian species, vitamin MK-4 seems to activate both human SXR and murine SXR (PXR). Later, it was shown that MK-2 and MK-3 also activate SXR [64]. Meanwhile, it was shown that vitamin K1 itself is not capable of activating SXR [16], suggesting vitamin K1 potentially contribute to this mechanism of action after being converted into MK-4. The fact that some forms of vitamin K2 could be ligands for SXR has opened up the possibility that vitamin K is involved in many physiological and pathological processes through the regulation of PXR target genes.

4. Other Modes of Vitamin K Actions

In 2005, another interactor of vitamin K2 was discovered. Otsuka et al. showed that vitamin K2 binds 17β-Hydroxysteroid dehydrogenase type 4 (17β-HSD4) by mass spectrometric analysis with a pull-down assay using biotinylated MK-4 [18] (Figure 2). It is known that 17β-HSD4 is an enzyme converting estradiol (E2) to estrone (E1). They showed a vitamin K2-dependent decrease of DNA binding of estrogen receptor α, suggesting 17β-HSD4-mediated inactivation of E2 by converting it into E1. This study proposed another mode of vitamin K action with a physical interaction with proteins other than GGCX or SXR/PXR. However, the precise mechanism of regulation on the enzymatic activity is not clarified. Since estrogen signal is shown to protect bone tissues [65] and supposed to promote muscular endurance [66], activating 17β-HSD4 by MK-4 may not explain the apparent beneficial functions of vitamin K on musculoskeletal tissues stated below.

In 2007, we proposed the fourth mechanism of vitamin K action. In osteoblastic cells, MK-4 induced the gene expression of growth differentiation factor 15 (*GDF15*) and stanniocalcin 2 (*STC2*). The induction of these genes was considered to be mediated by neither GGCX nor SXR because the induction was not suppressed by treatment with rifampicin nor siRNA against SXR. Further investigation revealed that MK-4 induced the phosphorylation of protein kinase A (PKA) and that the inhibition of PKA suppressed the expression of *GDF15* and *STC2* in osteoblastic cells [19] (Figure 2). Although the precise mechanism of PKA activation is unknown, these results suggested the fourth mechanism of vitamin K action.

In 2013, a surprising action of vitamin K was reported. Karasawa et al. showed that pro-apoptotic protein Bcl-2 antagonist killer 1 (Bak) was covalently modified by epoxide form of MK-4 at cysteine 166 in Bak [17] (Figure 2). This modification of Bak functionally regulated apoptosis induction in human promyelocytic cell HL60 [17]. Bak regulates apoptosis also in osteoblasts. Attenuation of apoptosis by genetic deletion of Bak and Bax in osteoblasts increased femoral cancellous bone mass, whereas it also increased cortical porosity in aged mice [67]. This report suggests that the covalent modification of Bak with MK-4 may affect bone metabolism. In addition, if the covalent modification of proteins with vitamin K is a general phenomenon, other proteins affecting aging-related musculoskeletal disorders might be involved.

5. Roles of Vitamin K on Osteoporosis

The relationship of vitamin K and bone metabolism was suggested from a long time ago. In 1960, Bouckaert and Said reported that vitamin K enhanced the healing of fracture in rabbits [68].

The discovery of γ-carboxylated osteocalcin from bone tissues [23,24] also suggested a relationship. In 1985, Hart et al. reported that circulating levels of vitamin K1 in patients who had spinal or femoral neck fractures were significantly lower than those of age-matched control subjects [69]. This research was made possible by the invention of electrochemical detection for a low concentration of vitamin K in plasma by using high-performance liquid chromatography (HPLC). At the turn of the century, several large-scale epidemiological studies on the relationship between fracture risk and bone fracture were conducted. The epidemiological study conducted in North America revealed low vitamin K intake to be associated with an increased risk of hip fracture [70]. Interestingly, the association of vitamin K intake and bone mineral density (BMD) was not significantly observed in this study [70], suggesting its contribution to bone quality. The relationship of low vitamin K intake and hip fracture was also observed in Japanese observational study [71,72].

In Japan, MK-4 was approved for a drug for osteoporosis treatment in 1995 based on domestic clinical trials showing the efficacy on bone mineral density. Now, MK-4 is in use for osteoporosis treatment in several Asian countries. For the last two decades, interventional clinical trials were conducted throughout the world. Many trials used MK-4 as vitamin K treatment, MK-7 or vitamin K1 was also used in some trials as well. According to the most recent meta-analysis, a favorable effect of vitamin K on clinical fractures was statistically significant, although the effect on vertebral or hip fractures was not statistically significant [73]. Among the clinical trials, the largest one was conducted in Japan [74]. This study involved more than 4000 Japanese women with three years of intervention and a one-year follow-up period. This study failed to demonstrate the fracture-preventive effect of vitamin K2 (MK-4) in the whole group of subjects. However, the significant effect on new vertebral fractures was observed in the subgroup analysis of high-risk patients with at least five pre-existing vertebral fractures.

GGCX-dependent mechanism may exist in the bone protective role of vitamin K. We found a single nucleotide polymorphism (SNP) in GGCX significantly correlated with bone mineral density in elderly Japanese women [75]. This SNP involves amino acid substitution, where GGCX with higher enzymatic activity was coded by a beneficial allele with a higher bone mineral density. This result suggested that part of the bone protective effect of vitamin K could be mediated by GGCX activity. However, it is still a difficult process to clarify which substrates of GGCX are responsible for this effect. Osteocalcin, one of the substrates of GGCX [23,24], is specifically expressed in osteoblastic lineage [25,26] and regulates mineralization of bone [27]. The concentration of undercarboxylated form of osteocalcin (ucOC) in serum is positively correlated with fracture risk [28] and used as a biomarker for the indication of vitamin K treatment in Japan. In these circumstances, we first hypothesized that some GGCX substrate in osteoblasts, especially osteocalcin, may be responsible for the bone protective effect. To test this hypothesis, we generated osteoblast-specific GGCX-deficient mice [29]. As expected, serum ucOC was increased and carboxylated osteocalcin (cOC) was decreased compared with control mice. Notably, the bone mineral density was even increased in osteoblast-specific GGCX-deficient mice and mechanical strength was not impaired compared with control mice [29]. This result implied that GGCX in osteoblast may not contribute to the bone protective effect of vitamin K in this mouse model, and that the γ-carboxylation of osteocalcin might not be responsible for the effect. It is possible to speculate that GGCX activity in other cell lineages or in other tissues is responsible for the bone protective effect of vitamin K. In terms of the role of osteocalcin, it is noteworthy that osteocalcin-deficient mice were shown to have mechanically stronger bone than wild type mice [30], suggesting a decrease of cOC rather than increase of ucOC may have a bone strengthening effect.

The bone protective role of vitamin K may be explained by transcriptional regulation mediated by SXR/PXR. We found three SXR-dependent vitamin K-responsive genes, *Tsukushi*, *Matrillin2*, and *CD14* in the human osteoblastic cell line, MG63 cells stably overexpressing SXR [76]. *Tsukushi* and *Matrilin2* encode proteins related with extracellular matrix [77,78], and *CD14* encodes protein regulating bone turnover by inducing differentiation of B cells [79–81]. The bone phenotype of systemic *Pxr* knockout mice suggested the roles of SXR/PXR in the bone metabolism. We analyzed 4-month-old female *Pxr* knockout mice and found decreased bone mineral density, enhanced bone resorption, suppressed bone formation, and weaker mechanical strength in femoral bone from *Pxr* knockout mice compared with wild type mice [82]. Konno et al. analyzed *Pxr* knockout mice from different origin and reported lower bone mineral density in *Pxr* knockout mice [83]. They showed that *Slc34a2* is a PXR responsive gene in intestine and that serum concentration of inorganic phosphate was significantly decreased in *Pxr* knockout mice. Meanwhile, the serum levels of inorganic phosphate in *Pxr* knockout mice were not decreased in our observation [82], suggesting the mechanisms depend on the mouse strains and/or environment. In the case of humans, we found an SNP in the first intron of the *SXR* gene associated with the total body BMD of postmenopausal Japanese women [84]. This suggests that vitamin K actions mediated by SXR may have clinical significance.

6. Roles of Vitamin K on Osteoarthritis

Epidemiological studies in North America and Japan revealed the association of low vitamin K intake and the prevalence of osteoarthritis [85–87], suggesting the cartilage protective effect of vitamin K. This effect was further examined by an interventional trial with negative results [88], possibly due to short study period or weak effect of vitamin K on established osteoarthritis.

A mechanism of the protective effect of vitamin K on articular cartilage was proposed that the abnormal γ-carboxylation of proteins was involved in the aberrant calcification of cartilage. In a genome-wide association study, an SNP significantly associated with hand osteoarthritis was found near matrix Gla protein (*MGP*) gene [32], coding one of the substrates of GGCX. The risk allele was significantly associated with a lower expression of MGP in subchondral bone. It is notable that *Mgp* knockout mice displayed inappropriate calcification of cartilages [33], and that human chondrocytes derived from patient of osteoarthritis produced less carboxylated MGP (cMGP) and more undercarboxylated MGP (ucMGP) [34]. Taken together it is likely that cMGP has a beneficial effect on preventing osteoarthritis by inhibiting the calcification of articular cartilage. Another candidate molecule which can explain protective effect of vitamin K on cartilage is Gla-rich protein (GRP). In osteoarthritic cartilage undercarboxylated GRP (ucGRP) was more evident than carboxylated GRP (cGRP), and both ucGRP and cGRP co-localized with ectopic calcification [48]. This observation suggested γ-carboxylation of GRP is important for inhibiting calcification of cartilage tissue.

The cartilage protective effect of vitamin K may also be explained by transcriptional regulation mediated by SXR/PXR. We found that *Pxr* knockout mice displayed aging-dependent wearing of articular cartilage of knee joints, resembling development of osteoarthritic lesion [89]. We identified an SXR-dependent vitamin K (MK-4)-responsive gene, *Fam20a* (family with sequence similarity 20a) using ATDC5 chondrocytic cells overexpressing human SXR [89]. Although the role of FAM20A in cartilage tissue is unknown, we speculate that FAM20A may regulate phosphorylation of certain extracellular matrix protein like other members of Fam20 family proteins [90,91].

7. Roles of Vitamin K on Sarcopenia

In 1988, the word 'sarcopenia' was invented by combining Greek words meaning 'muscle' and 'loss' [92]. However, it was not until 2010 when the operational definition of sarcopenia began to be proposed to familiarise people with pathological muscle loss [93]. Therefore, sarcopenia is an emerging clinical entity which requires attention to prevent locomotor disabilities. In 2016, sarcopenia was added to the list of International Classification of Diseases (ICD)-10, indicating that sarcopenia is now internationally regarded as a disease. In this decade, several definitions and diagnostic criteria have been proposed throughout the world, and clinical or basic studies on sarcopenia have been undertaken. Currently, more emphasis is put on muscle strength and physical performance rather than muscle mass [94], because muscle strength and physical performance are directly associated with disabilities of patients.

Some clinical observational studies suggest that vitamin K status is related to physical performance. One large clinical study conducted in the United States analyzed 1089 community-dwelling older adults, and reported that a higher plasma concentration of vitamin K1 was associated with higher SPPB (short physical performance battery; including the evaluation of gait speed, chair stand, and balance test) scores in both cross-sectional and longitudinal analyses [95]. More than half (67%) of the participants were female in this study, although the subgroup analysis of each gender was not performed. Another large observational study, in which 633 community-dwelling adults aged 55–56 years old participated, revealed that a higher vitamin K status was associated with a higher physical performance score (assessed with walk test, chair stand test, and cardigan putting on and taking off time) only in women [96]. Stronger handgrip power and larger calf circumference were associated with higher vitamin K status in both genders. According to a randomized controlled study originally aimed to evaluate the effect of vitamin K1 supplementation on bone loss and coronary artery calcification, three-year vitamin K1 supplementation did not change appendicular lean mass, which reflects muscle mass of arms and legs [97]. Unfortunately, physical performance was not assessed in this study. Another control study with six-month vitamin K2 (MK-7) supplementation did evaluate physical performance but showed no significant effect of vitamin K on handgrip strength and SPPB score [98].

Considering the results of several clinical studies introduced above, vitamin K may have a beneficial effect on muscle quality reflected by physical performance scores rather than muscle mass. As far as we know, there is no convincing basic study explaining the mechanisms of vitamin K functions in the skeletal muscle tissue. Further clinical and basic studies should be required for a detailed discussion on these matters.

8. Conclusions

In the present review, we described multiple mechanisms of vitamin K functions and their involvement in aging-related musculoskeletal disorders as examples for the biological significance of vitamin K beyond its roles in blood coagulation. In a super-aged society, musculoskeletal disorders are the leading cause of disabilities requiring health care. Therefore, osteoporosis, osteoarthritis and sarcopenia are becoming more important issues as obstacles to expanding a healthy life span in an aging society. We sincerely hope that studies on vitamin K lead to the discovery of new biological mechanisms and targets for disease prevention and treatment, and eventually contribute to human longevity and health by the clinical application of these discoveries.

Author Contributions: Writing—Original Draft Preparation, K.A.; Writing—Review & Editing, S.I.

References

1. Suttie, J.W.; Booth, S.L. Vitamin K. *Adv Nutr.* **2011**, *2*, 440–441. [CrossRef]
2. Tarvainen, M.; Fabritius, M.; Yang, B. Determination of vitamin K composition of fermented food. *Food Chem.* **2019**, *275*, 515–522. [CrossRef]
3. Fu, X.; Harshman, S.G.; Shen, X.; Haytowitz, D.B.; Karl, J.P.; Wolfe, B.E.; Booth, S.L. Multiple Vitamin K Forms Exist in Dairy Foods. *Curr. Dev. Nutr.* **2017**, *1*, e000638. [CrossRef] [PubMed]
4. Nakagawa, K.; Hirota, Y.; Sawada, N.; Yuge, N.; Watanabe, M.; Uchino, Y.; Okuda, N.; Shimomura, Y.; Suhara, Y.; Okano, T. Identification of UBIAD1 as a novel human menaquinone-4 biosynthetic enzyme. *Nature* **2010**, *468*, 117–121. [CrossRef] [PubMed]
5. Nakagawa, K.; Sawada, N.; Hirota, Y.; Uchino, Y.; Suhara, Y.; Hasegawa, T.; Amizuka, N.; Okamoto, T.; Tsugawa, N.; Kamao, M.; et al. Vitamin K2 biosynthetic enzyme, UBIAD1 is essential for embryonic development of mice. *PLoS ONE* **2014**, *9*, e104078. [CrossRef]
6. Dam, H. The antihemorrhagic vitamin of the chick: Occurrence and chemical nature. *Nature* **1935**, *135*, 652–653. [CrossRef]
7. Doisy, E.A.; Binkley, S.B.; Thayer, S.A.; McKee, R.W. VITAMIN K. *Science* **1940**, *91*, 58–62. [CrossRef] [PubMed]

8. Nelsestuen, G.L.; Zytkovicz, T.H.; Howard, J.B. The mode of action of vitamin K. Identification of gamma-carboxyglutamic acid as a component of prothrombin. *J. Biol. Chem.* **1974**, *249*, 6347–6350.
9. Stenflo, J.; Fernlund, P.; Egan, W.; Roepstorff, P. Vitamin K dependent modifications of glutamic acid residues in prothrombin. *Proc. Natl. Acad. Sci. USA* **1974**, *71*, 2730–2733. [CrossRef] [PubMed]
10. Czogalla, K.J.; Biswas, A.; Höning, K.; Hornung, V.; Liphardt, K.; Watzka, M.; Oldenburg, J. Warfarin and vitamin K compete for binding to Phe55 in human VKOR. *Nat. Struct. Mol. Biol.* **2017**, *24*, 77–85. [CrossRef] [PubMed]
11. Stafford, D.W. The vitamin K cycle. *J. Thromb Haemost.* **2005**, *3*, 1873–1878. [CrossRef] [PubMed]
12. Dissing, C.; Persson, E. Factor VII Tokushima (Cys22→Gly) is not -carboxylated due to a disrupted γ-carboxylase recognition site. *Thromb Res.* **2017**, *158*, 108–112. [CrossRef] [PubMed]
13. Bucher, D.; Nebelin, E.; Thomsen, J.; Stenflo, J. Identification of gamma-carboxyglutamic acid residues in bovine factors IX and X, and in a new vitamin K-dependent protein. *FEBS Lett.* **1976**, *68*, 293–296. [CrossRef]
14. Tabb, M.M.; Sun, A.; Zhou, C.; Grün, F.; Errandi, J.; Romero, K.; Pham, H.; Inoue, S.; Mallick, S.; Lin, M.; et al. Vitamin K2 regulation of bone homeostasis is mediated by the steroid and xenobiotic receptor SXR. *J. Biol. Chem.* **2003**, *278*, 43919–43927. [CrossRef] [PubMed]
15. Jones, S.A.; Moore, L.B.; Shenk, J.L.; Wisely, G.B.; Hamilton, G.A.; McKee, D.D.; Tomkinson, N.C.; LeCluyse, E.L.; Lambert, M.H.; Willson, T.M.; et al. The pregnane X receptor: A promiscuous xenobiotic receptor that has diverged during evolution. *Mol. Endocrinol.* **2000**, *14*, 27–39. [CrossRef] [PubMed]
16. Suhara, Y.; Hanada, N.; Okitsu, T.; Sakai, M.; Watanabe, M.; Nakagawa, K.; Wada, A.; Takeda, K.; Takahashi, K.; Tokiwa, H.; et al. Structure-activity relationship of novel menaquinone-4 analogues: Modification of the side chain affects their biological activities. *J. Med. Chem.* **2012**, *55*, 1553–1558. [CrossRef] [PubMed]
17. Karasawa, S.; Azuma, M.; Kasama, T.; Sakamoto, S.; Kabe, Y.; Imai, T.; Yamaguchi, Y.; Miyazawa, K.; Handa, H. Vitamin K2 covalently binds to Bak and induces Bak-mediated apoptosis. *Mol. Pharmacol.* **2013**, *83*, 613–620. [CrossRef] [PubMed]
18. Otsuka, M.; Kato, N.; Ichimura, T.; Abe, S.; Tanaka, Y.; Taniguchi, H.; Hoshida, Y.; Moriyama, M.; Wang, Y.; Shao, R.X.; et al. Vitamin K2 binds 17beta-hydroxysteroid dehydrogenase 4 and modulates estrogen metabolism. *Life Sci.* **2005**, *76*, 2473–2482. [CrossRef]
19. Ichikawa, T.; Horie-Inoue, K.; Ikeda, K.; Blumberg, B.; Inoue, S. Vitamin K2 induces phosphorylation of protein kinase A and expression of novel target genes in osteoblastic cells. *J. Mol. Endocrinol.* **2007**, *39*, 239–247. [CrossRef]
20. Tie, J.; Wu, S.M.; Jin, D.; Nicchitta, C.V.; Stafford, D.W. A topological study of the human gamma-glutamyl carboxylase. *Blood* **2000**, *96*, 973–978.
21. Kulman, J.D.; Harris, J.E.; Xie, L.; Davie, E.W. Identification of two novel transmembrane gamma-carboxyglutamic acid proteins expressed broadly in fetal and adult tissues. *Proc. Natl. Acad. Sci. USA* **2001**, *98*, 1370–1375. [CrossRef] [PubMed]
22. Morris, D.P.; Stevens, R.D.; Wright, D.J.; Stafford, D.W. Processive post-translational modification. Vitamin K-dependent carboxylation of a peptide substrate. *J. Biol. Chem.* **1995**, *270*, 30491–30498. [CrossRef] [PubMed]
23. Hauschka, P.V.; Lian, J.B.; Gallop, P.M. Direct identification of the calcium-binding amino acid, gamma-carboxyglutamate, in mineralized tissue. *Proc. Natl. Acad. Sci. USA* **1975**, *72*, 3925–3929. [CrossRef] [PubMed]
24. Price, P.A.; Otsuka, A.A.; Poser, J.W.; Kristaponis, J.; Raman, N. Characterization of a gamma-carboxyglutamic acid-containing protein from bone. *Proc. Natl. Acad. Sci. USA* **1976**, *73*, 1447–1451. [CrossRef] [PubMed]
25. Weinreb, M.; Shinar, D.; Rodan, G.A. Different pattern of alkaline phosphatase, osteopontin, and osteocalcin expression in developing rat bone visualized by in situ hybridization. *J. Bone Miner. Res.* **1990**, *5*, 831–842. [CrossRef]
26. Zhang, M.; Xuan, S.; Bouxsein, M.L.; von Stechow, D.; Akeno, N.; Faugere, M.C.; Malluche, H.; Zhao, G.; Rosen, C.J.; Efstratiadis, A.; et al. Osteoblast-specific knockout of the insulin-like growth factor (IGF) receptor gene reveals an essential role of IGF signaling in bone matrix mineralization. *J. Biol. Chem.* **2002**, *277*, 44005–44012. [CrossRef] [PubMed]
27. Hoang, Q.Q.; Sicheri, F.; Howard, A.J.; Yang, D.S. Bone recognition mechanism of porcine osteocalcin from crystal structure. *Nature* **2003**, *425*, 977–980. [CrossRef]

28. Szulc, P.; Chapuy, M.C.; Meunier, P.J.; Delmas, P.D. Serum undercarboxylated osteocalcin is a marker of the risk of hip fracture in elderly women. *J. Clin. Investig.* **1993**, *91*, 1769–1774. [CrossRef]
29. Azuma, K.; Shiba, S.; Hasegawa, T.; Ikeda, K.; Urano, T.; Horie-Inoue, K.; Ouchi, Y.; Amizuka, N.; Inoue, S. Osteoblast-Specific γ-Glutamyl Carboxylase-Deficient Mice Display Enhanced Bone Formation With Aberrant Mineralization. *J. Bone Miner. Res.* **2015**, *30*, 1245–1254. [CrossRef]
30. Ducy, P.; Desbois, C.; Boyce, B.; Pinero, G.; Story, B.; Dunstan, C.; Smith, E.; Bonadio, J.; Goldstein, S.; Gundberg, C.; et al. Increased bone formation in osteocalcin-deficient mice. *Nature* **1996**, *382*, 448–452. [CrossRef]
31. Price, P.A.; Urist, M.R.; Otawara, Y. Matrix Gla protein, a new gamma-carboxyglutamic acid-containing protein which is associated with the organic matrix of bone. *Biochem. Biophys. Res. Commun.* **1983**, *117*, 765–771. [CrossRef]
32. den Hollander, W.; Boer, C.G.; Hart, D.J.; Yau, M.S.; Ramos, Y.F.M.; Metrustry, S.; Broer, L.; Deelen, J.; Cupples, L.A.; Rivadeneira, F.; et al. Genome-wide association and functional studies identify a role for matrix Gla protein in osteoarthritis of the hand. *Ann. Rheum. Dis.* **2017**, *76*, 2046–2053. [CrossRef] [PubMed]
33. Luo, G.; Ducy, P.; McKee, M.D.; Pinero, G.J.; Loyer, E.; Behringer, R.R.; Karsenty, G. Spontaneous calcification of arteries and cartilage in mice lacking matrix GLA protein. *Nature* **1997**, *386*, 78–81. [CrossRef] [PubMed]
34. Wallin, R.; Schurgers, L.J.; Loeser, R.F. Biosynthesis of the vitamin K-dependent matrix Gla protein (MGP) in chondrocytes: A fetuin-MGP protein complex is assembled in vesicles shed from normal but not from osteoarthritic chondrocytes. *Osteoarthr. Cartil.* **2010**, *18*, 1096–1103. [CrossRef] [PubMed]
35. Varnum, B.C.; Young, C.; Elliott, G.; Garcia, A.; Bartley, T.D.; Fridell, Y.W.; Hunt, R.W.; Trail, G.; Clogston, C.; Toso, R.J.; et al. Axl receptor tyrosine kinase stimulated by the vitamin K-dependent protein encoded by growth-arrest-specific gene 6. *Nature* **1995**, *373*, 623–626. [CrossRef] [PubMed]
36. Nagata, K.; Ohashi, K.; Nakano, T.; Arita, H.; Zong, C.; Hanafusa, H.; Mizuno, K. Identification of the product of growth arrest-specific gene 6 as a common ligand for Axl, Sky, and Mer receptor tyrosine kinases. *J. Biol. Chem.* **1996**, *271*, 30022–30027. [CrossRef] [PubMed]
37. Nakamura, Y.S.; Hakeda, Y.; Takakura, N.; Kameda, T.; Hamaguchi, I.; Miyamoto, T.; Kakudo, S.; Nakano, T.; Kumegawa, M.; Suda, T. Tyro 3 receptor tyrosine kinase and its ligand, Gas6, stimulate the function of osteoclasts. *Stem Cells* **1998**, *16*, 229–238. [CrossRef]
38. Motomura, H.; Niimi, H.; Sugimori, K.; Ohtsuka, T.; Kimura, T.; Kitajima, I. Gas6, a new regulator of chondrogenic differentiation from mesenchymal cells. *Biochem. Biophys. Res. Commun.* **2007**, *357*, 997–1003. [CrossRef]
39. Stenflo, J.; Jönsson, M. Protein S, a new vitamin K-dependent protein from bovine plasma. *FEBS Lett.* **1979**, *101*, 377–381. [CrossRef]
40. Manfioletti, G.; Brancolini, C.; Avanzi, G.; Schneider, C. The protein encoded by a growth arrest-specific gene (gas6) is a new member of the vitamin K-dependent proteins related to protein S, a negative coregulator in the blood coagulation cascade. *Mol. Cell Biol.* **1993**, *13*, 4976–4985. [CrossRef]
41. Stitt, T.N.; Conn, G.; Gore, M.; Lai, C.; Bruno, J.; Radziejewski, C.; Mattsson, K.; Fisher, J.; Gies, D.R.; Jones, P.F.; et al. The anticoagulation factor protein S and its relative, Gas6, are ligands for the Tyro 3/Axl family of receptor tyrosine kinases. *Cell* **1995**, *80*, 661–670. [CrossRef]
42. Coutu, D.L.; Wu, J.H.; Monette, A.; Rivard, G.E.; Blostein, M.D.; Galipeau, J. Periostin, a member of a novel family of vitamin K-dependent proteins, is expressed by mesenchymal stromal cells. *J. Biol. Chem.* **2008**, *283*, 17991–18001. [CrossRef] [PubMed]
43. Rios, H.; Koushik, S.V.; Wang, H.; Wang, J.; Zhou, H.M.; Lindsley, A.; Rogers, R.; Chen, Z.; Maeda, M.; Kruzynska-Frejtag, A.; et al. Periostin null mice exhibit dwarfism, incisor enamel defects, and an early-onset periodontal disease-like phenotype. *Mol. Cell Biol.* **2005**, *25*, 11131–11144. [CrossRef] [PubMed]
44. Yu, H.; Wergedal, J.E.; Zhao, Y.; Mohan, S. Targeted disruption of TGFBI in mice reveals its role in regulating bone mass and bone size through periosteal bone formation. *Calcif Tissue Int.* **2012**, *91*, 81–87. [CrossRef] [PubMed]
45. Stewart, H.; Black, G.C.; Donnai, D.; Bonshek, R.E.; McCarthy, J.; Morgan, S.; Dixon, M.J.; Ridgway, A.A. A mutation within exon 14 of the TGFBI (BIGH3) gene on chromosome 5q31 causes an asymmetric, late-onset form of lattice corneal dystrophy. *Ophthalmology* **1999**, *106*, 964–970. [CrossRef]

46. Tagariello, A.; Luther, J.; Streiter, M.; Didt-Koziel, L.; Wuelling, M.; Surmann-Schmitt, C.; Stock, M.; Adam, N.; Vortkamp, A.; Winterpacht, A. Ucma–A novel secreted factor represents a highly specific marker for distal chondrocytes. *Matrix Biol.* **2008**, *27*, 3–11. [CrossRef]
47. Viegas, C.S.; Simes, D.C.; Laizé, V.; Williamson, M.K.; Price, P.A.; Cancela, M.L. Gla-rich protein (GRP), a new vitamin K-dependent protein identified from sturgeon cartilage and highly conserved in vertebrates. *J. Biol. Chem.* **2008**, *283*, 36655–36664. [CrossRef]
48. Rafael, M.S.; Cavaco, S.; Viegas, C.S.; Santos, S.; Ramos, A.; Willems, B.A.; Herfs, M.; Theuwissen, E.; Vermeer, C.; Simes, D.C. Insights into the association of Gla-rich protein and osteoarthritis, novel splice variants and γ-carboxylation status. *Mol. Nutr. Food Res.* **2014**, *58*, 1636–1646. [CrossRef]
49. Tew, B.Y.; Hong, T.B.; Otto-Duessel, M.; Elix, C.; Castro, E.; He, M.; Wu, X.; Pal, S.K.; Kalkum, M.; Jones, J.O. Vitamin K epoxide reductase regulation of androgen receptor activity. *Oncotarget* **2017**, *8*, 13818–13831. [CrossRef]
50. Kawano, H.; Sato, T.; Yamada, T.; Matsumoto, T.; Sekine, K.; Watanabe, T.; Nakamura, T.; Fukuda, T.; Yoshimura, K.; Yoshizawa, T.; et al. Suppressive function of androgen receptor in bone resorption. *Proc. Natl. Acad. Sci. USA* **2003**, *100*, 9416–9421. [CrossRef]
51. Falahati-Nini, A.; Riggs, B.L.; Atkinson, E.J.; O'Fallon, W.M.; Eastell, R.; Khosla, S. Relative contributions of testosterone and estrogen in regulating bone resorption and formation in normal elderly men. *J. Clin. Investig.* **2000**, *106*, 1553–1560. [CrossRef] [PubMed]
52. Bhasin, S.; Storer, T.W.; Berman, N.; Callegari, C.; Clevenger, B.; Phillips, J.; Bunnell, T.J.; Tricker, R.; Shirazi, A.; Casaburi, R. The effects of supraphysiologic doses of testosterone on muscle size and strength in normal men. *N. Engl. J. Med.* **1996**, *335*, 1–7. [CrossRef] [PubMed]
53. MacLean, H.E.; Chiu, W.S.; Notini, A.J.; Axell, A.M.; Davey, R.A.; McManus, J.F.; Ma, C.; Plant, D.R.; Lynch, G.S.; Zajac, J.D. Impaired skeletal muscle development and function in male, but not female, genomic androgen receptor knockout mice. *FASEB J.* **2008**, *22*, 2676–2689. [CrossRef] [PubMed]
54. Berkner, K.L.; Pudota, B.N. Vitamin K-dependent carboxylation of the carboxylase. *Proc. Natl. Acad. Sci. USA* **1998**, *95*, 466–471. [CrossRef] [PubMed]
55. Annis, D.S.; Ma, H.; Balas, D.M.; Kumfer, K.T.; Sandbo, N.; Potts, G.K.; Coon, J.J.; Mosher, D.F. Absence of Vitamin K-Dependent γ-Carboxylation in Human Periostin Extracted from Fibrotic Lung or Secreted from a Cell Line Engineered to Optimize γ-Carboxylation. *PLoS ONE* **2015**, *10*, e0135374. [CrossRef] [PubMed]
56. Sultana, H.; Watanabe, K.; Rana, M.M.; Takashima, R.; Ohashi, A.; Komai, M.; Shirakawa, H. Effects of Vitamin K_2 on the Expression of Genes Involved in Bile Acid Synthesis and Glucose Homeostasis in Mice with Humanized PXR. *Nutrients* **2018**, *10*, 982. [CrossRef]
57. Blumberg, B.; Sabbagh, W., Jr.; Juguilon, H.; Bolado, J., Jr.; van Meter, C.M.; Ong, E.S.; Evans, R.M. SXR, a novel steroid and xenobiotic-sensing nuclear receptor. *Genes Dev.* **1998**, *12*, 3195–3205. [CrossRef] [PubMed]
58. Zhou, C.; Verma, S.; Blumberg, B. The steroid and xenobiotic receptor (SXR), beyond xenobiotic metabolism. *Nucl. Recept. Signal.* **2009**, *7*, e001. [CrossRef]
59. Staudinger, J.L.; Goodwin, B.; Jones, S.A.; Hawkins-Brown, D.; MacKenzie, K.I.; LaTour, A.; Liu, Y.; Klaassen, C.D.; Brown, K.K.; Reinhard, J.; et al. The nuclear receptor PXR is a lithocholic acid sensor that protects against liver toxicity. *Proc. Natl. Acad. Sci. USA* **2001**, *98*, 3369–3374. [CrossRef]
60. Xie, W.; Radominska-Pandya, A.; Shi, Y.; Simon, C.M.; Nelson, M.C.; Ong, E.S.; Waxman, D.J.; Evans, R.M. An essential role for nuclear receptors SXR/PXR in detoxification of cholestatic bile acids. *Proc. Natl. Acad. Sci. USA* **2001**, *98*, 3375–3380. [CrossRef]
61. Synold, T.W.; Dussault, I.; Forman, B.M. The orphan nuclear receptor SXR coordinately regulates drug metabolism and efflux. *Nat. Med.* **2001**, *7*, 584–590. [CrossRef] [PubMed]
62. Miki, Y.; Suzuki, T.; Tazawa, C.; Blumberg, B.; Sasano, H. Steroid and xenobiotic receptor (SXR), cytochrome P450 3A4 and multidrug resistance gene 1 in human adult and fetal tissues. *Mol. Cell Endocrinol.* **2005**, *231*, 75–85. [CrossRef] [PubMed]
63. Albermann, N.; Schmitz-Winnenthal, F.H.; Z'graggen, K.; Volk, C.; Hoffmann, M.M.; Haefeli, W.E.; Weiss, J. Expression of the drug transporters MDR1/ABCB1, MRP1/ABCC1, MRP2/ABCC2, BCRP/ABCG2, and PXR in peripheral blood mononuclear cells and their relationship with the expression in intestine and liver. *Biochem. Pharmacol.* **2005**, *70*, 949–958. [CrossRef] [PubMed]

64. Suhara, Y.; Watanabe, M.; Motoyoshi, S.; Nakagawa, K.; Wada, A.; Takeda, K.; Takahashi, K.; Tokiwa, H.; Okano, T. Synthesis of new vitamin K analogues as steroid and xenobiotic receptor (SXR) agonists: Insights into the biological role of the side chain part of vitamin K. *J. Med. Chem.* **2011**, *54*, 4918–4922. [CrossRef] [PubMed]
65. Anderson, G.L.; Limacher, M.; Assaf, A.R.; Bassford, T.; Beresford, S.A.; Black, H.; Bonds, D.; Brunner, R.; Brzyski, R.; Caan, B.; et al. Effects of conjugated equine estrogen in postmenopausal women with hysterectomy: The Women's Health Initiative randomized controlled trial. *JAMA* **2004**, *291*, 1701–1712. [PubMed]
66. Nagai, S.; Ikeda, K.; Horie-Inoue, K.; Shiba, S.; Nagasawa, S.; Takeda, S.; Inoue, S. Estrogen modulates exercise endurance along with mitochondrial uncoupling protein 3 downregulation in skeletal muscle of female mice. *Biochem. Biophys. Res. Commun.* **2016**, *480*, 758–764. [CrossRef] [PubMed]
67. Jilka, R.L.; O'Brien, C.A.; Roberson, P.K.; Bonewald, L.F.; Weinstein, R.S.; Manolagas, S.C. Dysapoptosis of osteoblasts and osteocytes increases cancellous bone formation but exaggerates cortical porosity with age. *J. Bone Miner. Res.* **2014**, *29*, 103–117. [CrossRef]
68. Bouckaert, J.H.; Said, A.H. Fracture healing by vitamin K. *Nature* **1960**, *185*, 849. [CrossRef]
69. Hart, J.P.; Shearer, M.J.; Klenerman, L.; Catterall, A.; Reeve, J.; Sambrook, P.N.; Dodds, R.A.; Bitensky, L.; Chayen, J. Electrochemical detection of depressed circulating levels of vitamin K1 in osteoporosis. *J. Clin. Endocrinol. Metab.* **1985**, *60*, 1268–1269. [CrossRef]
70. Booth, S.L.; Tucker, K.L.; Chen, H.; Hannan, M.T.; Gagnon, D.R.; Cupples, L.A.; Wilson, P.W.; Ordovas, J.; Schaefer, E.J.; Dawson-Hughes, B.; et al. Dietary vitamin K intakes are associated with hip fracture but not with bone mineral density in elderly men and women. *Am. J. Clin. Nutr.* **2000**, *71*, 1201–1208. [CrossRef]
71. Kaneki, M.; Hodges, S.J.; Hosoi, T.; Fujiwara, S.; Lyons, A.; Crean, S.J.; Ishida, N.; Nakagawa, M.; Takechi, M.; Sano, Y.; et al. Japanese fermented soybean food as the major determinant of the large geographic difference in circulating levels of vitamin K2: Possible implications for hip-fracture risk. *Nutrition* **2001**, *17*, 315–321. [CrossRef]
72. Yaegashi, Y.; Onoda, T.; Tanno, K.; Kuribayashi, T.; Sakata, K.; Orimo, H. Association of hip fracture incidence and intake of calcium, magnesium, vitamin D, and vitamin K. *Eur. J. Epidemiol.* **2008**, *23*, 219–225. [CrossRef] [PubMed]
73. Mott, A.; Bradley, T.; Wright, K.; Cockayne, E.S.; Shearer, M.J.; Adamson, J.; Lanham-New, S.A.; Torgerson, D.J. Effect of vitamin K on bone mineral density and fractures in adults: An updated systematic review and meta-analysis of randomised controlled trials. *Osteoporos Int.* **2019**. [CrossRef] [PubMed]
74. Inoue, T.; Fujita, T.; Kishimoto, H.; Makino, T.; Nakamura, T.; Nakamura, T.; Sato, T.; Yamazaki, K. Randomized controlled study on the prevention of osteoporotic fractures (OF study): A phase IV clinical study of 15-mg menatetrenone capsules. *J. Bone Miner. Metab.* **2009**, *27*, 66–75. [CrossRef] [PubMed]
75. Kinoshita, H.; Nakagawa, K.; Narusawa, K.; Goseki-Sone, M.; Fukushi-Irie, M.; Mizoi, L.; Yoshida, H.; Okano, T.; Nakamura, T.; Suzuki, T.; et al. A functional single nucleotide polymorphism in the vitamin-K-dependent gamma-glutamyl carboxylase gene (Arg325Gln) is associated with bone mineral density in elderly Japanese women. *Bone* **2007**, *40*, 451–456. [CrossRef]
76. Ichikawa, T.; Horie-Inoue, K.; Ikeda, K.; Blumberg, B.; Inoue, S. Steroid and xenobiotic receptor SXR mediates vitamin K2-activated transcription of extracellular matrix-related genes and collagen accumulation in osteoblastic cells. *J. Biol. Chem.* **2006**, *281*, 16927–16934. [CrossRef]
77. Ohta, K.; Lupo, G.; Kuriyama, S.; Keynes, R.; Holt, C.E.; Harris, W.A.; Tanaka, H.; Ohnuma, S. Tsukushi functions as an organizer inducer by inhibition of BMP activity in cooperation with chordin. *Dev. Cell* **2004**, *7*, 347–358. [CrossRef]
78. Wagener, R.; Ehlen, H.W.; Ko, Y.P.; Kobbe, B.; Mann, H.H.; Sengle, G.; Paulsson, M. The matrilins–adaptor proteins in the extracellular matrix. *FEBS Lett.* **2005**, *579*, 3323–3329. [CrossRef]
79. Roman-Roman, S.; Garcia, T.; Jackson, A.; Theilhaber, J.; Rawadi, G.; Connolly, T.; Spinella-Jaegle, S.; Kawai, S.; Courtois, B.; Bushnell, S.; et al. Identification of genes regulated during osteoblastic differentiation by genome-wide expression analysis of mouse calvaria primary osteoblasts in vitro. *Bone* **2003**, *32*, 474–482. [CrossRef]
80. Filipp, D.; Alizadeh-Khiavi, K.; Richardson, C.; Palma, A.; Paredes, N.; Takeuchi, O.; Akira, S.; Julius, M. Soluble CD14 enriched in colostrum and milk induces B cell growth and differentiation. *Proc. Natl. Acad. Sci. USA* **2001**, *98*, 603–608. [CrossRef]

81. Manabe, N.; Kawaguchi, H.; Chikuda, H.; Miyaura, C.; Inada, M.; Nagai, R.; Nabeshima, Y.; Nakamura, K.; Sinclair, A.M.; Scheuermann, R.H.; et al. Connection between B lymphocyte and osteoclast differentiation pathways. *J. Immunol.* **2001**, *167*, 2625–2631. [CrossRef] [PubMed]
82. Azuma, K.; Casey, S.C.; Ito, M.; Urano, T.; Horie, K.; Ouchi, Y.; Kirchner, S.; Blumberg, B.; Inoue, S. Pregnane X receptor knockout mice display osteopenia with reduced bone formation and enhanced bone resorption. *J. Endocrinol.* **2010**, *207*, 257–263. [CrossRef] [PubMed]
83. Konno, Y.; Moore, R.; Kamiya, N.; Negishi, M. Nuclear xenobiotic receptor PXR-null mouse exhibits hypophosphatemia and represses the Na/Pi-cotransporter SLC34A2. *Pharm. Genom.* **2010**, *20*, 9–17. [CrossRef] [PubMed]
84. Urano, T.; Shiraki, M.; Ouchi, Y.; Inoue, S. Association of a single nucleotide polymorphism in the steroid and xenobiotic receptor (SXR) gene (IVS1-579A/G) with bone mineral density. *Geriatr. Gerontol. Int.* **2007**, *7*, 104–109. [CrossRef]
85. Neogi, T.; Booth, S.L.; Zhang, Y.Q.; Jacques, P.F.; Terkeltaub, R.; Aliabadi, P.; Felson, D.T. Low vitamin K status is associated with osteoarthritis in the hand and knee. *Arthritis Rheum.* **2006**, *54*, 1255–1261. [CrossRef] [PubMed]
86. Oka, H.; Akune, T.; Muraki, S.; En-yo, Y.; Yoshida, M.; Saika, A.; Sasaki, S.; Nakamura, K.; Kawaguchi, H.; Yoshimura, N. Association of low dietary vitamin K intake with radiographic knee osteoarthritis in the Japanese elderly population: Dietary survey in a population-based cohort of the ROAD study. *J. Orthop. Sci.* **2009**, *14*, 687–692. [CrossRef]
87. Misra, D.; Booth, S.L.; Tolstykh, I.; Felson, D.T.; Nevitt, M.C.; Lewis, C.E.; Torner, J.; Neogi, T. Vitamin K deficiency is associated with incident knee osteoarthritis. *Am. J. Med.* **2013**, *126*, 243–248. [CrossRef]
88. Neogi, T.; Felson, D.T.; Sarno, R.; Booth, S.L. Vitamin K in hand osteoarthritis: Results from a randomized clinical trial. *Ann. Rheum. Dis.* **2008**, *67*, 1570–1573. [CrossRef]
89. Azuma, K.; Casey, S.C.; Urano, T.; Horie-Inoue, K.; Ouchi, Y.; Blumberg, B.; Inoue, S. Pregnane X receptor knockout mice display aging-dependent wearing of articular cartilage. *PLoS ONE* **2015**, *10*, e0119177. [CrossRef] [PubMed]
90. Koike, T.; Izumikawa, T.; Tamura, J.; Kitagawa, H. FAM20B is a kinase that phosphorylates xylose in the glycosaminoglycan-protein linkage region. *Biochem. J.* **2009**, *421*, 157–162. [CrossRef]
91. Oya, K.; Ishida, K.; Nishida, T.; Sato, S.; Kishino, M.; Hirose, K.; Ogawa, Y.; Ikebe, K.; Takeshige, F.; Yasuda, H.; et al. Immunohistochemical analysis of dentin matrix protein 1 (Dmp1) phosphorylation by Fam20C in bone: Implications for the induction of biomineralization. *Histochem. Cell Biol.* **2017**, *147*, 341–351. [CrossRef] [PubMed]
92. Rosenberg, I.H. Sarcopenia: Origins and clinical relevance. *J. Nutr.* **1997**, *127*, 990S–991S. [CrossRef] [PubMed]
93. Cruz-Jentoft, A.J.; Baeyens, J.P.; Bauer, J.M.; Boirie, Y.; Cederholm, T.; Landi, F.; Martin, F.C.; Michel, J.P.; Rolland, Y.; Schneider, S.M.; et al. European Working Group on Sarcopenia in Older People. Sarcopenia: European consensus on definition and diagnosis: Report of the European Working Group on Sarcopenia in Older People. *Age Ageing* **2010**, *39*, 412–423. [CrossRef] [PubMed]
94. Cruz-Jentoft, A.J.; Bahat, G.; Bauer, J.; Boirie, Y.; Bruyère, O.; Cederholm, T.; Cooper, C.; Landi, F.; Rolland, Y.; Sayer, A.A.; et al. Writing Group for the European Working Group on Sarcopenia in Older People 2 (EWGSOP2), and the Extended Group for EWGSOP2. Sarcopenia: Revised European consensus on definition and diagnosis. *Age Ageing* **2019**, *48*, 16–31. [CrossRef] [PubMed]
95. Shea, M.K.; Loeser, R.F.; Hsu, F.C.; Booth, S.L.; Nevitt, M.; Simonsick, E.M.; Strotmeyer, E.S.; Vermeer, C.; Kritchevsky, S.B. Health ABC Study. Vitamin K Status and Lower Extremity Function in Older Adults: The Health Aging and Body Composition Study. *J. Gerontol. A Biol. Sci. Med. Sci.* **2016**, *71*, 1348–1355. [CrossRef] [PubMed]
96. Van Ballegooijen, A.J.; van Putten, S.R.; Visser, M.; Beulens, J.W.; Hoogendijk, E.O. Vitamin K status and physical decline in older adults-The Longitudinal Aging Study Amsterdam. *Maturitas* **2018**, *113*, 73–79. [CrossRef] [PubMed]
97. Shea, M.K.; Dawson-Hughes, B.; Gundberg, C.M.; Booth, S.L. Reducing Undercarboxylated Osteocalcin With Vitamin K Supplementation Does Not Promote Lean Tissue Loss or Fat Gain Over 3 Years in Older Women and Men: A Randomized Controlled Trial. *J. Bone Miner. Res.* **2017**, *32*, 243–249. [CrossRef] [PubMed]

98. Fulton, R.L.; McMurdo, M.E.; Hill, A.; Abboud, R.J.; Arnold, G.P.; Struthers, A.D.; Khan, F.; Vermeer, C.; Knapen, M.H.; Drummen, N.E.; et al. Effect of Vitamin K on Vascular Health and Physical Function in Older People with Vascular Disease—A Randomised Controlled Trial. *J. Nutr. Health Aging* **2016**, *20*, 325–333. [CrossRef]

2

Vitamin K in Chronic Kidney Disease

Mario Cozzolino [1,*], Michela Mangano [1], Andrea Galassi [1], Paola Ciceri [2], Piergiorgio Messa [2] and Sagar Nigwekar [3]

1 Renal Division, Department of Health Sciences, University of Milan, 20142 Milan, Italy; michelamangano91@gmail.com (M.M.); andrea.galassi@asst-santipaolocarlo.it (A.G.)

2 Renal Research Laboratory, Department of Nephrology, Dialysis and Renal Transplant, Fondazione IRCCS Ca' Granda, Ospedale Maggiore Policlinico & Fondazione D'Amico per la Ricerca sulle Malattie Renali, 20122 Milan, Italy; p.ciceri@hotmail.it (P.C.); piergiorgio.messa@unimi.it (P.M.)

3 Department of Medicine, Division of Nephrology, Massachusetts General Hospital, Boston, MA 02114, USA; SNIGWEKAR@mgh.harvard.edu

* Correspondence: mario.cozzolino@unimi.it

Abstract: Vitamin K is a composite term referring to a group of fat-soluble vitamins that function as a cofactor for the enzyme γ-glutamyl carboxylase (GGCX), which activates a number of vitamin K-dependent proteins (VKDPs) involved in haemostasis and vascular and bone health. Accumulating evidence demonstrates that chronic kidney disease (CKD) patients suffer from subclinical vitamin K deficiency, suggesting that this represents a population at risk for the biological consequences of poor vitamin K status. This deficiency might be caused by exhaustion of vitamin K due to its high requirements by vitamin K-dependent proteins to inhibit calcification.

Keywords: vitamin K; CKD; vascular calcification

---

1. Introduction

There are two forms of vitamin K: K1 (phylloquinone, PK) mainly found in green vegetables, and K2 (including different menaquinones, MKs) derived from intestinal bacteria and fermented food (cheeses and "natty", a Japanese soybean product) [1,2]. Liver is also a rich source of menaquinones [3]. We know about more than 12 different types of MKs, from MK-4 to MK-15, but the most common MKs in humans are the short-chain MK-4; it is the only MK produced by systemic conversion of phylloquinone to menaquinones [4].

Vitamin K is a non-polar molecule; after its intestinal absorption, vitamin k is solubilised by bile salt and pancreatic juice; vitamin K is then packaged into chylomicrons which are secreted into the lymphatic system [5]. For this reason lipids, in particular triglycerides, interfere with vitamin K measurement.

Vitamin K is as a substrate for an enzyme, the vitamin K-dependent carboxylase, that converts specific glutamic acid residues of a small number of proteins to glutamic carboxyl (Gla) residues by the addition of a CO_2. Vitamin K is necessary to introduce carboxyl groups into glutamic acid residues in blood coagulation factors (II, VII, IX, X) to yield Gla residues [6]; Gla-containing proteins include osteocalcin (OC), synthesized by the osteoblasts in bone, and matrix Gla protein (MGP), synthesized by chondrocytes and vascular smooth muscle cells (VSMCs), involved in bone mineralization and inhibition of vascular calcifications, respectively.

2. Vitamin K Deficiency

Indirect functional tests can be assessed to detect vitamin k levels, such as the prothrombin time or measurement of undercarboxylated proteins OC and MGP, which are more sensitive in detecting subclinical vitamin K deficiency than prothrombin time [6]. This measurement is possible because vitamin K-dependent proteins (VKDP) cannot attain their carboxylation status (and they remain undercarboxylated) in the presence of vitamin K deficiency; this condition causes the loss of their capacity to bind calcium, so that bone metabolism may be impaired and the process of vascular calcification enhanced [7]. A high percentage of undercarboxylated OC (uOC) reflects vitamin K intake and the long-term vitamin K status. Osteocalcin levels are also influenced by vitamin D, which is required for the production of uOC, and by parathyroid hormone (PTH), which is frequently elevated in CKD patients [6,8,9]. Therefore, chronic kidney disease (CKD) patients with hyperparathyroidism will present high serum uOC, but this does not necessarily mean that they are vitamin K deficient.

A good alternative to evaluate vitamin K status is through the inactive form of MGP, even if inactive MGP may only reflect the vitamin K status at the vascular level and not at bone or liver. Indeed, randomized controlled studies have shown that vitamin K therapy decreases undercarboxylated unphosphorylated MGP (uc-dp-MGP) levels [9–11]; in contrast, anti-vitamin K (AVK) treatment increased the amount of inactive uc-dp-MGP [12] and stopping that treatment decreased uc-dp-MGP [13]. All these data suggest that uc-dp-MGP could be a good marker of vitamin K status [6].

3. Vitamin K Status in CKD Patients

Evidence demonstrates that CKD patients suffer from subclinical vitamin K deficiency [14], suggesting that this population is at risk for any consequences of poor vitamin K status. This deficiency might be caused by exhaustion of vitamin K due to its high requirement by vitamin K-dependent proteins to inhibit calcification. However, dietary recommendations for CKD patients, such as diets low in potassium (fewer leafy green vegetables rich in K1) and low in phosphate (fewer dairy products rich in K2) could promote this deficiency.

Considering that vitamin K is essential for the activation of matrix Gla protein (MGP), a powerful inhibitor of tissue calcification, functional vitamin K deficiency may contribute to high vascular calcification (VC) burden in haemodialysis patients; this is process in which mineral is pathologically deposited in blood vessels, mainly in large elastic and muscular arteries such as the aorta and the coronary, carotid, and peripheral arteries. The presence of VC is directly related to increased cardiovascular morbidity and mortality in dialysis patients [15].

Circulating non-phosphorylated non-carboxylated MGP, which is formed as a result of vitamin K deficiency in CKD, is associated with cardiovascular disease and with overall survival [16]; in contrast, in older individuals without CKD, non-carboxylated MGP was linked to abnormal vitamin K status, but not to coronary artery calcium content [17]. Shea et al. [17] reported the latter condition, and these findings are in contrast with results of case–control studies reporting higher plasma ucMGP among patients with diseases characterized by vascular calcification and kidney disease; however, the prior studies did not measure CAC directly as they have. Furthermore, the ucMGP may be a marker for other risk factors, such as hyperlipidaemia and hypertension [17].

Schurgers et al. measured dpucMGP in a cohort of 107 patients ranging from CKD stages 2–5D, and reported that levels of plasma dp-ucMGP increased progressively with CKD stage. They showed, therefore, a decline in this biomarker with reduction in GFR [18]; the risk of vascular calcification is presumed higher if the calcification-inhibitory effect of MGP is impaired. Pre-clinical studies confirm that diminished vitamin K status influences the severity of arterial calcification in rats with CKD that can be prevented by a diet rich in vitamin K1 [19].

Holden et al., in a study of 172 stage 3–5 CKD patients, demonstrated that over 50% consumed less than the recommended adequate intake for vitamin K; moreover, 6% were vitamin K-insufficient according to low levels of serum phylloquinone (<0.4 ng/mL), 60% were insufficient according to high levels of ucOC (>20% ucOC), and 97% were insufficient according to high levels of protein-induced vitamin K absence or antagonist II (PIVKA-II) (>2 nmol/L) [20].

Several studies focused on the vitamin K status in haemodialysis (HD) patients [21]. On account of its lipophilic characteristics, vitamin K would not be expected to be removed via the dialysis procedure but there is a growing and consistent body of evidence supporting the notion that maintenance HD patients have a global poor vitamin K status; while the exact reason for the low intake is unknown, it is likely related to the dietary regimen prescribed for HD patients and overall poor nutrient intake.

As reported by Westenfeld et al., at baseline, haemodialysis patients had 4.5-fold higher dephosphorylated, uncarboxylated MGP and 8.4-fold higher uncarboxylated osteocalcin levels compared with controls [11]. Cranenburg et al. measured and assessed vitamin K1 and K2 intake and the vitamin K status in 40 haemodialysis patients: the intake was low in these patients (median 140 μg/day), especially on days of dialysis and the weekend as compared to intakes reported in a reference population of healthy adults (mean K1 and K2 intake 200 and 31 μg/day, respectively) [14]. In response to poor dietary intake, body stores of vitamin K are rapidly depleted. Undercarboxylated vitamin K-dependent bone and coagulation proteins were found to be elevated in 33 haemodialysis patients, indicating subclinical hepatic vitamin K deficiency. Very high non-carboxylated MGP levels, endemic to all patients, also strongly suggested vascular vitamin K deficiency.

Voong et al. reported that 29% and 93% of maintenance HD patients met criteria for sub-clinical vitamin K deficiency based on low levels of phylloquinone and high levels of ucOC, suggesting there is also vitamin K deficiency at the level of bone [22].

Some studies demonstrated that peritoneal dialysis (PD) patients have a similar degree of vitamin K insufficiency as maintenance HD patients: in a study of 28 PD patients, 46% had vitamin K deficiency as measured by elevated PIVKA II levels (>2 nM/L) [23]. In a cross-sectional study of 21 PD patients, it was demonstrated that 24% of them had vitamin K deficiency as assessed by serum K1 (<0.4 nM/L) and all patients had vitamin K deficiency as assessed by increased percentage of ucOC (>20% was the cut off for vitamin K deficiency, mean was 60%) [24].

Jansz et al. studied the influence of kidney transplantation and phosphate binder use on vitamin K status and found that kidney transplant recipients have substantially lower dp-ucMGP levels compared to patients on haemo- or peritoneal dialysis, indicating better vitamin K status after restoration of kidney function. In general, instead, phosphate binder use is not associated with dp-ucMGP levels except for sevelamer monotherapy. which is associated with significantly higher dp-ucMGP levels, suggesting a negative effect of sevelamer on vitamin K status [25].

4. Anti-Vitamin K Treatment and Effects—Warfarin

Warfarin is a vitamin K antagonist; its use represents a model of vitamin K insufficiency. It induces arterial calcification in experimental models, but whether this occurs in humans is unclear.

Tantisattamo et al. [26] examined breast arterial calcification identified on mammograms. Screening mammograms from women with current, past, or future warfarin use were examined for the presence of arterial calcification and compared with mammograms obtained in untreated women matched for age and diabetes mellitus. In 451 women with mammograms performed after ≥1 month of warfarin therapy, the prevalence of arterial calcification was 50% greater than in 451 untreated women (39.0% versus 25.9%; $p < 0.0001$). This study showed that the prevalence of breast arterial calcification is increased in women with current or past warfarin use independent of other risk factors and conditions predating warfarin use; this effect may be irreversible and appears to be cumulative.

McCabe at al. [19] wanted to determine whether modifying vitamin K status, either by increasing dietary vitamin K intake or by antagonism with therapeutic doses of warfarin, could alter the development of vascular calcification in male Sprague–Dawley rats with adenine-induced CKD. Pulse pressure and pulse wave velocity were increased after treatment with warfarin in CKD rats, as well as calcium concentrations in the thoracic aorta (3-fold), abdominal aorta (8-fold), renal artery (4-fold), and carotid artery (20-fold) were significantly increased. It is interesting to notice that therapeutic warfarin did not induce calcification in the blood vessels of healthy rats despite depletion of tissue vitamin K;

in contrast, compared with CKD alone, warfarin markedly increased the levels of vascular calcification in all vessels studied in the presence of CKD.

Thus, vitamin K has an important role in modifying mechanisms linked to the susceptibility of arteries to calcify in an experimental model of CKD.

As well as presenting a greater risk of development of vascular calcifications due to secondary hyperparathyroidism, haemodialysis patients are frequently treated with vitamin K antagonists, mainly to prevent stroke in atrial fibrillation, potentially compounding the cardiovascular risk in these already vulnerable patients. Warfarin may predispose to different side effect, such as bone fractures and vascular calcification, by different mechanisms: directly, by inhibition of carboxylation of OC and other bone matrix proteins; indirectly, because patients treated with warfarin may limit their dietary intake of foods rich in vitamin K [18,19].

4.1. Bone Fracture

Studies on bone fractures in CKD patients are limited. According to the available literature, the prevalence of vertebral fractures in dialysis patients appears to be similar to the general population, between 20.9% and 26.5% [27,28]; however Rodriguez-Garcia et al. [29] demonstrated a positive, significant correlation between vertebral fractures and vascular calcification in the dialysis population. This is probably due to underdiagnosis of vertebral fractures both in the general and in the dialysis population; this hypothesis was confirmed by the unpublished data of Fusaro et al., in which a vertebral fracture prevalence of 57% was found in a population of 68 haemodialysis patients [7]. Alem et al. studied the incidence of hip fractures and they found a considerably higher risk of hip fracture among dialysis patients than in general population [30].

Kohlmeier et al. were the first to demonstrate an independent association between poor vitamin K status and risk of bone fracture in patients in haemodialysis [31], while Fusaro et al. conducted an observational study of 387 prevalent HD, determining that over 50% of prevalent haemodialysis patients have vertebral fractures [32]. In this study, vitamin K1 deficiency (defined as a phylloquinone level adjusted for serum triglycerides <0.21 ng/mL), was the strongest predictor for the presence of a vertebral fracture (an adjusted odds ratio approaching 3).

In another study, Fusaro et al. found that haemodialysis patients treated with warfarin for greater than 1 year had an increased risk of vertebral fractures compared to those not on warfarin treatment [33]. With regard to vitamin K administration for the prevention of fractures, 13 randomized controlled studies with vitamin K1 and K2 treatment lasting for a minimum of 6 months were the subject of a meta-analysis [34]: 11 of these studies were from Japan, and seven reported fracture data. The subjects recruited in the studies were mainly menopausal women. All but one studies showed an advantage of vitamin K in reducing bone loss. All seven trials that reported fracture effects were from Japan and used vitamin K2 (menaquinone). Pooling the seven trials with fracture data in a meta-analysis, an odds ratio favouring menaquinone of 0.40 (95% confidence interval (CI), 0.25–0.65) for vertebral fractures, an OR of 0.23 (95% CI, 0.12–0.47) for hip fractures, and an OR of 0.19 (95% CI, 0.11–0.35) for all nonvertebral fractures were reported.

4.2. Cardiovascular Calcification

The first study [35] demonstrating strongly increased calcification of the aortic valves in patients taking oral anticoagulants—including warfarin and acenocoumarol—has been confirmed by many other researchers: Koos et al. demonstrated that subjects taking vitamin K antagonist anticoagulants had a significantly higher degree of arterial and aortic valve calcification than control subjects [36]. In a case report, Hristova et al. described a kidney transplant recipient exhibiting massive arterial calcification after the initiation of warfarin therapy [37]. Distal subcutaneous necrosis ultimately led to the patient's death. Rennenberg et al. showed rapid calcification of the femoral artery when patients are treated with oral anticoagulants, (OR 8.5; 95% confidence interval (CI) 2.01–35.95, for calcification in patients compared with controls) [38]. Similarly, patients taking oral anticoagulants showed significantly increased levels of coronary calcification [39].

4.3. Calciphylaxis

Approximately 1% of CKD patients develop calciphylaxis, a frequently fatal complication of end-stage renal disease. Notably, about 50% of patients with CKD stage 5D (CKD5D) who develop calciphylaxis are on vitamin K antagonists (VKAs) [40]. Compared to the dialysis patients worldwide, the overall number of calciphylaxis cases is minimal. However, in their case–control analysis, Hayashi et al. [41], calculated an 11.4-fold increased risk of developing calciphylaxis in Japanese dialysis patients on warfarin.

In the pilot case–control study by Nigwekar et al. the authors demonstrated that patients with calciphylaxis in end stage renal disease (ESRD) had proportionally higher plasma levels of the inactive ucMGP than dialysis controls. They investigated how MGP carboxylation influenced the risk of calciphylaxis in 20 patients receiving haemodialysis with calciphylaxis (cases) and 20 patients receiving haemodialysis without calciphylaxis (controls); case patients had higher plasma levels of ucMGP and carboxylated MGP (cMGP) than controls. However, the fraction of total MGP that was carboxylated (relative cMGP concentration = cMGP/(cMGP + uncarboxylated MGP)) was lower in cases than in controls (0.58 $\pm$ 0.02 versus 0.69 $\pm$ 0.03, respectively; $p = 0.003$). The authors concluded that a vitamin K deficiency-mediated reduction in relative cMGP concentration may have a role in the pathogenesis of calciphylaxis [42].

Krueger et al. believe that vitamin K, and especially vitamin K2, supplementation may become an important option in the standard treatment for calcification-prone CKD patients [43].

4.4. Arteriovenous Fistula Failure

Arteriovenous fistula (AVFs) is a frequently used vascular access type for CKD patients requiring haemodialysis (HD) [44]. AVF failure is a complication leading to high hospitalization rates and morbidity [45]. Whereas early AVF failure is caused by thrombosis or by inability of the vein to dilate, later course AVF failure is induced by stenosis and thrombosis resulting from neointimal hyperplasia (NIH) and calcification [46,47]. Recent work indicates that AVF calcification contributes to AVF failure [48]; in arterialized veins, calcification occurs in tunica media and intima. HD patients have a poor overall vitamin K status, and a high number of CKD patients at risk of arterial and venous thrombosis receive oral anticoagulants (vitamin K antagonists; VKAs) [49]. It has been shown that VSMCs from varicose veins increased calcification when treated with warfarin, indicating similar processes in venous and arterial VSMCs [50]. Vascular access calcification is an independent predictor of mortality, whereas nothing is known about effects of VKA on AVF, NIH, and calcification.

The objective of the study of Zaragatski et al. was to investigate the effects of vitamin K antagonists and vitamin K2 treatment on neointimal hyperplasia development and calcification in rats and in arterialized human veins [51]. AVF was generated in female rats while chronic kidney disease was induced using an adenine-enriched diet. Arterialization, CKD, and vitamin K antagonists all significantly enhanced venous neointimal hyperplasia. K2 treatment and vitamin K antagonists significantly reduced neointimal hyperplasia in arterialized veins in healthy rats but not in rats with CKD. Arterialization, CKD, and vitamin K antagonism all significantly increased, whereas K2 supplementation attenuated calcification in healthy rats and rats with CKD.

K2 significantly enhanced matrix Gla protein carboxylation in control rats and rats with CKD. Arterialized human vein samples contained inactive matrix Gla protein at calcification and neointimal hyperplasia sites, indicating local vitamin K deficiency. Thus, vitamin K antagonists have detrimental effects on AVF remodeling, whereas K2 reduced neointimal hyperplasia and calcification indicating vasoprotective effects. Hence, K2 administration may be useful to prevent neointimal hyperplasia and calcification in arterialized veins.

5. New Oral Anticoagulant vs. Warfarin

New oral anticoagulants (NOACs) are valid alternatives to vitamin K antagonists in the general population, but their use in dialysis has been limited by substantial renal clearance.

Dabigatran and rivaroxaban have not been studied in end-stage renal disease patients who were specifically excluded from two large randomized trials that were conducted in patients without renal failure [52,53]. In dialysis patients, prescription of these novel oral anticoagulant drugs (NOACs) is currently contraindicated because the drugs are cleared by kidneys and drug levels can bio-accumulate to precipitate bleeding; as demonstrated by Chan et al., the unadjusted event rate of major bleeding increased with drug dosage [54]. The study of Chan et al. is the first to evaluate these drugs in the dialysis population, and suggests concern given the increasing use of dabigatran and rivaroxaban in the ESRD population despite formal FDA warnings of caution in renal failure. In fact, their secondary analyses suggest excess morbidity and mortality from bleeding associatively higher with dabigatran and rivaroxaban when compared to warfarin [54].

Among the available NOACs, apixaban has the lowest renal elimination. Both dabigatran and rivaroxaban were associated with increased bleeding in dialysis patients but recently apixaban was non-inferior to warfarin in a large database study.

Siontis et al. [55] conducted a retrospective cohort study in patients with ESRD and atrial fibrillation (AF) in dialysis who initiated treatment with apixaban or warfarin. Standard dose of apixaban (5 mg twice a day) was associated with significantly lower risks of stroke/systemic embolism and death as compared with either reduced dose of apixaban (2.5 mg twice a day; n = 1317; HR 0.61, 95% CI 0.37–0.98, p = 0.04 for stroke/systemic embolism; and HR 0.64, 95% CI 0.45–0.92, p = 0.01 for death) or warfarin (HR 0.64, 95% CI 0.42–0.97, p = 0.04 for stroke/systemic embolism; and HR 0.63, 95% CI 0.46–0.85, p = 0.003 for death). The authors concluded that, among ESRD patients with AF on dialysis, apixaban use may be associated with lower risk of major bleeding compared with warfarin, with a standard 5 mg twice a day dose also associated with reductions in thromboembolic and mortality risk.

6. Phosphate Binders

Chronic kidney disease mineral bone disorders (CKD-MBD) is a complex syndrome in dialysis patients, which includes alterations of biochemical parameters of the mineral and bone metabolism, a clinically and histologically manifested bone disease and vascular calcifications associated with an increased risk of cardiovascular morbidity and mortality. One of its most frequent components is hyperphosphatemia, which has traditionally been treated with dietary restrictions and intestinal phosphorus binders [56].

It is unknown if the use of phosphate binders, especially calcium based binders, may actually be harmful [57]. There is some attenuation or delay of progression of VC by the noncalcium-based phosphate binders as compared to the calcium containing binders [58–60]. However VC frequently progresses despite adequate phosphate concentrations; probably due to chronic inflammation, increasing calcium load from calcium based binders and other factors such as vitamin K deficiency.

In their study, Neradova et al. set up a study in which vitamin K2 (menaquinone-7; MK-7) was mixed with five different phosphate binders, in presence or absence of phosphate, incubated at pH 6 and fixed temperature of 37 degrees Celsius. In particular, 1 mg of vitamin K2 was added to a medium with pH 6 containing 67 mg phosphate binder with either 7 mg of phosphate or no phosphate [61].

This experiment showed that sucroferric-oxyhydroxide and sevelamer carbonate were the only binders that did not bind vitamin K2 in vitro. This in vitro study demonstrated that calcium acetate/magnesium carbonate binds vitamin K2 strongly both in absence (p = 0.001) and presence of phosphate (p = 0.003). For Lanthanum carbonate this binding depends on the absence of phosphate, pointing to competitive binding between phosphate and vitamin K2 for this compound (p = 0.005) whereas no significant binding of vitamin K2 was observed in the solution containing vitamin K2 and phosphate (p = 0.462). Calcium carbonate binds vitamin K2 statistically and significantly in a solution with vitamin K2 and phosphate (p = 0.009), whereas without phosphate no significant binding of vitamin K2 was observed (p = 0.123). In the mixture with sevelamer carbonate a nominally lower concentration of K2 was shown as well, but this decline was not statistically significant. Addition of sucroferric-oxyhydroxide did not lead to any decline of vitamin K2 at all, irrespective of presence or absence of phosphate.

The authors did not study the chemical explanation for this feature, but possibly the formed calcium-phosphate salt itself binds K2 as well. In conclusion, the presence or absence of phosphate significantly interferes with vitamin K2 binding, so phosphate binders could potentially limit the bioavailability of vitamin K2.

According to these results, in HD patients, in which phosphorus levels are usually elevated, phosphate binders that do not bind vitamin K in the presence of phosphate should be selected.

7. Drug and Vitamin K-Dependent Protein (VKDP)

Fusaro et al. carried out a sub-analysis to evaluate associations between drug consumption and VKDP levels in 387 haemodialyzed patients [62]. The VIKI study was an observational study performed in 387 adult patients of both genders who had been on dialysis for more than 1 year at 18 centres in Italy between November 2008 and November 2009. It was designed primarily to assess the prevalence of deficiency of vitamin K1 and vitamin K2 in dialysis patients. In this sub-study the authors evaluated drug consumption, determined bone Gla proteins (BGP) and MGP levels, and verified the presence of any vertebral fractures (VF) and VC by spine radiographs. Regarding mineral and bone disorder treatment, the most common were oral calcitriol (45.7%) and sevelamer (42.1%).

Total BGP levels were twice as high with calcimimetics versus no calcimimetics (290 vs. 158.5 mcg/L, $p < 0.0001$) and 69% higher with vitamin D analogues (268 vs. 159 mcg/L, $p < 0.0001$). Total MGP was 19% higher with calcimimetics (21.5 vs. 18.1 mcg/L, $p = 0.04$) and 54% higher with calcium acetate (27.9 vs. 18.1 mcg/L, $p = 0.003$); no difference was found with vitamin D analogues. This finding of increased MGP in patients treated with calcimimetics is the first in humans and it is consistent with the results of in vitro and in vivo experimental studies, in which MGP was measured before and after the administration of the calcimimetic [63–65].

Median Total BGP level was 29% lower in patients with $\geq$1 VF (151 vs. 213 mcg/L, $p = 0.0091$) and 36% lower in patients with VC (164 vs. 262.1 mcg/L, $p = 0.0003$). In non-survivors, median BGP and MGP were lower, but this difference reached the statistical significance for MGP only (152 vs. 191 mcg/L, $p = 0.20$ and 15.0 vs. 19.7 mcg/L, $p = 0.02$, respectively). No significant association between MGP levels and VF or VC was found, despite an association between high MGP levels and survival.

Pending studies on vitamin K supplementation, calcimimetics, and vitamin D analogues may play a role in preserving vitamin K-dependent protein activity, thus contributing to bone and vascular health in CKD patients.

8. Vitamin K Supplementation

The question therefore arises of whether CKD patients might benefit from extra vitamin K intake. In the population-based Rotterdam study [66], dietary intake data including vitamin K were available for 4800 elderly patients. The authors assessed the risk of incident coronary heart disease, all-cause mortality, and aortic calcification based on tertiles of energy-adjusted vitamin K intake. They found that low vitamin K2 intake was associated with a higher incidence of severe aortic calcification and increased mortality. In line with this observation, a recent pilot study investigated whether daily vitamin K2 supplementation would improve the bioactivity of vitamin K-dependent proteins in CKD5D patients: after only 6 weeks of daily vitamin K2 supplementation, a significant decrease in dp-uc-MGP, ucOC, and uncarboxylated factor II (ucFII) levels was observed. This shows that vitamin K is able to reach tissues, including the vessel wall, and to correct the biochemical and local tissue consequences of vitamin K deficiency.

A supplementation in vitamin K in particular in HD an PD patients should be taken into account, considering the poor vitamin K status in CKD patients. One randomized controlled trial evaluated the response of biomarkers of vitamin K status (dp-uc-MGP, PIVKA-II and ucOC) to three doses of vitamin K2 (MK-7) administered over a period of 6 weeks in HD patients and the study reported that vitamin

K2 (MK-7) supplementation decreased dp-uc-MGP and PIVKA-II levels [11]. Shea et al. reported that supplementation with daily phylloquinone (0.5 mg) slowed the progression of cardiovascular calcification (CAC) over 3 years in healthy older adults with pre-existing CAC at baseline [67]; it is well established that patients with kidney failure have an increased risk for both vascular calcification and sub-clinical vitamin K deficiency but yet no trial that examines whether vitamin K supplementation prevents the progression of calcification in this population has been completed.

Furthermore, vitamin K status after kidney transplantation may play an important role. In a study made by Keyzer et al. [68], vitamin K deficiency was an important risk factor of overall mortality in kidney-transplanted patients.

Author Contributions: All Authors contributed in writing and reviewing the article.

References

1. Shearer, M.J.; Newman, P. Metabolism and cell biology of vitamin K. *Thromb Haemost* **2008**, *100*, 530–547. [PubMed]
2. Booth, S.L. Vitamin K: Food composition and dietary intakes. *Food Nutr. Res.* **2012**, *56*, 5505. [CrossRef] [PubMed]
3. Elder, S.J.; Haytowitz, D.B.; Howe, J.; Peterson, J.W.; Booth, S.L. Vitamin K contents of meat, dairy, and fast food in the US diet. *J. Agric. Food Chem.* **2006**, *54*, 463–467. [CrossRef] [PubMed]
4. Sakano, T.; Nagaoka, T.; Morimoto, A.; Hirauchi, K. Measurement of K vitamins in human and animal feces by high-performance liquid chromatography with fluorometric detection. *Chem. Pharm. Bull.* **1986**, *34*, 4322–4326. [CrossRef] [PubMed]
5. Ji, Y.; Li, X.; Tso, P. Intestinal fatty acid absorption. *Immununol. Endocr. Metab. Agents Med. Chem.* **2009**, *9*, 60–73. [CrossRef]
6. Fusaro, M.; Gallieni, M.; Rizzo, M.A.; Stucchi, A.; Delanaye, P.; Cavalier, E.; Moysés, R.M.A.; Jorgetti, V.; Iervasi, G.; Giannini, S.; et al. Vitamin K plasma levels determination in human health. *Clin. Chem. Lab. Med.* **2017**, *55*, 789–799. [CrossRef] [PubMed]
7. Fusaro, M.; Crepaldi, G.; Maggi, S.; Galli, F.; D'Angelo, A.; Calò, L.; Giannini, S.; Miozzo, D.; Gallieni, M. Vitamin K, bone fractures, and vascular calcifications in chronic kidney disease: An important but poorly studied relationship. *J. Endocrinol. Investig.* **2011**, *34*, 317–323. [CrossRef]
8. Buranasinsup, S.; Bunyaratavej, N. The intriguing correlation between undercarboxylated osteocalcin and vitamin D. *J. Med. Assoc. Thail.* **2015**, *98* (Suppl. 8), S16–S20.
9. Caluwé, R.; Vandecasteele, S.; Van Vlem, B.; Vermeer, C.; De Vriese, A.S. Vitamin K2 supplementation in haemodialysis patients: A randomized dose-finding study. *Nephrol. Dial. Transplant.* **2014**, *29*, 1385–1390. [CrossRef]
10. Boxma, P.Y.; van den Berg, E.; Geleijnse, J.M.; Laverman, G.D.; Schurgers, L.J.; Vermeer, C.; Kema, I.P.; Muskiet, F.A.; Navis, G.; Bakker, S.J.; et al. Vitamin K intake and plasma desphospho-uncarboxylated matrix Gla-protein levels in kidney transplant recipients. *PLoS ONE* **2012**, *7*, e47991. [CrossRef]
11. Westenfeld, R.; Krueger, T.; Schlieper, G.; Cranenburg, E.C.; Magdeleyns, E.J.; Heidenreich, S.; Holzmann, S.; Vermeer, C.; Jahnen-Dechent, W.; Ketteler, M.; et al. Effect of vitamin K2 supplementation on functional vitamin K deficiency in hemodialysis patients: A randomized trial. *Am. J. Kidney Dis.* **2012**, *59*, 186–195. [CrossRef] [PubMed]
12. Cranenburg, E.C.; Koos, R.; Schurgers, L.J.; Magdeleyns, E.J.; Schoonbrood, T.H.; Landewé, R.B. Characterisation and potential diagnostic value of circulating matrix Gla protein (MGP) species. *Thromb. Haemost.* **2010**, *104*, 811–822. [CrossRef]
13. Delanaye, P.; Dubois, B.E.; Lukas, P.; Peters, P.; Krzesinski, J.M.; Pottel, H.; Cavalier, E. Impact of stopping vitamin K antagonist therapy on concentrations of dephospho-uncarboxylated Matrix Gla protein. *Clin. Chem. Lab. Med.* **2015**, *53*, e191-3. [CrossRef] [PubMed]

14. Cranenburg, E.C.M.; Schurgers, L.J.; Uiterwijk, H.H.; Beulens, J.W.; Dalmeijer, G.W.; Westerhuis, R.; Magdeleyns, E.J.; Herfs, M.; Vermeer, C.; Laverman, G.D. Vitamin K intake and status are low in hemodialysis patients. *Kidney Int.* **2012**, *82*, 605–610. [CrossRef]
15. Bellasi, A.; Raggi, P. Vascular imaging in chronic kidney disease. *Curr. Opin. Nephrol. Hypertens.* **2012**, *21*, 382–388. [CrossRef] [PubMed]
16. Schlieper, G.; Westenfeld, R.; Krüger, T.; Cranenburg, E.C.; Magdeleyns, E.J.; Brandenburg, V.M.; Djuric, Z.; Damjanovic, T.; Ketteler, M.; Vermeer, C.; et al. Circulating nonphosphorylated carboxylated matrix gla protein predicts survival in ESRD. *J. Am. Soc. Nephrol.* **2011**, *22*, 387–395. [CrossRef] [PubMed]
17. Shea, M.K.; O'Donnell, C.J.; Vermeer, C.; Magdeleyns, E.J.; Crosier, M.D.; Gundberg, C.M.; Ordovas, J.M.; Kritchevsky, S.B.; Booth, S.L. Circulating uncarboxylated matrix gla protein is associated with vitamin K nutritional status, but not coronary artery calcium, in older adults. *J. Nutr.* **2011**, *141*, 1529–1534. [CrossRef]
18. Schurgers, L.J.; Barreto, D.V.; Barreto, F.C.; Liabeuf, S.; Renard, C.; Magdeleyns, E.J.; Vermeer, C.; Choukroun, G.; Massy, Z.A. The circulating inactive form of matrix gla protein is a surrogate marker for vascular calcification in chronic kidney disease: A preliminary report. *Clin. J. Am. Soc. Nephrol.* **2010**, *5*, 568–575. [CrossRef]
19. McCabe, K.; Booth, S.; Fu, X.; Shobeiri, N.; Pang, J.; Adams, M.; Holden, R. Dietary vitamin K and therapeutic warfarin alter the susceptibility to vascular calcification in experimental chronic kidney disease. *Kidney Int.* **2013**, *83*, 835–844. [CrossRef]
20. Holden, R.M.; Morton, A.R.; Garland, J.S.; Pavlov, A.; Day, A.G.; Booth, S.L. Vitamins K and D status in stages 3–5 chronic kidney disease. *Clin. J. Am. Soc. Nephrol.* **2010**, *5*, 590–597. [CrossRef]
21. McCabe, K.M.; Adams, M.A.; Holden, R.M. Vitamin K status in chronic kidney disease. *Nutrients* **2013**, *5*, 4390–4398. [CrossRef] [PubMed]
22. Voong, K.; Harrington, D.; Goldsmith, D. Vitamin K status in chronic kidney disease: A report of a study and a mini-review. *Int. Urol. Nephrol.* **2013**, *45*, 1339–1344. [CrossRef] [PubMed]
23. Stankowiak-Kulpa, H.; Krzyzanowska, P.; Koziol, L.; Grzymislawski, M.; Wanic-Kossowska, M.; Moczko, J.; Walkowiak, J. Vitamin K status in peritoneally dialyzed patients with chronic kidney disease. *Acta Biochim. Pol.* **2011**, *58*, 617–620. [PubMed]
24. Holden, R.M.; Iliescu, E.; Morton, A.R.; Booth, S.L. Vitamin K status of canadian peritoneal dialysis patients. *Perit. Dial. Int.* **2008**, *28*, 415–418. [PubMed]
25. Jansz, T.T.; Neradova, A.; van Ballegooijen, A.J.; Verhaar, M.C.; Vervloet, M.G.; Schurgers, L.J.; van Jaarsveld, B.C. The role of kidney transplantation and phosphate binder use in vitamin K status. *PLoS ONE* **2018**, *13*, e0203157. [CrossRef] [PubMed]
26. Tantisattamo, E.; Han, K.H.; O'Neill, W.C. Increased vascular calcification in patients receiving warfarin. *Arterioscler. Thromb. Vasc. Biol.* **2015**, *35*, 237–242. [CrossRef]
27. Rodriguez-Garcia, M.; Gomez-Alonso, C.; Naves-Diaz, M.; Díaz López, J.B.; Megido, J.; Gago, E.; Forascepi, R.; Cannata Andía, J.B. Prevalence of vertebral fractures and aortic calcifications in hemodialysis patients: Comparison with a population of the same age and sex. *Nefrologia* **2003**, *23* (Suppl. 2), 106–111. [PubMed]
28. Jamal, S.A.; Gilbert, J.; Gordon, C.; Bauer, D.C. Cortical pQCT measures are associated with fractures in dialysis patients. *J. Bone Miner. Res.* **2006**, *21*, 543–548. [CrossRef]
29. Rodriguez-Garcia, M.; Gomez-Alonso, C.; Naves-Diaz, M.; Diaz-Lopez, J.B.; Diaz-Corte, C.; Cannata-Andia, J.B.; Asturias Study Group. Vascular calcifications, vertebral fractures and mortality in haemodialysis patients. *Nephrol. Dial. Transplant.* **2009**, *24*, 239–246. [CrossRef]
30. Alem, A.M.; Sherrard, D.J.; Gillen, D.L.; Weiss, N.S.; Beresford, S.A.; Heckbert, S.R.; Wong, C.; Stehman-Breen, C. Increased risk of hip fracture among patients with end-stage renal disease. *Kidney Int.* **2000**, *58*, 396–399. [CrossRef] [PubMed]
31. Kohlmeier, M.; Saupe, J.; Shearer, M.J.; Schaefer, K.; Asmus, G. Bone health of adult hemodialysis patients is related to vitamin K status. *Kidney Int.* **1997**, *51*, 1218–1221. [CrossRef] [PubMed]
32. Fusaro, M.; Noale, M.; Viola, V.; Galli, F.; Tripepi, G.; Vajente, N.; Plebani, M.; Zaninotto, M.; Guglielmi, G.; Miotto, D.; et al. VItamin K Italian (VIKI) dialysis study investigators. Vitamin K, vertebral fractures, vascular calcifications, and mortality: Vitamin K Italian (VIKI) dialysis study. *J. Bone Miner. Res.* **2012**, *27*, 2271–2278. [CrossRef] [PubMed]

33. Fusaro, M.; Tripepi, G.; Noale, M.; Plebani, M.; Zaninotto, M.; Piccoli, A.; Naso, A.; Miozzo, D.; Giannini, S.; Avolio, M.; et al. Prevalence of vertebral fractures, vascular calcifications, and mortality in warfarin treated hemodialysis patients. *Curr. Vasc. Pharmacol.* **2013**, *13*, 248–258. [CrossRef]
34. Cockayne, S.; Adamson, J.; Lanham-New, S.; Shearer, M.J.; Gilbody, S.; Torgerson, D.J. Vitamin K and prevention of fractures: Systematic review and meta-analysis of randomized controlled trials. *Arch. Intern. Med.* **2006**, *166*, 1256–1261. [CrossRef] [PubMed]
35. Schurgers, L.J.; Aebert, H.; Vermeer, C.; Bultmann, B.; Janzen, J. Oral anticoagulant treatment: Friend or foe in cardiovascular disease? *Blood* **2004**, *104*, 3231–3232. [CrossRef]
36. Koos, R.; Mahnken, A.H.; Muhlenbruch, G.; Brandenburg, V.; Pflueger, B.; Wildberger, J.E.; Kuhl, H.P. Relation of oral anticoagulation to cardiac valvular and coronary calcium assessed by multislice spiral computed tomography. *Am. J. Cardiol.* **2005**, *96*, 747–749. [CrossRef] [PubMed]
37. Hristova, M.; van Beek, C.; Schurgers, L.J.; Lanske, B.; Danziger, J. Rapidly progressive severe vascular calcification sparing the kidney allograft following warfarin initiation. *Am. J. Kidney Dis.* **2010**, *56*, 1158–1162. [CrossRef]
38. Rennenberg, R.J.; van Varik, B.J.; Schurgers, L.J.; Hamulyak, K.; Ten Cate, H.; Leiner, T.; Vermeer, C.; de Leeuw, P.W.; Kroon, A.A. Chronic coumarin treatment is associated with increased extracoronary arterial calcification in humans. *Blood* **2010**, *115*, 5121–5123. [CrossRef]
39. Weijs, B.; Blaauw, Y.; Rennenberg, R.J.; Schurgers, L.J.; Timmermans, C.C.; Pison, L.; Nieuwlaat, R.; Hofstra, L.; Kroon, A.A.; Wildberger, J.; et al. Patients using vitamin K antagonists show increased levels of coronary calcification: An observational study in low-risk atrial fibrillation patients. *Eur. Heart J.* **2011**, *32*, 2555–2562. [CrossRef]
40. Chatrou, M.L.L.; Winckers, K.; Hackeng, T.M.; Reutelingsperger, C.P.; Schurgers, L.J. Vascular calcification: The price to pay for anticoagulation therapy with vitamin K-antagonists. *Blood Rev.* **2012**, *26*, 155–166. [CrossRef]
41. Hayashi, M.; Takamatsu, I.; Kanno, Y.; Yoshida, T.; Abe, T.; Sato, Y.; Japanese Calciphylaxis Study Group. A case-control study of calciphylaxis in Japanese end-stage renal disease patients. *Nephrol. Dial. Transplant.* **2012**, *27*, 1580–1584. [CrossRef] [PubMed]
42. Nigwekar, S.U.; Bloch, D.B.; Nazarian, R.M.; Vermeer, C.; Booth, S.L.; Xu, D.; Thadhani, R.I.; Malhotra, R. Vitamin K-dependent carboxylation of matrix Gla protein influences the risk of calciphylaxis. *J. Am. Soc. Nephrol.* **2017**, *28*, 1717–1722. [CrossRef] [PubMed]
43. Krueger, T.; Westenfeld, R.; Schurgers, L.; Brandenburg, V. Coagulation meets calcification: The vitamin K system. *Int. J. Artif. Organs* **2009**, *32*, 67–74. [CrossRef] [PubMed]
44. Pisoni, R.L.; Young, E.W.; Dykstra, D.M.; Greenwood, R.N.; Hecking, E.; Gillespie, B.; Wolfe, R.A.; Goodkin, D.A.; Held, P.J. Vascular access use in Europe and the United States: Results from the DOPPS. *Kidney Int.* **2002**, *61*, 305–316. [CrossRef] [PubMed]
45. Schwab, S.J.; Harrington, J.T.; Singh, A.; Roher, R.; Shohaib, S.A.; Perrone, R.D.; Meyer, K.; Beasley, D. Vascular access for hemodialysis. *Kidney Int.* **1999**, *55*, 2078–2090. [CrossRef] [PubMed]
46. Lemson, M.S.; Tordoir, J.H.; Daemen, M.J.A.P.; Kitslaar, P.J.E.H.M. Intimal hyperplasia in vascular grafts. *Eur. J. Vasc. Endovasc. Surg.* **2000**, *19*, 336–350. [CrossRef] [PubMed]
47. Goodman, W.G.; Goldin, J.; Kuizon, B.D.; Yoon, C.; Gales, B.; Sider, D.; Wang, Y.; Chung, J.; Emerick, A.; Greaser, L.; et al. Coronary-artery calcification in young adults with end-stage renal disease who are undergoing dialysis. *N. Engl. J. Med.* **2000**, *342*, 1478–1483. [CrossRef] [PubMed]
48. Balci, M.; Kirkpantur, A.; Turkvatan, A.; Mandıroglu, S.; Ozturk, E.; Afsar, B. Sclerostin as a new key player in arteriovenous fistula calcification. *Herz* **2013**, *40*, 289–297. [CrossRef]
49. Diener, H.C.; Hajjar, K.; Frank, B.; Perrey, M. New anticoagulants for stroke prevention in atrial fibrillation. *Herz* **2012**, *37*, 370–377. [CrossRef]
50. Cario-Toumaniantz, C.; Boularan, C.; Schurgers, L.J.; Le Cunff, M.; Léger, J.; Loirand, G.; Pacaud, P. Identification of differentially expressed genes in human varicose veins: Involvement of matrix gla protein in extracellular matrix remodeling. *J. Vasc. Res.* **2007**, *44*, 444–459. [CrossRef]
51. Zaragatski, E.; Grommes, J.; Schurgers, L.J.; Langer, S.; Kennes, L.; Tamm, M.; Koeppel, T.A.; Kranz, J.; Hackhofer, T.; Arakelyan, K.; et al. Vitamin K antagonism aggravates aggravates chronic kidney disease-induced neointimal hyperplasia and calcification in arterialized veins: Role of vitamin K tratment? *Kidney Int.* **2016**, *89*, 601–611. [CrossRef] [PubMed]

52. Connolly, S.J.; Ezekowitz, M.D.; Yusuf, S.; Eikelboom, J.; Oldgren, J.; Parekh, A.; Pogue, J.; Reilly, P.A.; Themeles, E.; Varrone, J.; et al. Dabigatran versus warfarin in patients with atrial fibrillation. *N. Engl. J. Med.* **2009**, *361*, 1139–1151. [CrossRef] [PubMed]
53. Patel, M.R.; Mahaffey, K.W.; Garg, J.; Pan, G.; Singer, D.E.; Hacke, W.; Breithardt, G.; Halperin, J.L.; Hankey, G.J.; Piccini, J.P.; et al. Rivaroxaban versus warfarin in nonvalvular atrial fibrillation. *N. Engl. J. Med.* **2011**, *365*, 883–891. [CrossRef] [PubMed]
54. Chan, K.E.; Edelman, E.R.; Wenger, J.B.; Thadhani, R.I.; Maddux, F.W. Dabigatran and rivaroxaban use in atrial fibrillation patients on hemodialysis. *Circulation* **2015**, *131*, 972–979. [CrossRef]
55. Siontis, K.C.; Zhang, X.; Eckard, A.; Bhave, N.; Schaubel, D.E.; He, K.; Tilea, A.; Stack, A.G.; Balkrishnan, R.; Yao, X.; et al. Outcomes Associated with Apixaban Use in End-Stage Kidney Disease Patients with Atrial Fibrillation in the United States. *Circulation* **2018**. [CrossRef] [PubMed]
56. Cozzolino, M.; Mangano, M.; Magagnoli, L.; Di Lullo, L.; Galassi, A.; Brancaccio, D.; Bellasi, A. Iron-based Phosphate Binders for ESRD Patients G Ital Nefrol. *Giornale italiano di nefrologia: Organo ufficiale della Societa italiana di nefrologia* **2016**, *33*, 27545638.
57. Palmer, S.C.; Gardner, S.; Tonelli, M.; Mavridis, D.; Johnson, D.W.; Craig, J.C.; French, R.; Ruospo, M.; Strippoli, G.F. Phosphate-binding agents in adults with CKD: A network meta-analysis of randomized trials. *Am. J. Kidney Dis.* **2016**, *68*, 691–702. [CrossRef]
58. Ohtake, T.; Kobayashi, S.; Oka, M.; Furuya, R.; Iwagami, M.; Tsutsumi, D.; Mochida, Y.; Maesato, K.; Ishioka, K.; Moriya, H.; et al. Lanthanum carbonate delays progression of coronary artery calcification compared with calcium-based phosphate binders in patients on hemodialysis: A pilot study. *J. Cardiovasc. Pharmacol. Ther.* **2013**, *18*, 439–446. [CrossRef]
59. Raggi, P.; Bommer, J.; Chertow, G.M. Valvular calcification in hemodialysis patients randomized to calcium-based phosphorus binders or sevelamer. *J. Heart Valve Dis.* **2004**, *13*, 134–141.
60. Chertow, G.M.; Burke, S.K.; Raggi, P.; Treat to Goal Working Group. Sevelamer attenuates the progression of coronary and aortic calcification in hemodialysis patients. *Kidney Int.* **2002**, *62*, 245–252. [CrossRef]
61. Neradova, A.; Schumacher, S.P.; Hubeek, I.; Lux, P.; Schurgers, L.J.; Vervloet, M.G. Phosphate binders affect vitamin K concentration by undesired binding, an in vitro study. *BMC Nephrol.* **2017**, *18*, 149. [CrossRef] [PubMed]
62. Fusaro, M.; Giannini, S.; Gallieni, M.; Noale, M.; Tripepi, G.; Rossini, M.; Messa, P.; Rigotti, P.; Pati, T.; Barbisoni, F.; et al. Calcimimetic and vitamin D analog use in hemodialyzed patients is associated with increasedlevels of vitamin K dependent proteins. *Endocrine* **2016**, *51*, 333–341. [CrossRef] [PubMed]
63. Rodriguez, M.; Aguilera-Tejero, E.; Mendoza, F.J.; Guerrero, F.; López, I. Effects of calcimimetics on extraskeletal calcifications in chronic kidney disease. *Kidney Int.* **2008**, *74* (Suppl. 111), S50–S54. [CrossRef] [PubMed]
64. Mendoza, F.J.; Martinez-Moreno, J.; Almaden, Y.; Rodriguez-Ortiz, M.E.; Lopez, I.; Estepa, J.C.; Henley, C.; Rodriguez, M.; Aguilera-Tejero, E. Effect of calcium and the calcimimetic AMG 641 on matrix-Gla protein in vascular smooth musclecells. *Calcif. Tissue Int.* **2011**, *88*, 169–178. [CrossRef] [PubMed]
65. Torbergsen, A.C.; Watne, L.O.; Wyller, T.B.; Frihagen, F.; Strømsøe, K.; Bøhmer, T.; Mowe, M. Vitamin K1 and 25(OH)D are independently and synergistically associated with a risk for hipfracture in an elderly population: A case control study. *Clin. Nutr.* **2015**, *34*, 101–106. [CrossRef] [PubMed]
66. Geleijnse, J.M.; Vermeer, C.; Grobbee, D.E.; Schurgers, L.J.; Knapen, M.H.; van der Meer, I.M.; Hofman, A.; Witteman, J.C. Dietary intake of menaquinone is associated with a reduced risk of coronary heart disease: The Rotterdam Study. *J. Nutr.* **2004**, *134*, 3100–3105. [CrossRef] [PubMed]
67. Shea, M.K.; O'Donnell, C.J.; Hoffmann, U.; Dallal, G.E.; Dawson-Hughes, B.; Ordovas, J.M.; Price, P.A.; Williamson, M.K.; Booth, S.L. Vitamin K supplementation and progression of coronary artery calcium in older men and women. *Am. J. Clin. Nutr.* **2009**, *89*, 1799–1807. [CrossRef]
68. Keyzer, C.A.; Vermeer, C.; Joosten, M.M.; Knapen, M.H.; Drummen, N.E.; Navis, G.; Bakker, S.J.; de Borst, M.H. Vitamin K status and mortality after kidney transplantation: A cohort study. *Am. J. Kidney Dis.* **2015**, *65*, 474–483. [CrossRef]

3

Nutrition Support in Liver Transplantation and Postoperative Recovery: The Effects of Vitamin D Level and Vitamin D Supplementation in Liver Transplantation

Junshi Doi [1,†], Amika Moro [1,†], Masato Fujiki [1], Bijan Eghtesad [1], Cristiano Quintini [1], K. V. Narayanan Menon [2], Koji Hashimoto [1] and Kazunari Sasaki [1,*]

[1] Department of General Surgery, Digestive Disease & Surgery Institute, Cleveland Clinic, Cleveland, OH 44195, USA; doij@ccf.org (J.D.); moroa2@ccf.org (A.M.); fujikim@ccf.org (M.F.); eghtesb@ccf.org (B.E.); quintic@ccf.org (C.Q.); hashimk@ccf.org (K.H.)

[2] Department of Gastroenterology and Hepatology, Cleveland Clinic, Cleveland, OH 44195, USA; menonk@ccf.org

* Correspondence: sasakik@ccf.org

† These authors contributed equally to this work.

Abstract: Vitamin D plays an important role in the arena of liver transplantation. In addition to affecting skeletal health significantly, it also clinically exerts immune-modulatory properties. Vitamin D deficiency is one of the nutritional issues in the perioperative period of liver transplantation (LT). Although vitamin D deficiency is known to contribute to higher incidences of acute cellular rejection (ACR) and graft failure in other solid organ transplantation, such as kidneys and lungs, its role in LT is not well understood. The aim of this study was to investigate the clinical implication of vitamin D deficiency in LT. LT outcomes were reviewed in a retrospective cohort of 528 recipients during 2014–2019. In the pre-transplant period, 55% of patients were vitamin-D-deficient. The serum vitamin D level was correlated with the model for end-stage liver disease (MELD-Na) score. Vitamin D deficiency in the post-transplant period was associated with lower survival after LT, and the post-transplant supplementation of vitamin D was associated with a lower risk of ACR. The optimal vitamin D status and vitamin D supplementation in the post-transplant period may prolong survival and reduce ACR incidence.

Keywords: vitamin D; liver transplant; rejection; vitamin D supplementation; survival

1. Introduction

Vitamin D plays an important role in bone metabolism, regulating gene expression in multiple tissues, and increasing the intestinal absorption of calcium. Recently, in addition to the well-known effects on musculoskeletal metabolism, it has been reported that vitamin D has anti-inflammatory and immune-modulatory properties [1–3]. Clinically low serum levels of vitamin D have been associated with a higher prevalence of infections, cancer, cardiovascular, and autoimmune disorders [4,5]. Vitamin D deficiency is one of nutrition issues that is addressed in liver transplantation (LT) patients [6]. Due to the end-stage liver disease (ESLD) of the LT patients, malabsorption, inadequate dietary intake, and impairment in hepatic activation of vitamins are major issues [7,8]. While LT has been reported to have positive effects in increasing serum vitamin D concentrations as well as the percentage of patients with sufficient vitamin D levels, immunosuppression-related metabolic disturbances cause vitamin D deficiency after LT [9,10]. These malnutrition/vitamin deficiencies are challenges in LT management and can cause debility and worse postoperative outcomes [11].

Previous reports show that vitamin D has a protective effect against rejection and infection in the clinical settings of solid organ transplantation, such as kidney and lung. In addition, vitamin D supplementation is reported to lower the risk of acute cellular rejection (ACR) [12,13]. According to one of the previous reports, which reviewed a small number of patients, vitamin D supplementation in the post-transplant period was recommended for better outcomes after LT including decreased incidence of ACR and infections [14]. However, in terms of immunological aspects, the clinical effects of vitamin D on the outcome of LT have not been fully understood. Furthermore, the optimal method of vitamin D supplementation in clinical settings remains unclear.

In this study, we focused on vitamin D as a part of nutritional management in LT. We conducted a retrospective study (1) to evaluate the relationship between vitamin D deficiency and ESLD, (2) to analyze the relationships between serum levels of vitamin D and LT outcomes, and (3) to discuss the clinical effects of vitamin D supplementation.

2. Materials and Methods

2.1. Study Design and Population

This study included patients who underwent LT between 2014 and 2019 at Cleveland Clinic, Cleveland, Ohio. Patients who were under 18 years old, died during the perioperative period, underwent multiple organ transplantations or living donor liver transplant, developed primary non-function, or diagnosed with fulminant/acute liver failure for LT were excluded from the cohort.

Patient demographic and clinic-pathological data were extracted for the recipients including age, sex, body mass index (BMI), cause of cirrhosis, received hepatocellular carcinoma (HCC) exception, medical condition at the time of LT, history of previous abdominal surgery, portal vein thrombosis, model for end-stage liver disease (MELD-Na) score [15], and waiting time. For the donor, in addition to the basic characteristics, race, graft type, cause of death, share type, and cold ischemic time were extracted. Crossmatches of T and B cell results were also investigated. Crossmatching of donors against transplant recipients are performed to determine the likelihood of donor-specific antibody-mediated responses [16]. The primary end point was overall survival (OS) after LT and incidence of ACR. The presence of ACR was defined by biopsy. Follow-up was conducted for ACR incidence until patient death or 12 months after LT. This study was conducted in accordance with the Declaration of Helsinki, and the protocol was approved by the Institutional Review Board of Cleveland Clinic (IRB# 20-1169).

2.2. Post-Transplant Management

The immunosuppression protocol was based on tacrolimus with its initial target blood level at 8–10 ng/mL. Dosing was adjusted to whole blood concentrations and occurrence of renal impairment and other adverse effects. Immunosuppression was started immediately after LT, and oral medication was given once gut function was restored. In most cases, it was combined with tapering doses of corticosteroids and mycophenolate mofetil (2000 mg/day) [17].

2.3. Vitamin D Measurement

The serum levels of 25-hydroxy vitamin D (25(OH)D) were measured at the time of listing and at the post-transplant period of <1 year after LT as a part of routine nutrition evaluation. The serum level of 25(OH)D was considered low when <20 ng/mL [18].

2.4. Statistical Analysis

Continuous variables were reported as median with interquartile ranges (IQRs), and categorical variables were presented as frequencies (%). Continuous variables were compared using Student's t-test or one/two-way ANOVA test, and categorical variables were compared using Fisher's Exact tests or Chi-square test. Pearson's rank correlation coefficient was used to test the association between calculated MELD-Na scores and serum levels of 25(OH)D. Kaplan–Meier curves were constructed and compared using a log-rank test. To evaluate the factors associated with survival after LT, Cox regression analysis was performed. Cumulative incidences of ACR were calculated using the Fine–Gray competing risk approach [19]. To evaluate the risk factors associated with ACR, Fine–Gray proportional hazards regression analysis was performed. Hazard ratio (HR) and subdistribution hazard ratio (sHR) are presented with 95% confidence intervals (95% CI). A p-value < 0.05 was considered statistically significant. All statistical analyses were performed with EZR (Saitama Medical Center, Jichi Medical University, Saitama, Japan), which is a graphical user interface for R (The R Foundation for Statistical Computing, Vienna, Austria) [20].

3. Results

3.1. Demographical Characteristics of Patients

A total of 528 patients were included in the analytic cohort (Table 1). The median recipient age at the time of LT was 58 years (IQR: 52–64), and more than half of the recipients were male (n = 350, 66.2%). Cause of cirrhosis was mainly alcohol (n = 154, 29.1%), NASH/Cryptogenic (n = 136, 25.9%), and viral hepatitis (n = 103, 19.5%). Half of the recipients received previous abdominal surgery (n = 266, 50.3%), and a minority of recipients had portal vein thrombosis at the time of LT (n = 104, 19.7%). The median laboratory MELD-Na score was 19 (IQR: 13–28). The median waiting time was 2.9 months (IQR: 0.8–7.4). The majority of the donor graft type was donor after brain dead (DBD) (n = 458, 86.8%). The median cold ischemic time was 6.2 h (IQR: 5.3–7.4). Figure 1A shows the distribution of vitamin D status prior to LT, showing 55% were vitamin-D-deficient. The characteristics of vitamin-D-deficient and -sufficient patients were compared (Table 2). Recipient characteristics including age >60 years, presence of HCC, alcohol consumption rate, MELD-Na score, and serum albumin level had a significant difference ($p < 0.05$). The relationship between the MELD-Na score and serum levels of vitamin D in the pre-transplant period was analyzed (Figure 1B). The correlation coefficient was −0.254 ($p < 0.01$; 95% CI: −0.34–−0.17).

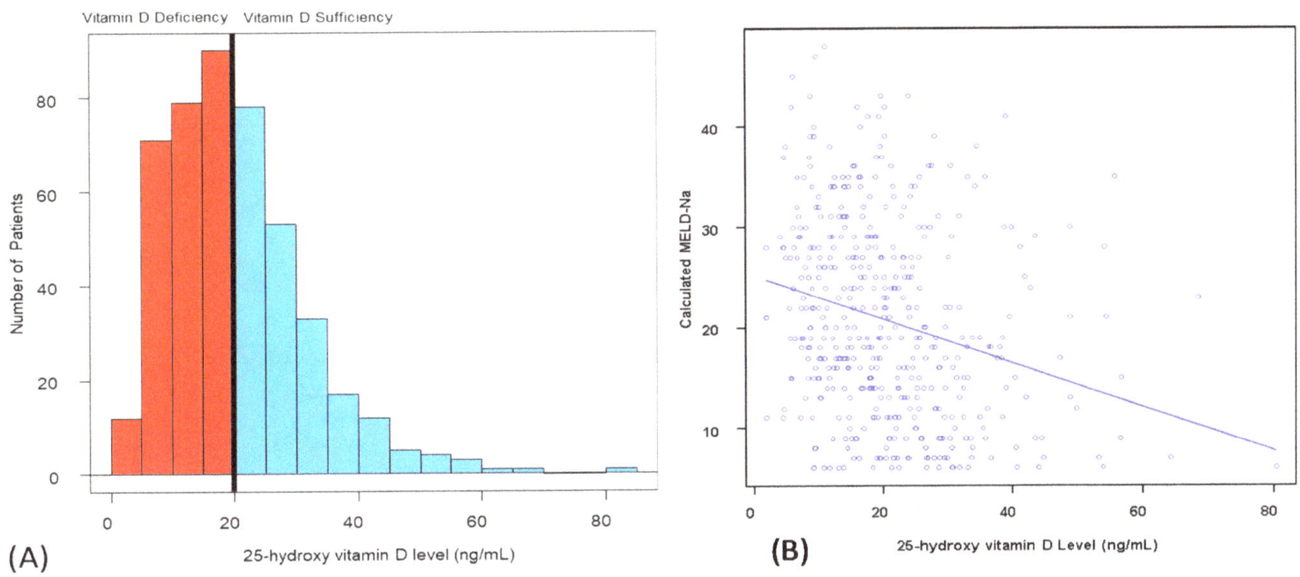

Figure 1. 25-hydroxy vitamin D levels in patients prior to LT. (**A**) Distribution of the 25-hydroxy vitamin D levels in the pre-transplant period. (**B**) Correlation between the 25-hydroxy vitamin D levels and MELD-Na score. Correlation coefficient r was −0.254 ($p < 0.01$; 95% CI: −0.34–−0.17). CI: confidence interval; MELD-Na: the model for end-stage liver disease. LT: liver transplantation.

Table 1. Recipient and donor characteristics. LT: liver transplantation.

Recipient Characteristics	
Age, years, Median (IQR)	58 (52–64)
Sex, male, Number (%)	350 (66.2)
Height, cm, Median (IQR)	174.0 (165.8–180.3)
Weight, kg, Median (IQR)	86.2 (72.3–101.3)
Body mass index, kg/m^2, Median (IQR)	28.7 (24.8–33.8)
Cause of cirrhosis, Number (%)	
Viral hepatitis	103 (19.5)
PBC/PSC/AIH	85 (16.1)
NASH/Cryptogenic	136 (25.9)
Alcohol	154 (29.1)
Other	50 (9.5)
Exception for HCC, Number (%)	202 (17.7)
Medical condition at the time of LT, Number (%)	
ICU	39 (7.4)
Hospitalized	207 (39.5)
Home	280 (53.1)
Previous abdominal surgery, Number (%)	266 (50.3)
Portal vein thrombosis, Number (%)	104 (19.7)
MELD-Na score, Median (IQR)	19 (13–28)
Waiting time, months, Median (IQR)	2.9 (0.8–7.4)
Donor Characteristics	
Age, years, Median (IQR)	42 (30–54)
Sex, male, Number (%)	317 (59.9)
Height, cm, Median (IQR)	173.0 (165.0–180.0)
Weight, kg, Median (IQR)	82.1 (69.9–99.4)
Body mass index, kg/m^2, Median (IQR)	28.1 (23.68–32.9)
Graft type, Number (%)	
DBD	429 (81.3)
DCD	65 (12.3)
Split	34 (6.4)
Race/Ethnicity, Number (%)	
White	410 (77.7)
African American	93 (17.6)
Others	25 (4.7)
Cause of death, Number (%)	
Head trauma	251 (47.6)
Anoxia	150 (28.4)
CVD	120 (22.7)
Others	7 (1.3)
Share type, Number (%)	
Local	300 (56.9)
Regional	180 (34.0)
National	48 (9.1)
Cold ischemic time, hours, Median (IQR)	6.2 (5.3–7.4)

IQR: interquartile range; PBC: primary biliary cirrhosis; PSC: primary sclerosing cholangitis; AIH: autoimmune hepatitis; NASH: non-alcoholic steatohepatitis; HCC: hepatocellular carcinoma; ICU: intensive care unit; MELD-Na: model for end-stage liver disease; DBD: donor after brain dead; DCD: donor after circulation death; CVD: cardiovascular disease.

Table 2. Characteristics of vitamin-D-deficient and -sufficient patients prior to liver transplantation.

	All Patients		
Characteristics	**Deficient (20 ng/mL<)**	**Sufficient (≥20 ng/mL)**	***p* Value**
Age >60 years, Number (%)	93 (37.1)	108 (51.7)	<0.01
Sex, Number (%)			0.37
Male	173 (68.9)	135 (64.6)	
Female	78 (31.1)	74 (35.4)	
Body mass index, kg/m^2, Median (IQR)	28.7 (24.7–34.1)	28.6 (25.0–33.3)	0.90
Main liver disease, Number (%)			0.08
HBV/HCV	37 (14.7)	49 (23.4)	
PBC/PSC/AIH	40 (15.9)	34 (16.3)	
NASH	68 (27.1)	54 (25.8)	
Alcohol	83 (33.1)	50 (23.9)	
Other	23 (9.2)	22 (10.5)	
Hepatocellular carcinoma, Number (%)	64 (25.5)	77 (36.8)	0.01
Diabetes mellitus, Number (%)	70 (27.9)	66 (31.6)	0.41
Alcohol consumption, Number (%)	83 (33.1)	50 (23.9)	0.04
MELD-Na score, Median (IQR)	22 (16–29)	16 (10–24)	<0.01
Albumin, g/dL, Median (IQR)	3.0 (2.6–3.5)	3.2 (2.8–3.7)	0.04
25(OH)D, Pre-transplant, ng/mL, Median (IQR)	12.9 (9.1–16.5)	27.0 (23.1–32.9)	<0.01
25(OH)D, Post-transplant, ng/mL, Median (IQR)	22.1 (14.4–29.0)	27.1 (20.3–35.5)	0.32
Crossmatch for T and B cell, Number (%)			0.24
T cell: −/B cell: −	154 (61.4)	129 (61.7)	
T cell: +/B cell: −	16 (6.4)	9 (4.3)	
T cell: −/B cell: +	47 (18.7)	51 (24.4)	
T cell: +/B cell: +	34 (13.5)	20 (9.6)	

IQR: interquartile range; HBV: hepatitis B virus; HCV: hepatitis C virus; PBC: primary biliary cirrhosis; PSC: primary sclerosing cholangitis; AIH: autoimmune hepatitis; NASH: non-alcoholic steatohepatitis; MELD-Na: model for end-stage liver disease; 25(OH)D: 25-hydroxy vitamin D.

3.2. Influence of Preoperative and Postoperative Serum Vitamin D Levels on Overall Survival

Differences in the long-term survival between patients who had vitamin D deficiency and sufficiency at pre- and post-transplant were compared (Figure 2A,B). There was no significant difference between the patients who had vitamin D deficiency and sufficiency in the pre-transplant period ($p = 0.64$) (Figure 2A). However, there was a significant difference between the two groups in the post-transplant period (Figure 2B).

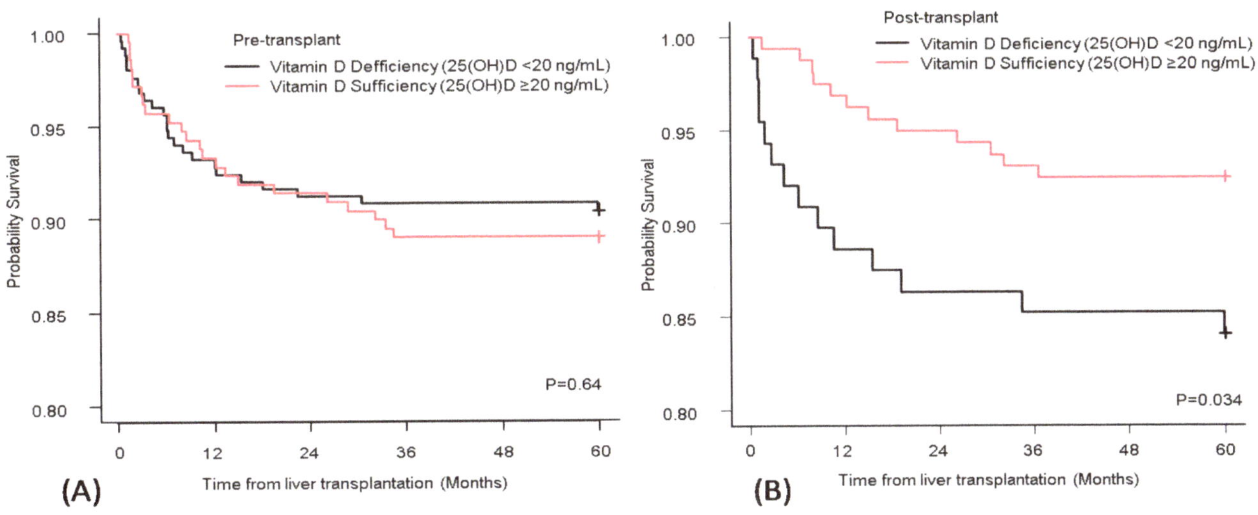

Figure 2. OS of recipients who had vitamin D deficiency and sufficiency at pre-transplant (**A**) and post-transplant (**B**). The Kaplan–Meier curve for OS of recipients who had vitamin D deficiency (black line) and sufficiency (red line). Vitamin D deficiency was defined as <20 ng/mL of the serum level of 25(OH)D. OS: overall survival; 25(OH)D: 25-hydroxy vitamin D.

A bivariate and multivariable Cox regression analysis was performed to assess the risk factors associated with the five-year OS (Table 3). Older age (>60 years old) (HR 3.47; 95% CI, 1.38–8.68, $p < 0.01$) and post-transplant vitamin D sufficiency (HR 0.31; 95% CI, 0.13–0.75, $p < 0.01$) were associated with five-year OS.

Table 3. Cox regression analysis of prognostic factors associated with overall survival.

Variable	Bivariate Analysis		Multivariable Analysis	
	HR (95% CI)	***p*-Value**	**HR (95% CI)**	***p* Value**
Age >60 years	2.84 (1.60–5.05)	<0.01	3.47 (1.38–8.68)	<0.01
Sex (Male)	0.79 (0.46–1.36)	0.39	0.65 (0.28–1.54)	0.33
Body mass index	0.87 (0.50–1.50)	0.61		
MELD-Na score >30	1.70 (0.94–3.04)	0.08	1.02 (0.97–1.06)	0.47
Hepatocellular carcinoma	1.48 (0.85–2.55)	0.16		
Alcohol-related cirrhosis	0.75 (0.47–1.19)	0.22		
Vitamin D sufficiency, Pre-transplant	1.15 (0.65–2.03)	0.63	1.02 (0.42–2.44)	0.97
Vitamin D sufficiency, Post-transplant	0.44 (0.21–0.96)	0.04	0.31 (0.13–0.75)	<0.01
Vitamin D supplementation, Pre-transplant	1.28 (0.71–2.32)	0.41		
Vitamin D supplementation, Post-transplant	0.92 (0.53–1.61)	0.78		
Crossmatch for T or B cell positive	1.26 (0.85–1.87)	0.26		

CI: confidence interval; HR: hazard ratio; MELD-Na: model for end-stage liver disease.

3.3. Influence of Preoperative and Postoperative Serum Vitamin D Levels on Acute Cellular Rejection

The incidence of ACR in LT recipients with pre- and post-transplant vitamin D deficiency was 19.1% and 22.0%, respectively. There was no significant difference in the cumulative incidence of ACR between vitamin D deficiency and sufficiency in both pre- and post-transplant periods (Figure 3A,B).

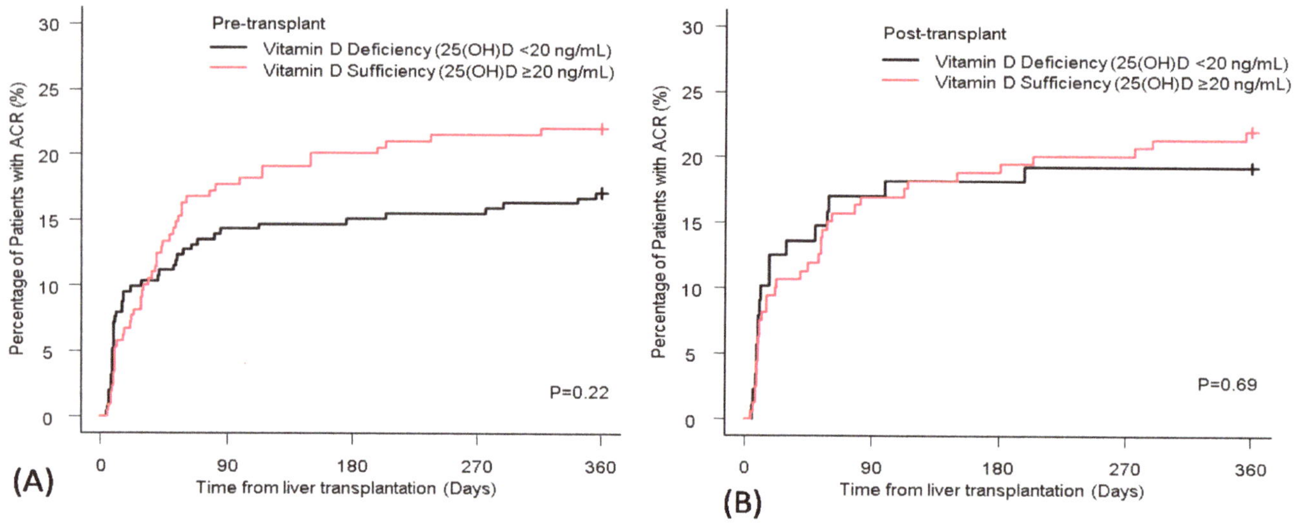

Figure 3. The cumulative incidence of ACR in liver transplant recipients with vitamin D deficiency and sufficiency at pre-transplant (**A**) and post-transplant (**B**). ACR: acute cellular rejection; 25(OH)D: 25-hydroxy vitamin D.

3.4. Comparison of Patient Characteristics Based on Vitamin D Supplementation Status

In examining the effect of vitamin D supplementation, four groups were investigated: (1) patients who did not receive supplementation (No Supplement), (2) patients who received supplementation during only pre-transplant (Pre), (3) patients who received supplementation during only post-transplant (Post), and (4) patients who received supplementation during both pre- and post- transplant (Pre/Post). The characteristics of the four groups were compared (Table 4). Among the four groups, there was a significant difference in the ratio of sex and 25(OH)D level at pre-transplant ($p < 0.05$).

Table 4. Comparison of patient characteristics among different vitamin D supplementation statuses.

Characteristics	All Patients (N = 528)				p Value
	No Supplementation N = 131	Pre N = 47	Post N = 41	Pre/Post N = 309	
Age >60 years, Number (%)	65 (49.6)	18 (38.3)	14 (34.1)	138 (44.7)	0.27
Sex, Number (%)					0.03
Male	98 (74.8)	29 (61.7)	31 (75.6)	191 (61.8)	
Female	33 (25.2)	18 (38.3)	10 (24.4)	118 (38.2)	
Body mass index, kg/m^2, Median (IQR)	28.7 (24.7–33.8)	28.5 (22.7–33.1)	29.0 (25.5–33.3)	28.7 (24.9–34.0)	0.98
Main liver disease, Number (%)					0.12
HBV/HCV	35 (26.7)	11 (23.4)	5 (12.2)	52 (16.8)	
PBC/PSC/AIH	15 (11.5)	8 (17.0)	3 (7.3)	59 (19.1)	
NASH	32 (24.4)	11 (23.4)	14 (34.1)	80 (25.9)	
Alcohol	38 (29.0)	14 (29.8)	11 (26.8)	90 (29.1)	
Other	11 (8.4)	3 (6.4)	8 (19.5)	28 (9.1)	
Hepatocellular carcinoma, Number (%)	44 (33.6)	15 (31.9)	11 (26.8)	88 (28.5)	0.70
Diabetes mellitus, Number (%)	40 (30.5)	17 (36.2)	9 (22.0)	87 (28.2)	0.49
Alcohol consumption, Number (%)	38 (29.0)	14 (29.8)	11 (26.8)	90 (29.1)	0.99
MELD-Na score, Median (IQR)	19 (13–28)	18 (11–27)	22 (15–28)	19 (14–28)	0.82
Albumin, g/dL, Median (IQR)	3.0 (2.6–3.5)	3.1 (2.8–3.5)	3.10 (2.4–3.8)	3.2 (2.7–3.6)	0.88
25(OH)D, Pre-transplant, ng/mL, Median (IQR)	18.1 (11.9–24.4)	14.3 (9.2–22.6)	17.65 (10.5–21.5)	20.2 (13.8–28.4)	<0.01
25(OH)D, Post-transplant, ng/mL, Median (IQR)	23.6 (19.4–33.6)	23.2 (13.1–29.3)	18.9 (11.4–23.9)	25.5 (18.2–34.1)	0.36
Crossmatch for T and B cell, Number (%)					0.12
T cell: −/B cell: −	83 (63.4)	26 (55.3)	32 (78.0)	180 (58.3)	
T cell: +/B cell: −	7 (5.3)	2 (4.3)	2 (4.9)	19 (6.1)	
T cell: −/B cell: +	30 (22.9)	15 (31.9)	7 (17.1)	66 (21.4)	
T cell: +/B cell: +	11 (8.4)	4 (8.5)	0 (0.0)	44 (14.2)	

IQR: interquartile range; HBV: hepatitis B virus; HCV: hepatitis C virus; PBC: primary biliary cirrhosis; PSC: primary sclerosing cholangitis; AIH: autoimmune hepatitis; NASH: non-alcoholic steatohepatitis; MELD-Na: model for end-stage liver disease; 25(OH)D: 25-hydroxy vitamin D.

3.5. *Effect of Vitamin D Supplementation on Overall Survival*

Differences in the long-term survival among the four patient groups (No Supplement, Pre, Post, Pre/Post) were compared using the Kaplan–Meier curve (Figure 4A). Regardless of the supplementation status, there were no significant differences in the OS (p = 0.60).

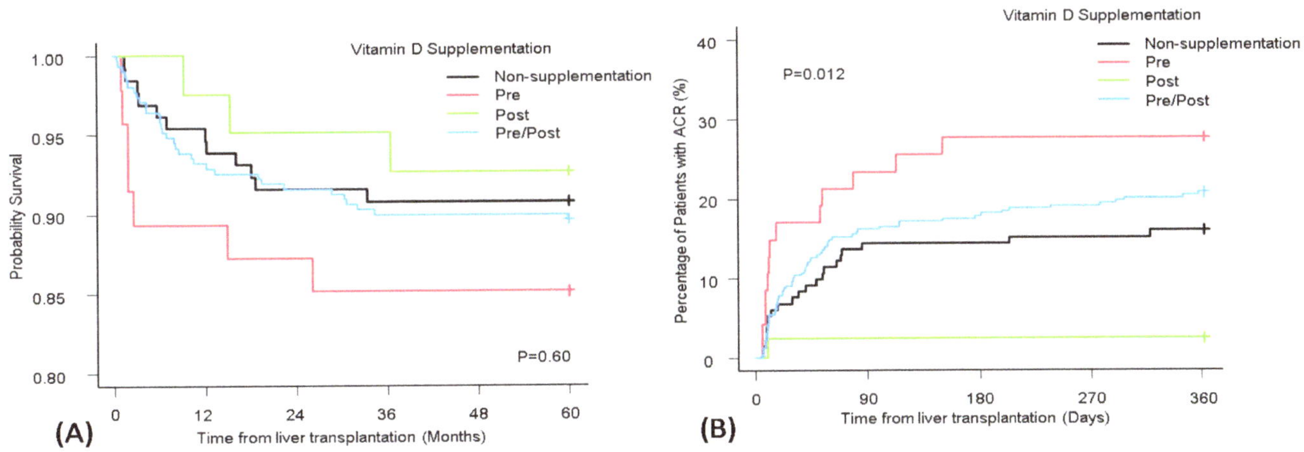

Figure 4. Comparison of vitamin D supplement status in OS (**A**) and the accumulate incidence of ACR (**B**). ACR: acute cellular rejection; OS: overall survival.

3.6. *Effect of Vitamin D Supplementation on Acute Cellular Rejection*

The cumulative incidence of ACR among the four groups (No Supplement, Pre, Post, Pre/Post) (Figure 4B) was compared. Interestingly, the incidence rate of ACR showed a significant difference based on the vitamin D supplementation status. The cumulative incidence was high in the Pre group and was low in the Post group.

The proportional subdistribution hazard model of the Fine and Gray method was used for ACR in the No Supplement group and Pre group (Table 5). From the bivariate and multivariable analysis, age (>60 years) was the only variable that was significant (sHR 0.30; 95% CI, 0.12–0.77, $p = 0.01$). In the same manner, the Fine and Gray method was used for ACR in the No Supplement group and Post group (Table 6). Among all variables, calculated MELD-Na score >30 (sHR < 0.01; 95% CI, <0.01–<0.01, $p < 0.01$) at the time of LT and vitamin D supplementation during post-transplant (sHR 0.09; 95% CI, 0.01–0.72, $p = 0.02$) were significant.

Table 5. Fine and Gray proportional subdistribution hazard model for ACR development in No Supplement and Pre group.

Variables	Bivariate Analysis		Multivariable Analysis	
	sHR (95% CI)	*p* Value	sHR (95% CI)	*p* Value
Age >60 years	1.03 (0.42–2.53)	0.95	0.30 (0.12–0.77)	0.01
Sex (Male)	1.02 (0.50–2.08)	0.95		
Calculated MELD-Na >30	0.34 (0.08–1.43)	0.14	0.28 (0.07–1.17)	0.08
Hepatocellular carcinoma	0.95 (0.47–1.94)	0.89		
Alcohol-related cirrhosis	1.00 (0.48–2.06)	0.99		
Vitamin D supplementation, Pre-transplant	1.39 (0.67–2.87)	0.38	1.05 (0.43–2.57)	0.92
Vitamin D sufficiency, Pre-transplant	1.23 (0.59–2.59)	0.58	1.38 (0.63–3.01)	0.42
Crossmatch for T or B cell positive	0.94 (0.48–1.86)	0.86		

CI: confidence interval; sHR: subdistribution hazard ratio; MELD-Na: model for end-stage liver disease.

Table 6. Fine and Gray proportional subdistribution hazard model for ACR development in No Supplement and Post group.

Variables	Bivariate Analysis		Multivariable Analysis	
	sHR (95% CI)	*p* Value	sHR (95% CI)	*p* Value
Age >60 years	0.42 (0.17–1.06)	0.07	0.38 (0.07–2.02)	0.26
Sex (Male)	0.91 (0.36–2.27)	0.84		
Calculated MELD-Na > 30	0.34 (0.08–1.43)	0.14	<0.01 (<0.01–<0.01)	<0.01
Hepatocellular carcinoma	1.24 (0.52–2.93)	0.63		
Alcohol-related cirrhosis	1.44 (0.61–3.40)	0.40		
Vitamin D supplementation, Post-transplant	0.14 (0.02–1.07)	0.06	0.09 (0.01–0.72)	0.02
Vitamin D sufficiency, Post-transplant	0.85 (0.18–4.04)	0.84	0.69 (0.14–3.48)	0.65
Crossmatch for T or B cell positive	1.71 (0.74–3.91)	0.21		

CI: confidence interval; sHR: subdistribution hazard ratio; MELD-Na: model for end-stage liver disease.

4. Discussion

Although previous studies have reported that vitamin D plays an important role in solid organ transplantation including kidney and lung [12,13], the clinical impact of vitamin D on LT outcomes and vitamin D supplementation is still unknown. The current study included 528 patients which is larger than any other previous studies of vitamin D in LT. Our study investigated the correlation of the pre-transplant vitamin D level and the MELD-Na score. Moreover, the current study is important because we were able to reveal how the perioperative vitamin D levels and vitamin D supplementation status affect long-term outcomes, such as OS and ACR all in the same cohort. Using the cutoff of 20 ng/mL of 25(OH)D [18], 55% of the patients had vitamin D deficiency before LT. The MELD-Na score and serum levels of 25(OH)D before LT showed a negative linear relationship. While there was no survival difference based on the vitamin D level during pre-transplant, patients who had vitamin D deficiency at post-transplantation had worse survival compared with vitamin-D-sufficient patients. The cumulative incidence of ACR was not affected by the perioperative 25(OH)D level. There was no difference in the OS when it was assessed based on the vitamin D supplementation status. However, the accumulated incidence of ACR was high in the Pre group and low in the Post group, showing a significant difference. Importantly, the risk factor of ACR in the Pre group and Post group was younger age and no vitamin D supplementation and higher MELD-Na score at the time of LT, respectively.

Vitamin D3 is taken in the body by diet (20%) or is synthesized by the skin (80%) from 7-dihydrocholesterol following UVB exposure. Vitamin D3 becomes biologically active after hydroxylation in the liver by the enzymes cytochrome P450 2R1 and cytochrome P450 27 becoming 25-hydroxyvitamin D3. The fully active metabolite 1,25-dihydroxyvitamin D3 is hydroxylated in the kidney [21]. ESLD patients have both impaired liver and kidney function that can alter calcium and vitamin D homeostasis [22,23]. Even when there were patients taking supplemental vitamin D during pre-transplant, more than half of the patients had vitamin D deficiency (Figure 1A). In addition, we found that there was a negative correlation between MELD-Na scores and serum levels of 25(OH)D in the pre-transplant period, which was compatible with the vitamin D physiology since the MELD-Na score incudes both hepatic and renal components [15].

Vitamin-D-sufficient status in the post-transplant period was associated with five-year survival after LT. The optimal vitamin D status prolonged survival. This indicated that post-transplant nutritional support including the correction of vitamin D deficiency will support better OS. These results are consistent with a study from Lowery et al., showing that the mortality of lung transplant recipients who remained vitamin-D-deficient at one-year post-transplant was higher than that of recipients who maintained normal vitamin D levels [13]. In the current study, the six-month mortality rate of vitamin-D-deficient patients in the post-transplant period was 8.0% while that in vitamin-D-sufficient patients was 0.63% ($p < 0.01$) (Figure 2B). Post-transplant vitamin-D-deficient status had larger effects on mortality in the early period after LT compared with the late period. Even though early mortality after LT can be caused by different conditions such as early allograft dysfunction and infections [24], these complications might be related to decreased immune-modulatory properties because of the low vitamin D level [1–3]. On the other hand, low vitamin D can be a result of the malnourished condition of LT recipients. Malnutrition itself could also negatively affect mortality [25,26]. Thus, serum levels of 25(OH)D in the post-transplant period can be a prognostic factor or a predictive factor for survival. Further investigation to determine how the vitamin D status contributes to OS is needed.

Pre-transplant vitamin D status was not associated with the long-term accumulated incidence of ACR after LT in this study (Figure 3A). Although focusing on the short term after LT, the vitamin D deficiency group had a higher rate of ACR compared to the sufficiency group. Similar findings were seen in a paper from Zhou et al. showing that high pre-transplant 25(OH)D level (>25 ng/mL) prior to LT significantly decreased the incidence of ACR in 30 days after LT [27]. Another report from Bitetto et al. also confirmed that low pre-transplant 25(OH)D level (<5 ng/mL) was independently associated with moderate to severe ACR episodes within two months after LT [28]. After the early period of LT, the incidence of ACR in the vitamin D sufficiency group tended to be higher than the deficiency group. This implies that the vitamin D sufficiency in the pre-transplant period contributed to reduced risks for ACR in the early post-transplant period and smoothly boosted the immune system of recipients through the recovery phase from LT-related surgical procedures in the late post-transplant period. The vitamin D status during the post-transplant period had no significant relationship with the incidence of ACR (Figure 3B).

As such, pre-transplant vitamin D levels may be associated with ACR in the early period after LT, and it can be hypothesized that optimization of vitamin-D-deficient status by supplementation in the pre-transplant period may contribute to reducing the incidence of ACR.

The clinical effects of vitamin D supplementation on LT outcomes remained unclear. We demonstrated that vitamin D supplementation in the post-transplant period has positive effects in decreasing the incidence of ACR during one year after LT. A previous study showed similar findings that vitamin D supplementation for the first one month significantly decreased the incidence of ACR in 30 days after LT [27]. Vitamin D supplementation is assumed to increase the components of suppressor T cells/T memory cells, decrease the C3 co-stimulatory molecule expression (HLA-DR, CD28), and expand T naïve cells/cytotoxic T cells [27,29]. Our comparison between the No Supplement and the Post groups clarified the anti-rejection effects of the post-transplant vitamin D supplementation. From these results, we propose that vitamin D supplementation should be considered, especially to reduce the incidence of ACR. Yet, our result does not demonstrate that vitamin D supplementation in the pre-transplant period could reduce the incidence of ACR. Thus, prospective studies should be conducted to elucidate the importance of vitamin D supplementation in LT, including the relationship between vitamin D supplementation and modification of vitamin D levels.

This study had several limitations. Since this was a retrospective study, information bias was possible given that the data were manually abstracted from the medical records. Additionally, there was potential for unmeasured confounders of the relationship between vitamin D status and hepatic graft status. The multivariable analysis of all four groups (No Supplement, Pre, Post, Pre/Post) showed that sex is not a significant factor regulating the incidence of ACR (Tables 5 and 6) or five-year survival (data not shown), although there were gender differences among groups (Table 4). In this study, more female patients tended to be on vitamin D supplementation compared with male patients. We assume it was because of the higher incidence of bone-related disorders in female groups, such as osteoporosis. Future research is needed to elucidate the gender effects on outcomes after LT.

Finally, it should be noted that there are no guidelines for screening or supplementation of vitamin D in LT recipients. Further investigation is needed to clarify the importance of screening for vitamin D status and the effectiveness of vitamin D supplementation for patients in the peri-transplant period.

5. Conclusions

Vitamin D deficiency in the post-transplant period was associated with lower survival after LT, and the post-transplant supplementation of vitamin D was associated with a lower risk of ACR. Vitamin D levels in the pre-transplant period may be an important factor of ACR. Nutritional support with vitamin D supplementation might be contributing to improving LT outcomes.

Author Contributions: Conceptualization, A.M. and K.S.; methodology, A.M. and K.S.; software, K.S. and J.D.; validation, M.F., K.V.N.M., B.E., C.Q., and K.H.; formal analysis, K.S. and J.D.; investigation, M.F. and K.V.N.M.; resources, K.V.N.M, B.E., C.Q., and K.H.; data curation, J.D., K.S., and K.V.N.M.; writing—original draft preparation, J.D.; writing—review and editing, A.M. and K.S.; visualization, K.S. and A.M.; supervision, K.S.; project administration, K.S., A.M., M.F., and K.H. All authors have read and agreed to the published version of the manuscript.

References

1. Gorman, S.; Judge, M.A.; Hart, P.H. Topical 1,25-dihydroxyvitamin D3 subverts the priming ability of draining lymph node dendritic cells. *Immunology* **2010**, *131*, 415–425. [CrossRef] [PubMed]
2. Pludowski, P.; Holick, M.F.; Pilz, S.; Wagner, C.L.; Hollis, B.W.; Grant, W.B.; Shoenfeld, Y.; Lerchbaum, E.; Llewellyn, D.J.; Kienreich, K.; et al. Vitamin D effects on musculoskeletal health, immunity, autoimmunity, cardiovascular disease, cancer, fertility, pregnancy, dementia and mortality-a review of recent evidence. *Autoimmun. Rev.* **2013**, *12*, 976–989. [CrossRef] [PubMed]
3. Vanherwegen, A.-S.; Cook, D.P.; Ferreira, G.B.; Gysemans, C.; Mathieu, C. Vitamin D-modulated dendritic cells delay lethal graft-versus-host disease through induction of regulatory T cells. *J. Steroid Biochem. Mol. Biol.* **2019**, *188*, 103–110. [CrossRef] [PubMed]
4. Covic, A.; Vervloet, M.; Massy, Z.A.; Torres, P.U.; Goldsmith, D.; Brandenburg, V.; Mazzaferro, S.; Evenepoel, P.; Bover, J.; Apetrii, M.; et al. Bone and mineral disorders in chronic kidney disease: Implications for cardiovascular health and ageing in the general population. *Lancet Diabetes Endocrinol.* **2018**, *6*, 319–331. [CrossRef]
5. Charoenngam, N.; Holick, M.F. Immunologic Effects of Vitamin D on Human Health and Disease. *Nutrients* **2020**, *12*, 2097. [CrossRef] [PubMed]

6. Guichelaar, M.M.J.; Schmoll, J.; Malinchoc, M.; Hay, J.E. Fractures and avascular necrosis before and after orthotopic liver transplantation: Long-term follow-up and predictive factors. *Hepatology* **2007**, *46*, 1198–1207. [CrossRef]
7. Abbott-Johnson, W.; Kerlin, P.; Clague, A.; Johnson, H.; Cuneo, R. Relationships between blood levels of fat soluble vitamins and disease etiology and severity in adults awaiting liver transplantation. *J. Gastroenterol. Hepatol.* **2011**, *26*, 1402–1410. [CrossRef]
8. Venu, M.; Martin, E.; Saeian, K.; Gawrieh, S. High prevalence of vitamin A deficiency and vitamin D deficiency in patients evaluated for liver transplantation. *Liver Transpl.* **2013**, *19*, 627–633. [CrossRef]
9. Wiśniewska, H.; Bander, M.; Bander, D.; Biront, A.; Zeair, S.; Wawrzynowicz-Syczewska, M. Vitamin D Status before and after Liver Transplantation. *Int. J. Transplant. Res. Med.* **2019**. [CrossRef]
10. Rabinovitz, M.; Shapiro, J.; Lian, J.; Block, G.D.; Merkel, I.S.; Van Thiel, D.H. Vitamin D and osteocalcin levels in liver transplant recipients. Is osteocalcin a reliable marker of bone turnover in such cases? *J. Hepatol.* **1992**, *16*, 50–55. [CrossRef]
11. Anastácio, L.R.; Correia, M.I.T.D. Nutrition therapy: Integral part of liver transplant care. *World J. Gastroenterol.* **2016**, *22*, 1513–1522. [CrossRef] [PubMed]
12. Lee, J.R.; Dadhania, D.; August, P.; Lee, J.B.; Suthanthiran, M.; Muthukumar, T. Circulating Levels of 25-Hydroxyvitamin D and Acute Cellular Rejection in Kidney Allograft Recipients. *Transplantation* **2014**, *98*, 292–299. [CrossRef] [PubMed]
13. Lowery, E.M.; Bemiss, B.; Cascino, T.; Durazo-Arvizu, R.A.; Forsythe, S.M.; Alex, C.; Laghi, F.; Love, R.B.; Camacho, P. Low vitamin D levels are associated with increased rejection and infections after lung transplantation. *J. Heart Lung Transplant.* **2012**, *31*, 700–707. [CrossRef]
14. Grant, C. A vitamin D protocol post-liver transplantation. *J. Am. Assoc. Nurse Pract.* **2017**, *29*, 658–666. [CrossRef] [PubMed]
15. Biggins, S.W.; Kim, W.R.; Terrault, N.A.; Saab, S.; Balan, V.; Schiano, T.; Benson, J.; Therneau, T.; Kremers, W.; Wiesner, R.; et al. Evidence-based incorporation of serum sodium concentration into MELD-NA. *Gastroenterology* **2006**, *130*, 1652–1660. [CrossRef] [PubMed]
16. Mulley, W.R.; Kanellis, J. Understanding crossmatch testing in organ transplantation: A case-based guide for the general nephrologist. *Nephrology* **2011**, *16*, 125–133. [CrossRef]
17. Hashimoto, K.; Aucejo, F.; Quintini, C.; El-Gazzaz, G.; Hodgkinson, P.; Fujiki, M.; Diago, T.; Kelly, D.; Winans, C.; Vogt, D.; et al. Liver transplantation at Cleveland Clinic. *Liver* **2010**, *2*, 3.
18. Holick, M.F.; Binkley, N.C.; Bischoff-Ferrari, H.A.; Gordon, C.M.; Hanley, D.A.; Heaney, R.P.; Murad, M.H.; Weaver, C.M. Evaluation, treatment, and prevention of vitamin D deficiency: An Endocrine Society clinical practice guideline. *J. Clin. Endocrinol. Metab.* **2011**, *96*, 1911–1930. [CrossRef]
19. Fine, J.P.; Gray, R.J. A Proportional Hazards Model for the Subdistribution of a Competing Risk. *J. Am. Stat. Assoc.* **1999**, *94*, 496–509. [CrossRef]
20. Kanda, Y. Investigation of the freely available easy-to-use software 'EZR' for medical statistics. *Bone Marrow Transplant.* **2013**, *48*, 452–458. [CrossRef]
21. Sassi, F.; Tamone, C.; D'Amelio, P. Vitamin D: Nutrient, Hormone, and Immunomodulator. *Nutrients* **2018**, *10*, 1656. [CrossRef] [PubMed]
22. Jean, G.; Souberbielle, J.C.; Chazot, C. Vitamin D in Chronic Kidney Disease and Dialysis Patients. *Nutrients* **2017**, *9*, 328. [CrossRef] [PubMed]
23. Arteh, J.; Narra, S.; Nair, S. Prevalence of vitamin D deficiency in chronic liver disease. *Dig. Dis. Sci.* **2010**, *55*, 2624–2628. [CrossRef] [PubMed]
24. Bolondi, G.; Mocchegiani, F.; Montalti, R.; Nicolini, D.; Vivarelli, M.; de Pietri, L. Predictive factors of short term outcome after liver transplantation: A review. *World J. Gastroenterol.* **2016**, *22*, 5936–5949. [CrossRef]
25. Englesbe, M.J.; Patel, S.P.; He, K.; Lynch, R.J.; Schaubel, D.E.; Harbaugh, C.; Holcombe, S.A.; Wang, S.C.; Segev, D.L.; Sonnenday, C.J. Sarcopenia and Mortality after Liver Transplantation. *J. Am. Coll. Surg.* **2010**, *211*, 271–278. [CrossRef]
26. Mazurak, V.C.; Tandon, P.; Montano-Loza, A.J. Nutrition and the transplant candidate. *Liver Transpl.* **2017**, *23*, 1451–1464. [CrossRef]
27. Zhou, Q.; Li, L.; Chen, Y.; Zhang, J.; Zhong, L.; Peng, Z.; Xing, T. Vitamin D supplementation could reduce the risk of acute cellular rejection and infection in vitamin D deficient liver allograft recipients. *Int. Immunopharmacol.* **2019**, *75*. [CrossRef]

28. Bitetto, D.; Fabris, C.; Falleti, E.; Fornasiere, E.; Fumolo, E.; Fontanini, E.; Cussigh, A.; Occhino, G.; Baccarani, U.; Pirisi, M.; et al. Vitamin D and the risk of acute allograft rejection following human liver transplantation. *Liver Int.* **2010**, *30*, 417–444. [CrossRef]
29. Xing, T.; Qiu, G.; Zhong, L.; Ling, L.; Huang, L.; Peng, Z. Calcitriol reduces the occurrence of acute cellular rejection of liver transplants: A prospective controlled study. *Pharmazie* **2013**, *68*, 821–826.

4

Development and Characterization of an Orodispersible Film for Vitamin D3 Supplementation

Irma Elisa Cupone, Eleonora Dellera, Fabio Marra and Andrea Maria Giori *

IBSA Farmaceutici Italia, 26900 Lodi, Italy; irma.cupone@ibsa.it (I.E.C.); eleonora.dellera@ibsa.it (E.D.); fabio.marra@ibsa.it (F.M.)

* Correspondence: andrea.giori@ibsa.it

Academic Editors: Mihai Brebu and Elena Stoleru

Abstract: Vitamin D plays a crucial and very well-known role in regulation of calcium homeostasis and bone metabolism and mineralization. However, a huge and more recent body of evidence supports the positive influence of vitamin D on the regulation of immune response, ranging from protection against respiratory tract infections to prevention and management of asthma. Nevertheless, vitamin D deficiency is a very common condition and there is an increasing need for suitable products for proper supplementation, allowing good compliance also in specific populations. Orally disintegrating tablets (ODT) were first developed to overcome the difficulty experienced by pediatric and geriatric patients of swallowing traditional oral dosage forms and, recently, orodispersible films (ODF) are gaining popularity as novel dosage form for assuming active pharmaceutical ingredients, vitamins, and ingredients for food supplements. This study describes a 2000 IU Vitamin D3 ODF for daily intake, consisting of hydrophilic polymers and suitable excipients, manufactured by film-casting process. Elongation-at-break (E%), Young's modulus (Y), and tensile strength (TS) were investigated using a dynamometer. Chemical stability was evaluated assaying the vitamin D3 in the films stored at different environmental conditions. In addition, in vitro disintegration and dissolution studies were performed. Correlation existed between the mechanical properties of the film and the residual water, acting as plasticizer. The stability study showed that vitamin D3 assay was ≥90% also after 3 months at 40 °C. The film disintegrated in less than 1 min and the vitamin D3 released was ≥75% after 15 min. An ODF with suitable properties can be manufactured and used as innovative dosage form for vitamin D3 food supplements.

Keywords: vitamin D3; immune system; food supplement; orodispersible film; innovative dosage form; mechanical properties

1. Introduction

Vitamin D has for a long time been known for its activity carried out in bone health, by promoting calcium absorption in the gut and maintenance of serum calcium and phosphate concentration [1]. As vitamin D is a central regulator of calcium homeostasis and bone metabolism, vitamin D deficiency in adults results in poorly mineralized skeletal matrix, a symptom known as osteomalacia, and is known to cause osteoporosis and muscle weakness, increasing the risk for fractures due to falls, especially in the elderly [2].

More recently, the role of vitamin D as regulator of the immune system was investigated. Vitamin D acts as an important stimulant for innate immunity and supports the adaptive immune system [3]. Vitamin D3 has been recognized as an important mediator of innate immune responses, enhancing the antimicrobial activity of immune cell, such as monocytes and macrophages [2].

Moreover, vitamin D can increase T regulatory lymphocytes, that are the principal defense against uncontrolled inflammation and against viral infection in general. Low levels of vitamin D are also associated with an increase in inflammatory cytokines [4].

Vitamin D can reduce risk of infections through several mechanisms, such as the induction of cathelicidins and defensins that can lower viral replication rates.

Recent data reported the direct antiviral effects of vitamin D, which hinders viral replication. Vitamin D can also be effective in an anti-inflammatory and immunomodulatory way, reducing concentrations of pro-inflammatory cytokines, responsible for the damage to the lining of the lungs, which leads to pneumonia, as well as increasing concentrations of anti-inflammatory cytokines. Vitamin D could be an effective means of preventing respiratory tract infection [5]. Analysis indicated that daily or weekly intake of Vitamin D showed protective effects against acute respiratory tract infection especially in person with vitamin D deficiency. In clinical studies, low levels of serum vitamin D were associated with acute respiratory tract infections including epidemic influenza. Some recent reviews hypothesized that vitamin D insufficiency may compromise respiratory immune function, increasing the risk of COVID-19 severity and mortality [6].

Vitamin D deficiency (serum level <50 nmol/L or 20 ng/mL) is present in 24% of US population, 37% of Canada population, and 40% of Europeans. In addition, even more severe deficiency defined as serum level <30 nmol/L or 12 ng/mL) is reported in 5.9% in US, 7.4% in Canada, and 13% in Europe. Vitamin D deficiency may vary by age, with lower levels in childhood and the elderly, and also ethnicity in different regions [7].

In humans, vitamin D can be obtained from two distinct sources, either from diet or by endogenous production, whereby solar UV-B irradiates 7-dehydrocholesterol present in the skin to generate cholecalciferol (also named vitamin D3), which is subsequently activated in the liver and kidney [8].

Since sunlight exposure and dietary intake alone is usually insufficient in most individuals to maintain optimal vitamin D status, there is an increasing need of suitable products for proper supplementation, allowing good compliance also in specific populations at risk, such as the elderly and children.

Currently, there is no international consensus on the optimal level for vitamin D supplementation. Recommendations differ in many countries, and range from 400 to 2000 IU daily (10–50 μg). The European Food and Safety Authority recommend staying below 4000 IU/day (100 μg). Most countries have prudently set the safe upper level at 50 μg daily (2000 IU) for adults [7].

The aim of this study is to develop a 2000 IU Vitamin D3 orodispersible film (ODF) for daily supplementation that is easy to use and characterized by an improved compliance when compared to the existing oral dosage forms.

ODF is a novel dosage form for taking active pharmaceutical ingredients, vitamins and ingredients for food supplements.

According to the European Pharmacopoeia (Ph. Eur.), ODFs are defined as "single or multilayered sheets of suitable materials, to be placed in the mouth where they disperse rapidly". ODFs require only a small amount of saliva to dissolve within a few minutes and water is not necessary for administration. The advantage is the improvement of acceptance and patient compliance with no risk of choking, associated with better safety and efficacy in comparison with conventional dosage forms [9]. ODFs allow overcoming the difficulty in swallowing conventional oral dosage forms among pediatric, geriatric, and psychiatric patients with dysphagia. Their convenience, superior dosing accuracy, and rapid onset of action contribute to strong patient preference over conventional solid dosage forms across a wide range of patient groups [10].

Moreover, orodispersible films have advantages over orally disintegrating tablet formulations, which may require more complicated and expensive manufacturing processes, have issues of hardness and friability during manufacturing, storage, handling, and administration.

Orodispersible films are thin and flexible, can be manufactured in a wide range of sizes and shapes, and are easily transported and stored.

Essential excipients of ODFs are polymers, which are the backbone of film formulations (40–50% of film mass) and plasticizers, usually added up to 20% of dry polymer weight. Film forming polymers have to disintegrate or dissolve rapidly in contact with saliva, have to guarantee suitable mechanical properties, and avoid stickiness. Plasticizers reduce glass transition temperature of the polymer, reduce brittleness, improve mechanical properties of films, and improve flexibility. Other components can be: taste masking agents and sweeteners that mask bitter and unpleasant taste that characterized the majority of drug substances; surfactants that act as solubilizing, dispersing, and wetting agents and improve coating step during manufacturing of ODFs by casting methods.

Due to their moderate size and thickness, ODFs can typically be loaded only with limited active substance amounts per unit volume and surface area. Therefore, oral films are not generally suitable for treatments requiring high dosages (i.e., >100–150 mg), although up to 50% drug loading in an ODF has been reported [11]. Drug dose can be modulated modifying the size and the thickness of the film and the high drug loading capacity of ODF allows the reduction of excipients intake.

ODFs can be manufactured by different methods: solvent casting, hot melt extrusion, semisolid casting method, rolling method, or electrospinning [12].

Ideal ODFs should exhibit adequate elasticity, flexibility, softness, mechanical properties to facilitate their production, packaging, and application, good stability, short disintegration time, and pleasant taste.

The flexibility and toughness of the film affect manufacturing process of films such as cutting, film formation, and packaging. Oral film should be flexible to be handled without failure and at the same time should exhibit a tensile strength that guarantees a suitable toughness to allow films to be self-supporting. Elongation at break should be low to avoid deformation of films during manufacturing process.

Taste is an important factor in the development of ODF to ensure patient acceptability and compliance and is one of the prime factors determining market penetration and commercial success. Palatability and pleasant taste are necessary for fast dissolving films, and various techniques are available to mask drug taste. Flavors and sweeteners can be added to the formulation, generally in association with other taste-masking components. Mouthfeel and texture are also considered key characteristics, potentially affecting the acceptability of ODFs, particularly with regards to the presence of residual particles following disintegration.

This work describes the development of a new vitamin D3 orodispersible film and the study to scale up the product to the manufacturing plant. The new vitamin D3 ODF was conceived as food supplement, consisting of hydrophilic polymers and suitable excipients, and manufactured by film-casting process. Critical quality attributes—such as vitamin D assay, mechanical properties, moisture content, disintegration time, dissolution profile, and stability—were investigated.

2. Results and Discussion

2.1. Selection of Components and Formulation Development

The main ingredient of Vitamin D3 oral film is maltodextrin. We started the development of the product considering the patent EP1689347 "Self supporting film for pharmaceutical and food use" and the patent WO2014/049548 "Orodispersible films having quick dissolution times for therapeutic and food use" [13,14], that required the use of maltodextrin as the only film forming ingredient. This polymer provides advantages in terms of palatability, physical properties, and stability. This ingredient was successfully used previously to design a pharmaceutical oral film formulation containing Sildenafil Citrate. In vivo study showed that such formulation was safe, efficacious, and bioequivalent to the conventional branded film-coated tablets [10]. Starting from this positive experience in the pharmaceutical field, we decided to apply for the first time the same technology to a food supplement. Maltodextrins (MDXs) are natural, safe, and cheap polymers widely used both in pharmaceutical and food applications. They are water soluble film forming biopolymers and, according to the patents, an amount of maltodextrins ranging between 40% and 80% allows to obtain a rapidly dissolving self-supporting and edible film. MDXs are a non-sweet, nutritive saccharide mixture of polymers that consists of D-glucose units, with a dextrose equivalent (DE) less than 20. MDXs are obtained by partial hydrolysis of a food grade starch with suitable acids and/or enzymes. DE is defined as the measure of the total reducing power of all sugars present in the hydrolysate material relative to glucose as 100 and expressed on a dry weight basis. DE is an indicator of the degree of depolymerization of starch: the DE value of the MDXs increases as the average molecular weight decreases. Several physical and functional characteristics are affected by the DE value. The solubility, sweetness, and hygroscopicity increase with increasing DE, whereas the viscosity, the anti-crystallizing power, and the freezing temperature decrease as the DE increases. DE value of 6 was selected, as it guarantees film formation ability and suitable tensile properties.

To improve the mechanical properties of the orodispersible film, the addition of plasticizers and surfactants is mandatory.

Glycerol and mannitol are below to the chemical group of polyols and are used as plasticizers. Plasticizers improve the flexibility and reduce the brittleness of orodispersible films, reducing the polymer glass transition temperature. They help to overcome brittleness after the step in the drying tunnel and the following punching and pouching in the primary packaging. In addition, residual water also acts as a plasticizer.

Glyceryl monolinoleate and polysorbate 80 were the surfactants chosen. Glyceryl monolinoleate consists of mono-, di-, and triglycerides of mainly linoleic (C18:2) and oleic (C18:1) acids, is a liquid water insoluble surfactant with an HLB = 1. Polysorbate 80 is a non-ionic surfactant, it is a viscous water-soluble yellow liquid with an HLB = 15. In the formulation of vitamin D3 orodispersible film a mixture of glyceryl monolinoleate: Polysorbate 80, 75:25% *w/w*, was used and the calculated value of HLB is 4.5.

An equilibrated HLB was selected to improve the spreadability of the water-based mass on the silicone/PET release liner during coating step and to avoid the foaming during the mixing.

Surfactants have also an important role in dissolution of Vitamin D3, acting as dissolution enahncers. To improve the homogeneity of the bulk, it is recommended to solubilize the active substance before mixing. However, vitamin D3 is a very lipophilic substance, insoluble in the water used as solvent for MDXs and other hydrophilic excipients. To overcome these problems, extra virgin olive oil was used as solubilizing agent for vitamin D3. Vitamin D3 is then added to the mixture as oil solution and the surfactants comprised in the formula allowed the complete and homogeneous dispersion of vitamin D3 solution in the aqueous mass. Therefore, even if vitamin D3 is a poorly water soluble substance, the use of organic solvent to obtain a homogeneous mixture is not necessary [15], with advantages in terms of safety of both manufacturing process and finished product.

Copovidone and alginate were also introduced as film forming agents able to improve the mechanical properties of the films. Copovidone was introduced in the film formulation according to the patent WO 2014/049548: this patent teaches that it is possible to avoid hardening of the films, based on maltodextrins and plasticizer, adding a homopolymer or copolymer of vinyl acetate to the composition.

Alginate acts also as a thickener, and was add to the formulation mainly for this role. Alginate is a hydrocolloid, explicitly excluded by both patents of reference on maltodextrins platform. The addition of alginate improved the physical stability of the mixture (data not shown). That is the main difference between the formula described in this paper and the ones claimed by the cited patents.

The low concentration of vitamin D3 in the film does not affect the pleasantness, but, in order to improve the organoleptic characteristics and to make the product more agreeable, low amounts of sweetener and flavor were added to the formula. Sucralose was selected as sweetener while orange, apricot, and peach flavors were tested. Among them, after an expert panel evaluation, orange flavor was considered the most suitable for this kind of formulation.

Titanium dioxide is a white pigment used to improve film aspect and was combined with yellow iron oxide and red iron oxide to obtain a light orange colored film.

Vitamin D3 is sensitive to air, heat, humidity, and light and accordingly ascorbic acid and DL-alfa tocopherol are introduced as antioxidant agent to improve stability of Vitamin D3. Vitamin C and Vitamin E acted synergically in combination [16,17]. The two vitamins were added in 1:1 weight ratio.

An overage of Vitamin D3 was loaded in the product (+20%) in compliance with the European regulation on food supplement. Vitamin D3 film with labeled strength of 2000 IU, corresponding to 50 μg, contains a nutrient level of 60 μg. Such amount of Vitamin D3 was loaded on a film of 6 cm^2, with a concentration of active ingredient of 0.06% *w/w*.

Final composition and function of each ingredient of developed vitamin D3 orodispersible film are reported in Table 1.

Table 1. Composition and excipients function of vitamin D3 orodispersible films.

Ingredients	Function	Composition (%, *w/w*)
Main ingredients:		
Vitamin D3	Active substance	0.06
Maltodextrin	Film polymer	60.45
Glycerol	Plasticizer	12.00
Purified water	Plasticizer	9.00
Mannitol	Plasticizer	7.50
Extra virgin olive oil	Solubilizing agent	3.00
Other ingredients:		
Orange flavor	Flavor	
Copovidone	Bulking agent	
Vitamin C	Antioxidant	
Vitamin E	Antioxidant	
Glycerol monolinoleate	Emulsifier	
Polysorbate 80	Emulsifier	
Titanium dioxide	Opacifier/pigment	
Sucralose	Sweetener	
Yellow iron oxide	Colour	
Red iron oxide	Colour	
Alginate	Thickener	

2.2. *Manufacturing Process Development*

The manufacturing of Vitamin D3 orodispersible films was performed according to an IBSA standard process developed and validated for the manufacturing of other orodispersible film already on the market.

Zhang et al. [18] has already described an oral fast dissolving film containing Vitamin D3 obtained by microemulsifying; these films were prepared in laboratory on a bench and no evidence of feasibility of industrial manufacturing was provided.

Manufacturing process of vitamin D3 ODF was previously studied in laboratory, then the process was scaled up to the industrial plant. Water content and viscosity of the mass were identified as two important quality attributes of the mass in the scale up of the process and were investigated during laboratory studies in order to obtain a mass suitable for industrial process. Previous studies on orodispersible films demonstrated that the suitable viscosity value has to be in the range 2000–5000 cP. Vitamin D3 mass was formulated to have a viscosity of about 3500 cP: this value is suitable for industrial coating process and is the result of a mixture containing the 39.0% of water.

Mass manufacturing process was developed in laboratory using 5 L mixer equipped with anchor and high disk speed: order of addition of components and time of mixing necessary to obtain a homogeneous mixture were identified as critical process parameters

Industrial mixture was prepared in a 50 L stainless steel mixer equipped with anchor and high disk speed and critical process parameters were set on the basis of lab scale.

The mixture, homogeneous and without bubble and clumps, was spread on a support, a siliconized PET sheet moving along the oven, that at the end is coiled up onto a jumbo roll (Figure 4a). According to our knowledge, temperature of ovens was set between 90–110 °C and coating speed at 0.5 m/min. These conditions were suitable to remove the excess of water and the industrial continuous process allowed the production of a film with a homogeneous and smooth surface, a weight of 167 g/m^2, and a thickness in the range 125 μm ± 5% (Table 2). The size and the strengths of the orodispersible film are defined by the consecutive processes of slitting (Figure 4b) and formation. In the first step, jumbo rolls were cut in 7 reels of 30 ± 1 mm. The 30 mm reels are cut by a single rotary die blade with a cutting pitch of 20 mm originating the 2000 IU orodispersible film (20 × 30 mm).

During the film formation, the support is removed.

Each orodispersible film was individually inserted between two packaging foils that were sealed by two sealing stations. A rotating knife cuts the single packaging unit after sealing. The variable data are printed on the sachet on the line. Secondary packaging is the last step of manufacturing process.

The industrial manufacturing process allows to obtain the following theoretical quantities of intermediate and films:

- Wet mixture: 50 Kg
- Coated laminate: 200 m^2
- Reel: about 6000 linear meter
- Films: about 300,000 films of 2000 IU (3 × 2 cm)

Figure 1 shows Vitamin D3 orodispersible films obtained on industrial scale and manufacturing for sale.

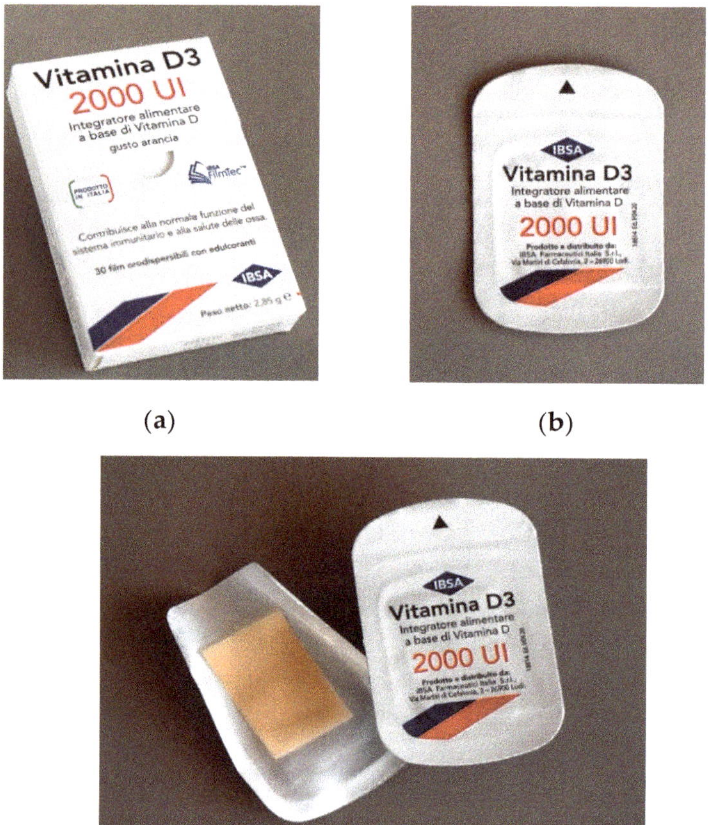

(a) (b)

(c)

Figure 1. Vitamin D3 orodispersible films: secondary packaging (**a**), primary packaging (**b**), and an oral film in the sachet (**c**).

2.3. Characterization of Vitamin D3 Orodispersible Films

The critical issues in the development the formulation of an orodispersible film are represented by the time of disintegration in the oral cavity, the tensile properties required for packaging and handling procedures, and the taste of the ingredients.

At the end of the development, the formulation selected was suitable for the industrial manufacturing process. The films were characterized and results are described below.

A thin and flexible light orange film was obtained, the color was homogeneous and it was characterized by a pleasant odor and taste of orange fruit. Orodispersible films containing 2000 IU of vitamin D3 measured 20 × 30 mm and weighed 100.0 mg. Average vitamin D3 content is 60.3 μg/film, corresponding to 120.7% of label content.

ODF disintegrated within 1 min therefore making vitamin D3 immediately available to dissolve. As shown in Figure 2, vitamin D3 dissolved completely (>90%) within 30 min, but already after 15 min the dissolved amount of vitamin D3 was greater than 85%, satisfying the requirements for the immediate release dosage forms. Vitamin D3 can be promptly bioavailable to be absorbed.

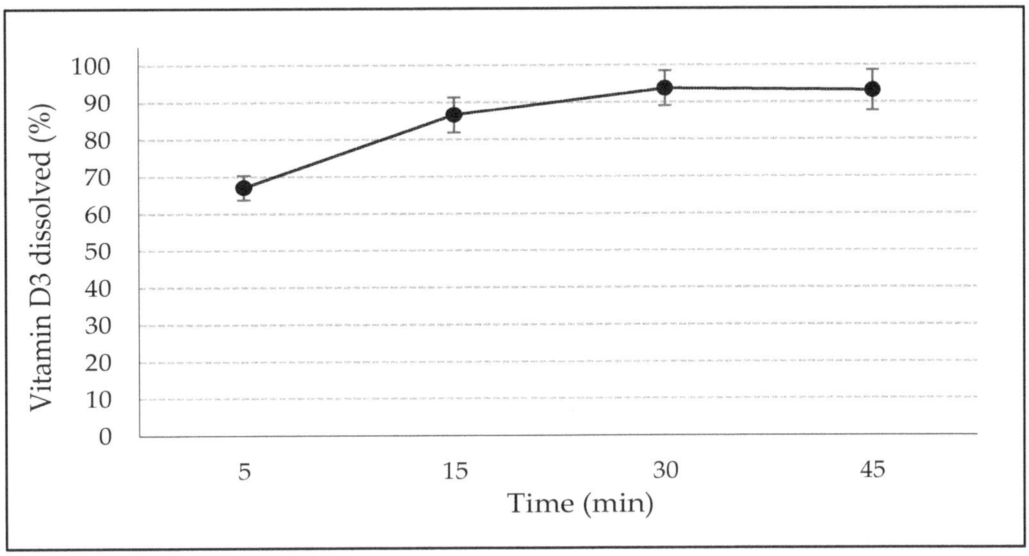

Figure 2. Dissolution profile of vitamin D3 ODF.

2.4. Evaluation of Mechanical Properties

The flexibility and stiffness of the film could affect cutting, film formation and packaging during the manufacturing process.

To facilitate the handling, oral film should be flexible and exhibit a tensile strength (TS) that guarantees a suitable stiffness. Elongation at break (E%) should be low to avoid deformation of films during manufacturing process.

The main responsible of the mechanical properties of the film is the film forming polymers, while the amount of plasticizers modulated the mechanical properties. Glycerol is the main plasticizer, but also the residual water, the amount of water remaining after the drying, acted as a plasticizer in the formulation. We studied the relation between the water content and the mechanical properties of the film.

Table 2 reports the water content and the tensile properties of ten different vitamin D ODF prepared in laboratory modifying slightly the drying time. Water content ranged between 8.1 and 10.6%. All tested films were flexible, handy, and not brittle. A correlation between tensile properties and water content was proved: TS decreased and E% increased proportionally to water content.

The Figure 3a–c show correlation between tensile properties of vitamin D3 orodispersible films and water content. Linear correlations between elongation at break and water content ($R2 = 0.945$) and tensile strength and water content (R2 = 0.902) and elastic modulus and water content (R2 = 0.811) can be determined. The water content is a parameter that can predict the tensile properties of film: a residual amount of water ranging between the 8.0–11.0%, was necessary to provide the film with the suitable plasticity and tensile strength. Thus, the drying step of the manufacturing process was tuned to comply with this specification, allowing the handling of the dried film during slitting, film formation, and packaging steps on industrial plants.

Table 2. Mechanical properties.

Sample	Residual Water (%)	Thickness (μm)	TS (Mpa)	E% (%)	Y (Mpa)
1	8.1	130	5.93	14.0	284
2	8.9	122	4.50	31.9	172
3	8.9	126	5.58	22.0	220
4	8.9	125	4.70	29.9	169
5	9.1	127	4.73	29.4	223
6	9.3	125	4.21	38.1	191
7	9.6	127	2.85	56.0	93
8	9.6	123	2.96	58.7	112
9	10.3	128	2.22	71.7	74
10	10.6	124	1.87	84.4	80

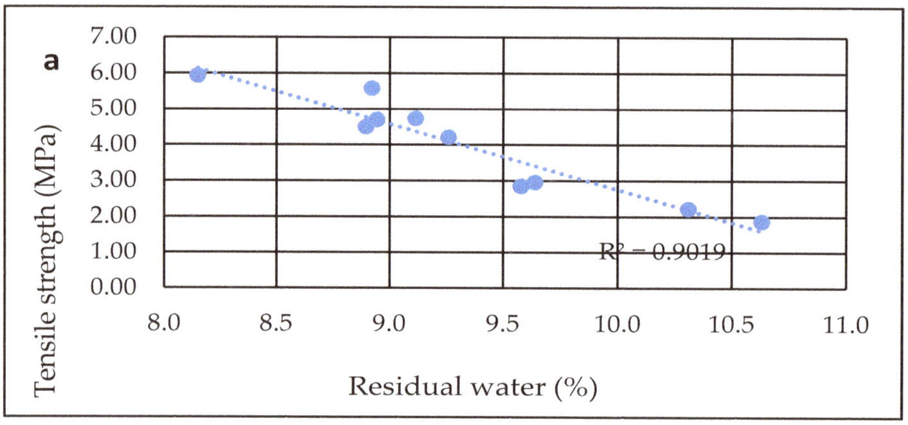

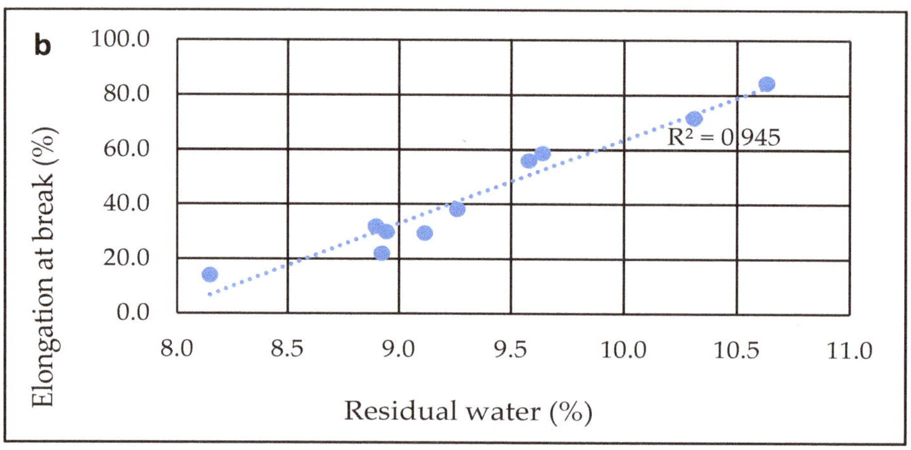

Figure 3. *Cont.*

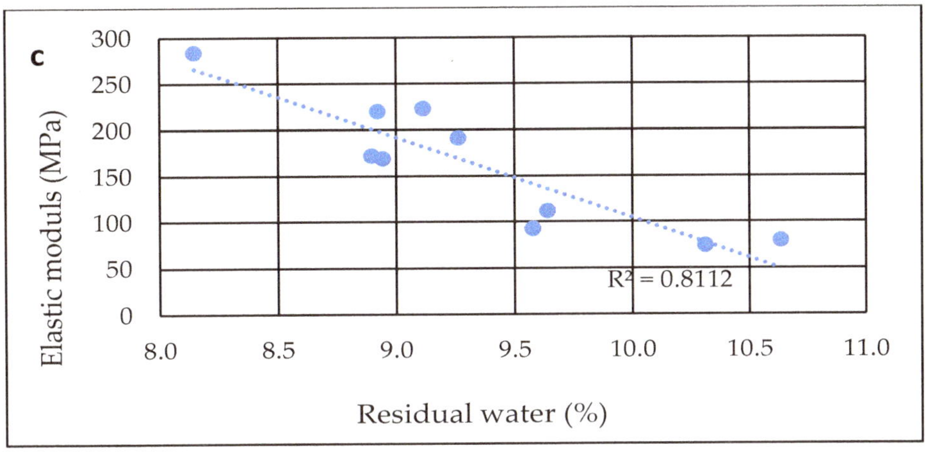

Figure 3. Correlation between water content and mechanical properties of films. (**a**) Tensile strength and water content correlation; (**b**) elongation at break and water content correlation; (**c**) elastic modulus and water content correlation.

2.5. Stability Data of Vitamin D3 Orodispersible Films

Stability data of industrial batch of film kept at the different ICH conditions are reported in Table 3. Several parameters were monitored: residual water, vitamin D3 assay, the weight, the water activity, and microbiology. The residual water remained in the range 8.0–11.0%, that guaranteed suitable mechanical properties as demonstrated above, throughout the examined period.

The weight of the films remained in the range 90–110% and weighs of films at three months are not significantly different from T0. Stability specification for vitamin D3 assay was set to 80.0 ÷ 135.0% of theoretical amount in accordance with European regulations for food supplements. Vitamin D3 assay did not decrease after three months: it remained 122.1% of the claimed value also after three months at 40 °C. Vitamin C and vitamin E protected vitamin D3 from degradation.

Water activity measures the vapor pressure of free water, a key parameter in the quality control of moisture sensitive products or materials. Free water is the water available to chemical reactions and to support microbial growth in pharmaceutical and food products, that can reduce shelf life. Water activity value 0.600 is recognized to be the critical value acceptable to prevent microbial contamination. The results of the analysis of water activity on the samples stored at 25 °C ± 2 °C/60% RH ± 5% RH and 40 °C ± 2 °C/75% RH ± 5% RH were below 0.600 and not significantly different from T0, granting the unlikelihood of a microbiological contamination during the shelf life, as confirmed by microbiological data, reported in the Table 3. Water activity is a useful and fast method to establish microbial stability.

Table 3. Stability data of vitamin D3 ODF.

Test		T0 (at the Start of Stability Study)	Three-Month Stability Point	
			25 °C ± 2 °C/ 60% RH ± 5% RH	40 °C ± 2 °C/ 75% RH ± 5% RH
Average weight (mg)		106.1 ± 3.5	106.5 ± 5.6	106.9 ± 2.2
Residual water (%)		9.6 ± 0.3	8.7 ± 0.6	9.4 ± 0.3
Vitamin D3 assay	μg/film	60.3	62.7	61.1
	% of theoretical amount	120.7	125.3	122.1
Water activity		0.538 ± 0.026	0.554 ± 0.017	0.579 ± 0.009
TAMC (CFU/film) TYMC (CFU/film) *E. Coli* (unit/film)		<10 CFU/film <10 CFU/film Absent/film	<10 CFU/film <10 CFU/film Absent/film	<10 CFU/film <10 CFU/film Absent/film

3. Material and Methods

3.1. Materials

Vitamin D3 (DSM, Village Neuf, France), maltodextrin and mannitol (Roquette, Lestrem, France), glycerol, (Oleon, Ertvelde, Belgium), orange flavor (Sensient, Milwaukee, WI, USA), extra virgin olive oil (Balestrini, Milano, Italy), copovidone and polysorbate 80 (Eigenmann & Veronelli, Rho, Italy), vitamin C (ACEF, Fiorenzuola d'Arda, Italy), vitamin E (BASF, Ludwigshafen, Germany), glycerol monolinoleate (Gattefossè, Saint-Priest, France), titanium dioxide (Brenntag, Essen, Germany), sucralose (Sunvision Sweet, Xintai City, China), yellow iron oxide and red iron oxide (Aromata Group, Bresso, Italy), and alginate (FMC Corporation, Philadelphia, PA, USA).

All ingredients used are food grade in accordance with European Regulation.

All the solvents for the analysis were of analytical grade, unless specified, purchased from VWR (VWR, Milano, Italy).

Cholecalciferol reference standard is supplied by EDQM (European Pharmacopoeia Chemical Reference Substances).

3.2. Methods

3.2.1. Film Preparation

Vitamin D3 orodispersible film was manufactured according to the casting method consisting of different steps. Generally, at first, a water-based mixture was prepared, under the control of the temperature and the stirring speed of the mixer. Afterwards, the mixture was spread on the intermediate liner and dried in a drying tunnel, controlling temperature, air circulation, and coating speed. The roll of dry mass was submitted to the slitting process, to cut the roll in the reels with the first dimension of the final surface of the films. In the last step, the films are punched, pouched, and sealed in suitable single-dose sachets, using pouch-forming and sealing machine. Figure 4 shows pictures of coating and slitting manufacturing steps.

The flow chart (Figure 5) briefly describes the steps for the manufacture of orodispersible films containing vitamin D3.

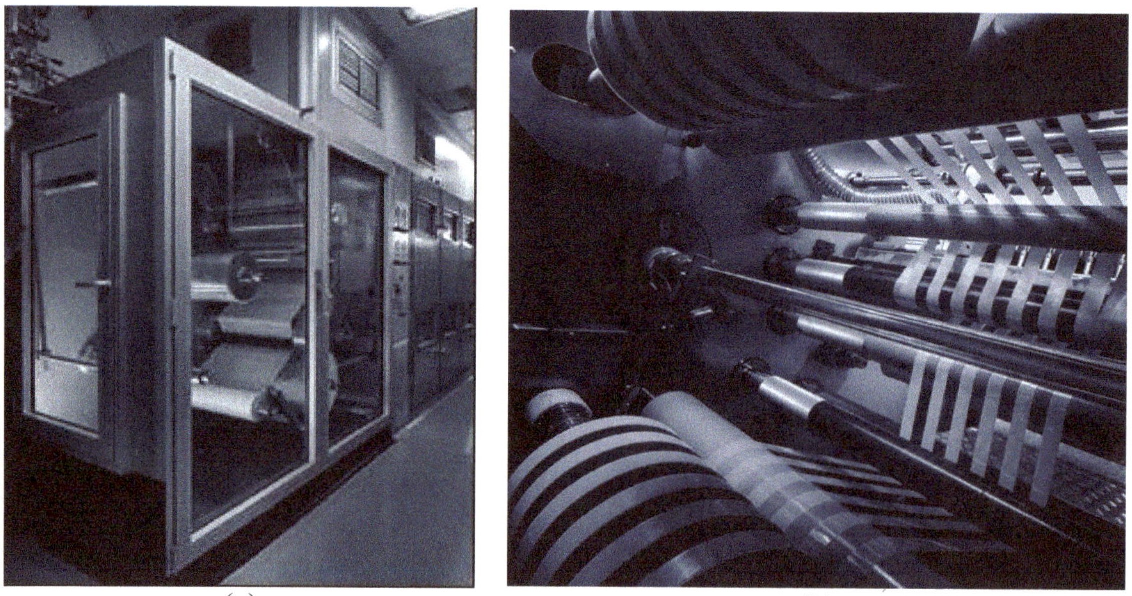

(a) (b)

Figure 4. Coating (**a**) and slitting (**b**) process.

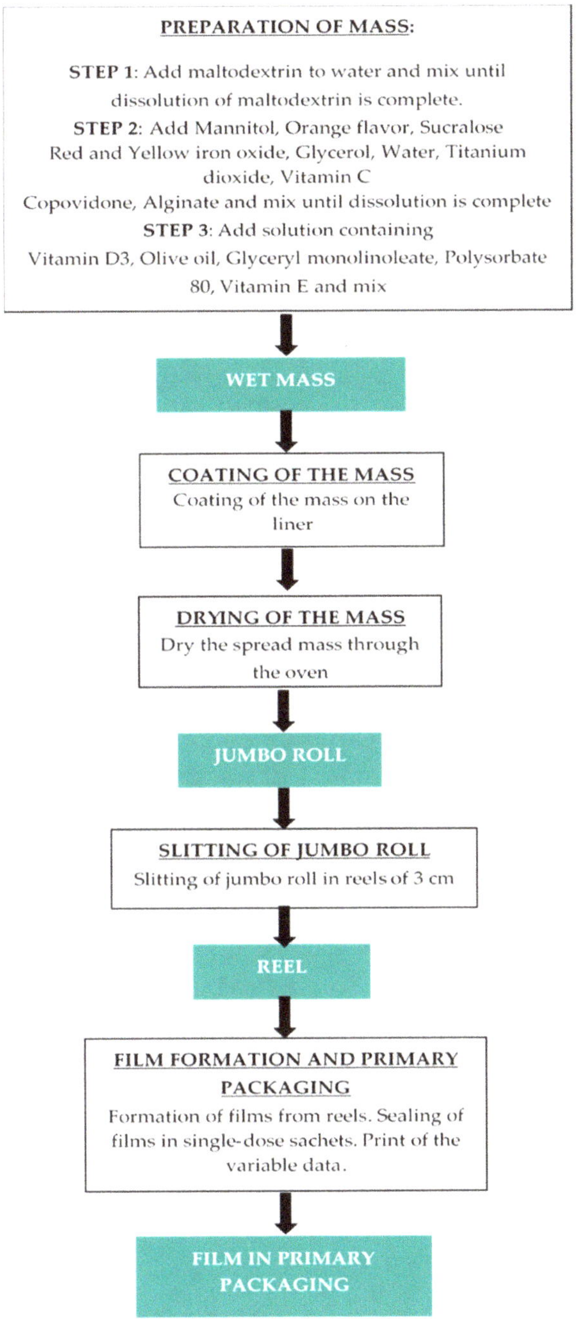

Figure 5. Flow chart of manufacturing steps of vitamin D3 ODF.

3.2.2. Characterization of Vitamin D3 ODF

Aspect, Dimension, and Weight

Orodispersible films were evaluated by visual and organoleptic inspection. The area of films was determined by multiplying length and width of each film and weight of films (n = 10) was evaluated.

Vitamin D3 Content

The determination of Vitamin D3 assay was carried out by a reversed phase HPLC method.

HPLC method: A 15 μL volume of the sample was injected. A reverse-phase column (KINETEX EVO C18, 150 × 4.6 mm–5 μm) was selected as stationary phase. The mobile phase was prepared mixing 90 volumes of acetonitrile and 10 volumes of water. Flow rate was set at 2.0 mL/min and column temperature at 40 °C. Vitamin D3 was detected at 265 nm. Runtime was set up to 12 min and vitamin D3 retention time was 5 min.

Preparation of Sample solution for assay–2000 IU: Five orodispersible films were accurately weighed and transferred together in a 100 mL amber glass bottle and were dissolved with 10 mL of purified water (exactly measured) stirring for 30 min. 100 mL of MeOH were added with a calibrated pipette, the solution was stirred for 60 min, then filtered with a 0.22 μm PTFE syringe filter and injected in HPLC system.

Each solution was carefully protected from actinic light and air.

Disintegration and Dissolution Test

Disintegration test was performed using the Apparatus for disintegration test of tablets (Tecnogalenica, Cernusco sul Naviglio, I), provided with cylindrical discs, described in Ph. Eur. current edition (2.9.1). Dissolution test was performed by a Sotax AT7 Smart dissolution testing unit (Sotax, Aesch, CH), equipped with paddle according to Apparatus 2 of European Pharmacopoeia, current edition (2.9.3). 2000 IU Vitamin D3 orodispersible films were attached to sinkers to avoid floating of the dosage unit. The dissolution medium was 250 mL solution of Triton X-100 0.025% in purified water, maintained at 37.0 ± 0.5 °C. Paddle speed was set up to 50 rpm. 1 mL samples were collected at 5, 15, 30, and 45 min and analyzed by HPLC. Disintegration and dissolution tests were performed on six samples.

Loss on Drying

Three orodispersible films were individually weighed and placed in the oven at 105 °C. After 1 h films were taken out of the oven, cooled at room temperature and weighed again. The water content of the films was calculated with the formula

$$\text{Loss on drying\%} = \frac{weight\ 1 - weight\ 2}{weight\ 1} \times 100$$

where:

weight 1: weight of the film before the test (mg)
weight 2: weight of the film after the test, in the oven at 105 °C for 1 h (mg)

Water Activity

Water activity was determined using Rotronic HW4 instrument (Rotronic Italia, I) on three films.

Tensile Properties

Mechanical test was performed using a texture analyzer H5K-T (Tinius Olsen, Horsham, PA, USA) equipped with a 100 N load cell, according to ASTM International Test Method for Thin Plastic Sheeting (D 882-02). Each test strip was longitudinal placed in the tensile grips on the texture analyzer. Initial grip separation was 20 mm and crosshead speed was 50 mm/min. The test was considered concluded at the film break. Tensile strength (TS), elongation at break (EB), and elastic modulus or Young's modulus (E%) were computed to evaluate the tensile properties of the films.

Tensile strength (TS): was calculated by dividing the maximum load by the original cross-sectional area of the specimen, it was expressed in force per unit area (MPa).

Percent elongation at break (E%): was calculated by dividing the extension at the moment of rupture of the specimen by the initial gage length of the specimen and multiplying by 100.

Elastic modulus or Young's modulus (Y): was calculated as the slope of the linear portion of the stress strain curve. The results were expressed in force per unit area (Mpa).

Before the test, film thickness of each specimen was measured by using an electronic micrometer (ChemInstruments, Fairfield, OH, USA). Results are the average value of five tests.

Microbial Control

The methods to evaluate the total viable aerobic count and the presence of *Escherichia coli* are described in paragraphs 2.6.12 and 2.6.13 of European Pharmacopoeia current edition. The limits of the total count satisfy the requirements of the European Pharmacopoeia current edition, par. 5.1.4 for preparation for oral use. The acceptance criteria are: for total aerobic microbial count (TAMC) $\leq 10^2$ colony forming units (CFU)/film, for total yeast and molds count (TYMC) ≤ 10 CFU/film, and absence of *Escherichia coli*.

3.2.3. Stability Study

Stability of 2000 IU Vitamin D3 ODF was studied at long and accelerated term conditions: 25 ± 2 °C and 60% ± 5% relative humidity (RH) and 40 ± 2 °C and 75% ± 5% RH. Each orodispersible film was individually packed in a PET/foil extrusion laminate sachet and it was stored in the climatic chambers in the primary packaging. After three months of vitamin D3 ODFs were evaluated for average weight, vitamin D3 assay, residual water (%), water activity, and microbiology.

3.2.4. Statistical Analysis

The results were expressed as the mean value ± SD. Stability data were analyzed by a *t*-test. A statistical *p*-value of less than 0.05 was considered significant.

4. Conclusions

Orodispersible film is an innovative dosage form, currently well investigated at laboratory scale but with few large-scale applications. Most of the existing published literature refers to formulations prepared, for instance, on a petri dish, and are thus almost useless to understand suitability for industrial production. Regarding vitamin D, Zhang et al. [18] has already described an oral fast dissolving film containing vitamin D3 obtained by microemulsifying, but again these films were prepared in laboratory on a bench and no evidence of feasibility of industrial manufacturing was provided.

InTo our knowledge, current work is the first paper reporting industrial preparation of vitamin D in ODF form. An orodispersible film with suitable properties and containing 2000 IU of vitamin D3 was developed and manufactured as innovative dosage form for vitamin D3 supplementation. The food grade ingredients selected for the development of the formula, including the main component maltodextrins, are suitable for manufacturing orodispersible films at industrial scale. Manufacturing process was successfully transferred from lab scale to industrial scale and feasibility of industrial manufacturing for ODF was demonstrated. Residual water content is directly correlated to mechanical properties and a water content in the range 8.0–11.0% *w*/*w* guarantees the suitable mechanical properties of vitamin D3 ODF for production on industrial continuous equipment. Batches of vitamin D3 ODF are chemically and microbiologically stable in the tested period. The selected packaging material guarantees a proper shelf-life of the product and the single pouch is an easy to use packaging. The manufactured films are flexible and can be easily handled, have a pleasant taste and aspect, and are free of organic solvent. The ODFs are homogeneous for vitamin D3 content, disintegrate rapidly in the mouth without water and with no risk of choking, and vitamin D3 is immediately released for quick absorption. Such properties allow good compliance also for specific group populations, such as children and the elderly.

Author Contributions: Conceptualization, A.M.G. and F.M.; investigation, I.E.C. and E.D.; writing—original draft preparation, I.E.C.; writing—review and editing, F.M.; supervision, A.M.G. All authors have read and agreed to the published version of the manuscript.

Acknowledgments: The authors would like to acknowledge Lollini Roberta and Simona Gianella for their contribution to the analytical support.

References

1. Gil, A.; Diaz, J.P.; Mesa, M.D. Vitamin D: Classic and novel actions. *Ann. Nutr. Metab.* **2018**, *72*, 87–95. [CrossRef] [PubMed]
2. Baeke, F.; Takiishi, T.; Korf, H.; Gysemans, C.; Mathieu, C. Vitamin D: Modulator of the immune system. *Curr. Opin. Pharmacol.* **2010**, *10*, 482–496. [CrossRef] [PubMed]
3. Prietl, B.; Treiber, G.; Pieber, T.R.; Amrein, K. Vitamin D and immune function. *Nutrients* **2013**, *5*, 2502–2521. [CrossRef] [PubMed]
4. Weir, E.K.; Thenappan, T.; Bhargava, M.; Chen, Y. Does vitamin D deficiency increase the severity of COVID-19? *Clin. Med.* **2020**, *20*, 107–108. [CrossRef] [PubMed]
5. Bergman, P.; Lindh, A.U.; Bjorkhem-Bergman, L.; Lindh, J.D. Vitamin D and Respiratory Tract Infections: A SystematicReview and Meta-Analysis of Randomized ControlledTrials. *PLoS ONE* **2013**, *8*, e65835. [CrossRef] [PubMed]
6. Nurshad, A. Role of vitamin D in preventing of COVID-19 infection, progression and severity. *J. Infect. Public Health* **2020**. [CrossRef]
7. Amrein, K.; Scherkl, M.; Hoffmann, M.; Sommeregger, S.N.; Kostenberger, M.; Berish, A.T.; Martucci, G.; Pinz, S.; Malle, O. Vitamin D deficiency 2.0: An update on the current status worldwide. *Eur. J. Clin. Nutr.* **2020**. [CrossRef] [PubMed]
8. Calton, E.K.; Keane, K.N.; Newsholme, P.; Soares, M.J. The Impact of Vitamin D Levels on inflammatory status: A systematic review of immune cell studies. *PLoS ONE* **2015**, *10*, e0141770. [CrossRef] [PubMed]
9. Irfan, M.; Rabel, S.; Bukhtar, Q.; Imran Qadir, M.I.; Jabeen, F.; Khan, A. Orally disintegrating films: A modern expansion in drug delivery system. *Saudi Pharm. J.* **2015**, *24*, 537–546. [CrossRef] [PubMed]
10. Radicioni, M.; Castiglioni, C.; Giori, A.; Cupone, I.; Frangione, V.; Rovati, S. Bioequivalence study of a new sildenafil 100 mg orodispersible film compared to the conventional film-coated 100 mg tablet administered to healthy male volunteers. *Drug Des. Dev. Ther.* **2017**, *11*, 1183–1192. [CrossRef] [PubMed]
11. Scarpa, M.; Stegemann, S.; Hsiao, W.K.; Pichler, H.; Gaisford, S.; Bresciani, M.; Paudel, A.; Orlu, M. Orodispersible films: Towards drug delivery in special population. *Int. J. Pharm.* **2017**, *523*, 327–335. [CrossRef] [PubMed]
12. Wasilewska, K.; Winnicka, K. How to assess orodispersible film quality? A review of applied methods and their modifications. *Acta Pharm.* **2019**, *69*, 155–176. [CrossRef] [PubMed]
13. Cilurzo, F.; Montanari, L.; Minghetti, P. Self Supporting Film for Pharmaceutical and Food Use. Patent EP1689347, 27 October 2004.
14. Cilurzo, F.; Di Grigoli, M.; Minghetti, P.; Pagani, S. Orodispersible Films Having Quick Dissolution Times for Therapeutic and Food Use. Patent WO2014/049548, 3 April 2014.
15. Thabet, Y.; Breitkreutz, J. Orodispersible films: Product transfer from lab-scale to continuous manufacturing. *Int. J. Pharm.* **2018**, *535*, 285–292. [CrossRef] [PubMed]
16. Cuomo, F.; Cinelli, G.; Chirascu, C.; Marconi, E.; Lopez, F. Antioxidant effect of vitamins in olive oil emulsion. *Colloids Interfaces* **2020**, *4*, 23. [CrossRef]
17. Im, S.; Nam, T.G.N.; Lee, S.G.; Kim, Y.J.; Chun, O.K.; Kim, D.O. Additive Antioxidant Capacity of Vitamin C and Tocopherols in combination. *Food Sci. Biotecnol.* **2014**, *23*, 693–699. [CrossRef]
18. Zhang, M.; Zhang, T.; Zou, Y.; Han, P.; Liu, K. Self-microemulsifying oral fast dissolving films of vitamin D3 for infants: Preparation and characterization. *Food Sci. Nutr.* **2019**, *7*, 2577–2583. [CrossRef]

5

The Inhibitory Roles of Vitamin K in Progression of Vascular Calcification

Atsushi Shioi [1,*], Tomoaki Morioka [2], Tetsuo Shoji [1] and Masanori Emoto [2]

1 Department of Vascular Medicine and Vascular Science Center for Translational Research, Osaka City University Graduate School of Medicine, Osaka 545-8585, Japan; t-shoji@med.osaka-cu.ac.jp
2 Department of Metabolism, Endocrinology, and Molecular Medicine, Osaka City University Graduate School of Medicine, Osaka 545-85858, Japan; m-tomo@med.osaka-cu.ac.jp (T.M.); memoto@med.osaka-cu.ac.jp (M.E.)
* Correspondence: as@med.osaka-cu.ac.jp

Abstract: Vitamin K is a fat-soluble vitamin that is indispensable for the activation of vitamin K-dependent proteins (VKDPs) and may be implicated in cardiovascular disease (CVD). Vascular calcification is intimately associated with CV events and mortality and is a chronic inflammatory process in which activated macrophages promote osteoblastic differentiation of vascular smooth muscle cells (VSMCs) through the production of proinflammatory cytokines such as IL-1β, IL-6, TNF-α, and oncostatin M (OSM) in both intimal and medial layers of arterial walls. This process may be mainly mediated through NF-κB signaling pathway. Vitamin K has been demonstrated to exert anti-inflammatory effects through antagonizing NF-κB signaling in both in vitro and in vivo studies, suggesting that vitamin K may prevent vascular calcification via anti-inflammatory mechanisms. Matrix Gla protein (MGP) is a major inhibitor of soft tissue calcification and contributes to preventing both intimal and medial vascular calcification. Vitamin K may also inhibit progression of vascular calcification by enhancing the activity of MGP through facilitating its γ-carboxylation. In support of this hypothesis, the procalcific effects of warfarin, an antagonist of vitamin K, on arterial calcification have been demonstrated in several clinical studies. Among the inactive MGP forms, dephospho-uncarboxylated MGP (dp-ucMGP) may be regarded as the most useful biomarker of not only vitamin K deficiency, but also vascular calcification and CVD. There have been several studies showing the association of circulating levels of dp-ucMGP with vitamin K intake, vascular calcification, mortality, and CVD. However, additional larger prospective studies including randomized controlled trials are necessary to confirm the beneficial effects of vitamin K supplementation on CV health.

Keywords: atherosclerosis; matrix Gla protein; oncostatin M; vascular calcification

1. Introduction

Vitamin K is a fat-soluble vitamin that is composed of a 2-methyl-1,4-naphthoquinone ring and a side chain at the 3-carbon position varying in length and degree of saturation [1]. Vitamin K naturally occurs in two forms: vitamin K1 (phylloquinone) and vitamin K2 (menaquinones (MKs)). Vitamin K1 is predominantly found in green leafy vegetables and plant oils such as soybean, canola, and olive, whereas vitamin K2 is present in small amounts in fermented foods, milk products, meat, and cheese. Vitamin K2 is the most potent form and has a longer half-life compared with vitamin K1 [2]. Moreover, MK-4 is the most prevalent form of vitamin K in human and animal tissues and can be formed from menadione through the action of UbiA prenyltranferase domain-containing protein 1 (UBIAD1) [3].

The most important function of vitamin K is to serve as a cofactor in the synthesis of vitamin K-dependent coagulation factors II, VII, IX, and X in the liver [4,5]. Activation of vitamin K-dependent proteins (VKDPs) is mediated through the conversion of glutamic acid (Glu) residue of their molecules to γ-carboxyglutamic acid (Gla) by the action of γ-glutamyl carboxylase (GGCX). This process proceeds by the oxidation of vitamin K hydroquinone (KH_2) to vitamin K epoxide (KO) in the vitamin K cycle. KO is reduced to KH2 by vitamin K epoxide reductase (VKOR). Vitamin K antagonists such as warfarin exert their anti-coagulative effects by inhibiting VKOR activities.

Two natural anticoagulants, protein C and protein S, are the vitamin K-dependent plasma proteins that regulate blood coagulation by inhibiting activated factors Va and VIIIa (FVa and FVIIIa) [6]. In addition to its anticoagulant activity, activated protein C (APC) exhibits anti-inflammatory and anti-apoptotic effects by its binding to endothelial cell protein C receptor (EPCR), leading to activation of protease-activated receptor 1 (PAR1) [7]. Protein S functions as a cofactor for APC in the degradation of FVa and FVIIIa. Protein S also exerts anti-inflammatory effect through its binding to the Tyro3/Axl/Mer (TAM) family of receptor tyrosine kinases [8].

Other extra-hepatic VKDPs such as matrix Gla protein (MGP), osteocalcin, and Gas6, and Gla-rich protein (GRP) have been identified. Osteocalcin (also called bone Gla protein) is mainly secreted by osteoblasts and facilitates the deposition of calcium into bone matrix [9,10]. Matrix Gla protein (MGP) is predominantly produced by chondrocytes and vascular smooth muscle cells and functions as a potent calcification inhibitor within the arterial walls [10,11]. Growth arrest-specific 6 (Gas6) is known to be a ligand for the TAM family of receptor tyrosine kinases and prevents endothelial cells and vascular smooth muscle cells (VSMCs) from undergoing apoptosis and inhibits vascular calcification through its anti-apoptotic effect on VSMCs [10,12]. Gla-rich protein (GRP) was identified in sturgeon cartilage as a novel VKDP containing many Gla residues in the molecule (16 Gla residues among 74 amino acids) and may serve as an inhibitor of vascular calcification [10,13].

Vitamin K has been shown to function as an anti-inflammatory factor, independent of its activity as a cofactor for GGCX. Vitamin K status was inversely associated with circulating inflammatory markers such as IL-6 and C-reactive protein (CRP) [14]. Vitamin K attenuated lipopolysaccharide (LPS)-induced inflammatory responses by blocking nuclear factor κB (NF-κB) signal transduction [15–17].

Cardiovascular disease (CVD) is the leading cause of morbidity and mortality all over the world. Vascular calcification is a striking feature of chronic inflammatory diseases such as atherosclerosis, type 2 diabetes, and chronic kidney disease (CKD) and is associated with increased risk of adverse CV events [18–21]. Vitamin K has been proposed to show a protective effect against CVD through the action of VKDPs such as MGP to inhibit vascular calcification [22,23]. Furthermore, anti-inflammatory effects of vitamin K may be involved in preventing progression of atherosclerotic plaque calcification. In this review, we will describe the inhibitory roles of vitamin K and MGP in vascular calcification and the clinical significance of inactive MGP (dephospho-uncarboxylated MGP: dp-ucMGP) as a novel biomarker of vascular calcification and CVD.

2. Vascular Calcification and CVD

Vascular calcification is a hallmark of atherosclerosis especially in coronary arteries. Particularly in patients with diabetes mellitus and CKD, coronary artery calcification (CAC) is strikingly accelerated and predicts future CV events and all-cause mortality [19,24].

Morphologically, two types of vascular calcification have been described. Intimal calcification usually develops in accordance with progression of atherosclerosis and may cause coronary ischemic events. On the other hand, medial calcification is independent of atherosclerosis and predominantly develops along elastic fibers. Consequently, medial calcification promotes arterial stiffness and increases pulse pressure as well as systolic blood pressure, resulting in left ventricular hypertrophy, diastolic dysfunction, and heart failure [25].

VSMCs play a pivotal role in vascular calcification. Under procalcifying conditions, VSMCs undergo osteoblastic differentiation and express Runx2, the master transcription factor for osteogenesis along with other bone-related proteins such as alkaline phosphatase (ALP) and bone sialoprotein II (BSP-II) [26]. These transdifferentiated osteoblast-like cells generate matrix vesicles and exosomes that initiate the mineralization process and deposit bone-like matrix within the arterial wall. These processes are promoted by loss of calcification inhibitors, oxidative stress, endoplasmic reticulum stress, apoptosis, and DNA damage response signaling [26].

3. Inflammation and Vascular Calcification

Vascular calcification is an inflammation-mediated process where macrophages promote osteoblastic differentiation and mineralization of VSMCs via secreting proinflammatory cytokines such as interleukin (IL)-1β, IL-6, tumor necrosis factor-α (TNF-α), and oncostatin M (OSM) [27–30]. In intimal vascular calcification, plaque inflammation evoked by infiltrated macrophages precedes active calcification [31,32], while an increased number of CD68-positive macrophages are localized in the vascular wall associated with medial calcification in CKD [33,34]. Moreover, it has been suggested that pro-inflammatory cytokines such as TNF-α may play an important role in the development of medial calcification associated with diabetes and CKD [35].

It has been shown that NF-κB activation by TNF-α and LPS promotes osteogenic differentiation of human adipose tissue-derived mesenchymal stromal/stem cells [36,37]. Moreover, TNF-α also enhanced osteogenic differentiation of both human bone marrow-derived mesenchymal stem cells and human dental pulp stem cells through activation of NF-κB signaling pathway [38,39]. Furthermore, NF-κB signaling stimulated by various stimuli such as high glucose, high phosphate, and oxidative stress as well as proinflammatory cytokines has also been involved in osteogenic differentiation of VSMCs [40–44]. Therefore, NF-κB signaling play a pivotal role in osteogenic differentiation of not only mesenchymal stem cells, but also VSMCs.

4. Anti-Inflammatory Effects of Vitamin K

Anti-inflammatory action of vitamin K has been shown in several in vitro and in vivo studies. MK-4 suppressed LPS-induced expression of inflammatory cytokines such as IL-6 in macrophage-like cells and MG-6 mouse microglia-derived cells through the inhibition of NF-κB signaling pathway [16,45]. Pretreatment with MK-7 inhibited the production of TNF-α after the toll-like receptor (TLR) activation in human monocyte-derived macrophages [17]. LPS-induced production of IL-6 in human fibroblasts is intensively inhibited by naphthoquinone compounds [46]. In an in vivo study utilizing rats, vitamin K1 supplementation suppresses the inflammation induced by LPS as evidenced by plasma levels of transaminases and hepatic mRNA levels of macrophage migration inhibitory factor [15]. Vitamin K1 also attenuates streptozotocin-induced diabetes in rats by reducing free radical stress and suppressing NF-κB activation [47]. Clinical studies have showed that vitamin K status is negatively associated with circulating levels of inflammatory markers. Plasma K1 levels were inversely associated with IL-6 and C-reactive protein (CRP) in a cross-sectional study conducted with 379 healthy men and women [48]. However, no significant changes of the levels of inflammatory biomarkers were observed in the 3-year follow-up of patients supplemented with vitamin K1 [48]. In another cross-sectional analysis of the Framingham Offspring Study (n = 1381), plasma levels of phylloquinone (vitamin K1) and its intake were inversely associated with overall circulating markers of inflammation, including CD40 ligand and IL-6 [14]. Higher serum phylloquinone levels were associated with several serum inflammatory markers such as IL-6, soluble intercellular adhesion molecule-1 (ICAM-1), and CRP in a cross-sectional study conducted with 662 community-dwelling adults from the Multi-Ethnic Study of Atherosclerosis (MESA) [49]. Therefore, it is likely that vitamin K may prevent inflammatory vascular diseases including atherosclerosis and vascular calcification through its anti-inflammatory actions on vascular cells.

5. Matrix Gla Protein and other VKDPs in Vascular Calcification

Matrix Gla protein (MGP) is an 84-amino acid VKDP that is secreted by chondrocytes and VSMCs and is expressed in not only bone, but also the heart, vessels, kidneys, and cartilage. MGP contains five glutamic acid residues and three serine residues and this molecule is activated through two post-translational modifications as follows: vitamin K-dependent carboxylation of glutamate and serine phosphorylation [50]. After these maturation steps, activated MGP serves as a potent calcification inhibitor.

Mice lacking MGP developed extensive arterial calcification and die within six to eight weeks due to rupture of the aorta [51]. Histological analyses clarified extensive calcification along with elastic fibers and the presence of chondrocyte-like cells in the media. Interestingly, restoration of MGP expression in VSMCs rescued the arterial calcification phenotype in MGP-deficient mice, while raising circulating levels of MGP through overexpression of MGP transgene in the liver did not affect vascular calcification, suggesting that only expression of MGP in VSMCs can inhibit vascular calcification [52]. MGP expression in VSMCs was inversely regulated by the development of VSMC calcification [53]. In humans, mutations in the gene encoding MGP causes Keutel syndrome, a rare autosomal recessive disorder characterized by severe calcification of soft tissues [54,55]. The possible mechanisms have been suggested for the inhibitory actions of MGP on calcification. Firstly, MGP binds hydroxyapatite crystals thereby inhibiting crystal growth [56]. Secondly, MGP has the capacity to bind bone morphogenetic protein-2 (BMP-2) and to attenuate its activity [57,58]. BMP-2 promotes transdifferentiation of VSMCs into osteoblast-like cells. MGP has been shown to be localized in not only calcified atherosclerotic plaques, but also medial calcified lesions [59–63]. Thus, MGP has been recognized as a major inhibitor of both intimal and medial vascular calcification.

As mentioned in the previous section, VKDPs other than MGP may also function as inhibitors of vascular calcification. Gas6 exerts its inhibitory effect on vascular calcification through its binding to the Axl receptor. Interaction between Gas6 and Axl activates the PI3K/Akt pathway resulting in stimulation of cell survival pathway [64]. Therefore, apoptosis-mediated VSMC calcification can be inhibited by the Gas6/Axl-PI3K/Akt pathway activated by statin and vitamin K2 [65,66]. GRP also function as an inhibitor of vascular calcification. GRP is immunohistochemically localized at the site of mineral deposition in human aorta and aortic valve tissues [67]. The gene expression of GRP is also significantly upregulated in calcified aortic valve tissues compared with non-calcified aortic valve tissues [68]. VSMCs derived from GRP-deficient mice exhibit an increased capacity of in vitro calcification and expression of osteogenic markers such as Runx2, ALP, and OCN [68]. Protein C and protein S deficiency may be involved in the pathogenesis of calcific uremic arteriolopathy (also known as calciphylaxis) characterized by skin ulcer and tissue necrosis [69].

6. Vitamin K and CAC

CAC is closely related to the overall plaque burden of coronary artery atherosclerosis. Higher CAC score is associated with a greater risk of adverse CV events and all-cause mortality [70–72]. A preventive role for vitamin K against CAC progression has been proposed through the inhibitory action of MGP on mineral deposition within the arterial wall [22,73]. Once MGP is activated through vitamin K-dependent γ-carboxylation and subsequent serine phosphorylation, it potently suppresses arterial calcification [50]. Anti-inflammatory effects of vitamin K, independent of γ-carboxylation, may also contribute to the inhibition of CAC as mentioned above.

6.1. Vitamin K Status and CAC

There have been several observational studies assessing the relationship between vitamin K status and CAC. Vitamin K status has been assessed by vitamin K intake, circulating levels of phylloquinone (PK) or menaquinone (MK), and measuring uncarboxylated fractions of certain VKDPs such as MGP [2,74]. In an observational study among U.S. military personnel at low CVD risk, phylloquinone intake was not associated with CAC [75]. In a case-cohort study conducted on MESA subjects, low levels of serum vitamin K1 were significantly associated with CAC progression in patients treated with antihypertensive drugs [76]. In a cross-sectional study of 564 post-menopausal women to examine the association of PK and MK intake with CAC, PK intake was not associated with CAC [RR (95% CI):1.17 (0.96–1,42); the highest versus lowest quartile], while MK intake was associated with reduced CAC [RR (95% CI):0.80 (0.65–0.98); the highest versus lowest quartile] [77]. In an observational study to investigate the association of CAC and circulating levels of PK, MK-4, and MK-7, there was no significant correlation of CAC with plasma levels of PK, MK-4, and MK-7 [78]. In another cross-sectional study among 40 hemodialysis (HD) patients, circulating uc-MGP levels as a vitamin K status marker were inversely associated with the severity of CAC [79].

6.2. Vitamin K Supplementation and CAC

There are a few studies examining the effect of vitamin K supplementation on coronary artery calcification. A 3-year prospective randomized controlled trial (RCT) revealed that PK supplementation significantly reduced CAC progression compared to control supplementation in a subgroup of participants who were ≥ 85% adherent to the intervention [80]. In another RCT including 42 nondialyzed patients with CKD stages 3–5 for 270 days, the increase of common carotid intima-media thickness (CCA-IMT) was significantly lower in the supplementation group with MK-7 at a dose of 90 μg together with 10 μg of cholecalciferol (vitamin D) (K + D group) compared with the D group [81]. The increase of CAC was slightly lower in the K + D group than in the D group, but the difference was not significant [81]. In a single arm study of 26 patients supplemented with 45 mg MK-4 for 1 year, the annual increase of CAC was 14%, but brachial ankle pulse wave velocity was not significantly changed [82]. In a recent RCT among 68 patients with type 2 diabetes and CVD for 6 months, MK-7 supplementation (360 μg/day) did not significantly change calcification mass score of both femoral arteries compared with placebo treatment [83]. RCTs designed to assess the effect of PK and MK-7 on CAC in HD patients are ongoing [84–86].

6.3. Vitamin K Antagonists and CAC

Vitamin K antagonists (VKAs) including coumarins (warfarin, acenocoumarol, and phenprocoumon, etc.) and indandiones (fluindione, etc.) are oral anticoagulants utilized for the treatment of thromboembolic diseases [87]. VKAs exert their anticoagulant effect by interfering with vitamin K cycle [88]. VKAs inhibit the action of VKOR to deplete the reduced (hydroquinone) form of vitamin K, thereby suppressing hepatic γ-carboxylation of VKDPs such as coagulation factors II, VII, IX, and X. In addition to the inhibitory effect on coagulation factors in the liver, warfarin also affects peripheral γ-carboxylation of VKDPs including MGP in vascular tissues [4]. Blocking γ-carboxylation of MGP in VSMCs by warfarin has been shown to contribute to its inhibitory effect on VSMC calcification [89]. Experimental studies using animal models have demonstrated that warfarin induces arterial calcification. In a rat model, warfarin caused acute medial calcification of major arteries and markedly increased the expression levels of MGP mRNA and protein in calcified arteries and decreased serum levels of MGP [90]. ApoE-deficient mice treated with warfarin developed atherosclerotic plaque calcification associated with features of plaque vulnerability [91]. Moreover, high doses of vitamin K reversed warfarin-induced medial vascular calcification in rats [92].

There are several clinical studies investigating the pro-calcific effect of warfarin on arterial calcification. In a cross-sectional study including 133 VKA users and 133 age, gender and the Framingham Risk Score (FRS) matched non-VKA users, the mean coronary calcification score (Agatston score) and the fraction of calcified coronary plaques significantly increased according increasing the duration of drug use in VKA users compared with non-VKA users [91]. In another cross-sectional study of 236 patients, use of VKA was significantly associated with the presence of ascending and descending aorta calcification compared with no anticoagulation treatment [93]. In a retrospective matched cohort study, a higher prevalence of lower extremity arterial calcification was found in patients receiving warfarin compared with those with no treatment [94]. The prevalence of breast arterial calcification was greater in women currently or in the past treated with warfarin compared with those without warfarin treatment [95]. The long-term effect of VKA use on coronary artery calcification has been investigated in 43 patients receiving VKA with metallic prosthetic valves and 65 control patients. CAC score assessed by CT was significantly higher in long-term VKA users compared with the control group [96]. In serial coronary intravascular ultrasound (IVUS) examinations performed during an

18- to 24-month period, a post hoc analysis of 8 prospective trials revealed that warfarin therapy was associated with progressive coronary plaque calcification independent of changes in atheroma volume [97].

7. dp-ucMGP as a Marker of Vitamin K Status

Active MGP is formed through sequential post-translational modification processes [50]. While carboxylation affords the capacity to bind calcium ions, phosphorylation may facilitate the cellular secretion process of MGP. After translation in the endoplasmic reticulum, MGP is firstly carboxylated by the action of GGCX requiring vitamin K as a cofactor, forming dephospho-carboxylated MGP (dp-cMGP). Next, a Golgi casein kinase phosphorylates dp-cMGP to p-cMGP (phosphorylated-carboxylated MGP), thereby facilitating secretion. p-cMGP is secreted into the extracellular space where it acts as an inhibitor of tissue calcification. Inactive dp-ucMGP is also released from cells into the bloodstream. Subsequently, three forms of MGP, that is, dp-ucMGP, dp-cMGP, and p-cMGP are present in the circulation. Vitamin K deficiency may impair the activity of MGP. Among these three conformations, dp-ucMGP is recognized as the best single biomarker of vitamin K deficiency [98]. In the general population, circulating levels of dp-ucMGP increase with age and with deterioration of renal function [50].

There are several studies to investigate whether vitamin K supplementation could decrease plasma levels of dp-ucMGP and subsequently reduce the risk of CV events. In a randomized, double-blind, placebo-controlled trial of 60 participants from the general population for 12 weeks, plasma levels of dp-ucMGP were dose-dependently decreased in the 180 μg and 360 μg menaquinone-7 (MK-7) supplementation groups by 31% and 46%, respectively, whereas dp-ucMGP levels remained unchanged in the placebo group [99]. In another double-blind, placebo-controlled trial of 244 healthy postmenopausal women for 3 years, MK-7 supplementation reduced dp-ucMGP levels by 50% in comparison with the placebo group [100]. A prospective, randomized, single-blind intervention study conducted with 200 chronic HD patients for 8 weeks showed that MK-7 supplementation dose-dependently decreased dp-ucMGP levels in the groups with 360, 720, 1080 μg thrice weekly by 17, 33, and 46%, respectively [101]. These data suggest that MK-7 supplementation may reduce the circulating levels of dp-ucMGP through enhancement of MGP activation. Therefore, it is likely that vitamin K2 intake might be beneficial for prevention of future CV events.

8. dp-ucMGP as a Novel Marker of VC

The association between blood levels of MGP including its inactive forms and vascular calcification has been investigated in various populations [102–109]. In a prospective cohort study of 571 women aged 57.3 years, plasma levels of dp-ucMGP were borderline significantly associated with the presence of CAC [106]. A cross-sectional study conducted with 198 type 2 diabetes mellitus (DM) patients with normal or slightly impaired kidney function revealed that circulating dp-ucMGP was independently associated with below-knee arterial calcification score [107]. Plasma levels of dp-ucMGP were positively associated with the aortic calcification score in a cohort consisting of 107 patients with CKD stages 2–5 [108]. An observational cohort study of 136 hemodialysis (HD) patients indicated that plasma levels of dp-ucMGP were significantly associated with the vascular calcification score [109]. These studies on various populations, including healthy subjects and patients with high risks of CV, suggest that plasma dp-ucMGP may be a useful marker of VC.

9. The Association of dp-ucMGP with CV Events and Mortality

Vascular calcification is independently associated with an increased risk of CV events and mortality [110–116]. Since there are accumulating evidence suggesting that plasma dp-ucMGP is a useful marker of VC, several investigators have explored the possible association of dp-ucMGP with CV events and mortality in various populations. In a study among 577 older adults of the Longitudinal Aging Study Amsterdam study (LASA) with no history of previous CVD, there was a more than 2-fold higher risk of CVD in the highest tertile of dp-ucMGP group (HR: 2.69, 95% CI: 1.09–6.62) compared with the lowest tertile after a follow-up period of 5.6 years [111]. In a Flemish population study of 2318 participants, higher concentrations of dp-ucMGP were an independent predictor of total, non-cancer, CV mortality after a follow-up period of 14.1 years [115]. In a prospective cohort study consisting of 518 type 2 DM patients, high dp-ucMGP levels were associated with increased risk for CVD, especially with peripheral artery disease (PAD) and heart failure after a follow-up of 11.2 years [110]. In a prospective cohort study conducted with 799 patients with history of myocardial infarction, stroke, or coronary artery disease, there was a higher risk of all-cause and CV mortality in the highest quartile of dp-ucMGP (HR 1.89, 95% CI: 1.32–2.72 and HR 1.88, 95% CI: 1.22–2.90, respectively) [116]. These data suggest that plasma dp-ucMGP may be a novel biomarker for CV events and mortality.

10. Conclusion

Vascular calcification is an inflammation-mediated process in which activated transdifferentiation of VSMCs into osteoblastic cells was induced by the action of cytokines such as TNF-α and OSM secreted from macrophages infiltrated in intimal and medial tissues of arterial wall. Vitamin K may prevent vascular calcification through an anti-inflammatory mechanism as well as promotion of γ-carboxylation of MGP. The preventive role of active MGP in vascular calcification has been proven by several clinical studies demonstrating the procalcific effect of warfarin, a vitamin K antagonist in arteries. Various clinical studies have revealed that higher vitamin K intake may reduce the risk of vascular calcification and CVD and higher plasma concentrations of dp-ucMGP may predict future risk of death or CV events. High-quality prospective cohort studies and RCTs are still required to establish the role of vitamin K in CV health.

Author Contributions: A.S. wrote the manuscript. T.M. searched the literature and selected the referenced papers. T.S. and M.E. critically reviewed and corrected all versions of the manuscript. All authors have read and agreed to the published version of the manuscript.

Acknowledgments: The authors would like to thank Asako Sawada for her secretarial assistance.

References

1. Shearer, M.J.; Okano, T. Key Pathways and Regulators of Vitamin K Function and Intermediary Metabolism. *Annu. Rev. Nutr.* **2018**, *38*, 127–151. [CrossRef]
2. van Ballegooijen, A.J.; Beulens, J.W. The Role of Vitamin K Status in Cardiovascular Health: Evidence from Observational and Clinical Studies. *Curr. Nutr. Rep.* **2017**, *6*, 197–205. [CrossRef]
3. Nakagawa, K.; Hirota, Y.; Sawada, N.; Yuge, N.; Watanabe, M.; Uchino, Y.; Okuda, N.; Shimomura, Y.; Suhara, Y.; Okano, T. Identification of UBIAD1 as a novel human menaquinone-4 biosynthetic enzyme. *Nature* **2010**, *468*, 117–121. [CrossRef]
4. Danziger, J. Vitamin K-dependent proteins, warfarin, and vascular calcification. *Clin. J. Am. Soc. Nephrol.* **2008**, *3*, 1504–1510. [CrossRef]
5. Halder, M.; Petsophonsakul, P.; Akbulut, A.C.; Pavlic, A.; Bohan, F.; Anderson, E.; Maresz, K.; Kramann, R.; Schurgers, L. Vitamin K: Double Bonds beyond Coagulation Insights into Differences between Vitamin K1 and K2 in Health and Disease. *Int. J. Mol. Sci.* **2019**, *20*, 896. [CrossRef]
6. Rezaie, A.R. Regulation of the protein C anticoagulant and antiinflammatory pathways. *Curr. Med. Chem.* **2010**, *17*, 2059–2069. [CrossRef] [PubMed]
7. Mohan Rao, L.V.; Esmon, C.T.; Pendurthi, U.R. Endothelial cell protein C receptor: A multiliganded and multifunctional receptor. *Blood* **2014**, *124*, 1553–1562. [CrossRef] [PubMed]
8. Suleiman, L.; Negrier, C.; Boukerche, H. Protein S: A multifunctional anticoagulant vitamin K-dependent protein at the crossroads of coagulation, inflammation, angiogenesis, and cancer. *Crit. Rev. Oncol. Hematol.* **2013**, *88*, 637–654. [CrossRef] [PubMed]

9. Hauschka, P.V.; Lian, J.B.; Cole, D.E.; Gundberg, C.M. Osteocalcin and matrix Gla protein: Vitamin K-dependent proteins in bone. *Physiol. Rev.* **1989**, *69*, 990–1047. [CrossRef] [PubMed]
10. Wen, L.; Chen, J.; Duan, L.; Li, S. Vitamin Kdependent proteins involved in bone and cardiovascular health (Review). *Mol. Med. Rep.* **2018**, *18*, 3–15. [PubMed]
11. Theuwissen, E.; Smit, E.; Vermeer, C. The role of vitamin K in soft-tissue calcification. *Adv. Nutr.* **2012**, *3*, 166–173. [CrossRef]
12. Azuma, K.; Inoue, S. Multiple Modes of Vitamin K Actions in Aging-Related Musculoskeletal Disorders. *Int. J. Mol. Sci.* **2019**, *20*, 2844. [CrossRef] [PubMed]
13. Viegas, C.S.; Herfs, M.; Rafael, M.S.; Enriquez, J.L.; Teixeira, A.; Luis, I.M.; van 't Hoofd, C.M.; Joao, A.; Maria, V.L.; Cavaco, S.; et al. Gla-rich protein is a potential new vitamin K target in cancer: Evidences for a direct GRP-mineral interaction. *BioMed Res. Int.* **2014**, *2014*, 340216. [CrossRef]
14. Shea, M.K.; Booth, S.L.; Massaro, J.M.; Jacques, P.F.; D'Agostino, R.B., Sr.; Dawson-Hughes, B.; Ordovas, J.M.; O'Donnell, C.J.; Kathiresan, S.; Keaney, J.F., Jr.; et al. Vitamin K and vitamin D status: Associations with inflammatory markers in the Framingham Offspring Study. *Am. J. Epidemiol.* **2008**, *167*, 313–320. [CrossRef] [PubMed]
15. Ohsaki, Y.; Shirakawa, H.; Hiwatashi, K.; Furukawa, Y.; Mizutani, T.; Komai, M. Vitamin K suppresses lipopolysaccharide-induced inflammation in the rat. *Biosci. Biotechnol. Biochem.* **2006**, *70*, 926–932. [CrossRef] [PubMed]
16. Ohsaki, Y.; Shirakawa, H.; Miura, A.; Giriwono, P.E.; Sato, S.; Ohashi, A.; Iribe, M.; Goto, T.; Komai, M. Vitamin K suppresses the lipopolysaccharide-induced expression of inflammatory cytokines in cultured macrophage-like cells via the inhibition of the activation of nuclear factor κB through the repression of IKKα/β phosphorylation. *J. Nutr. Biochem.* **2010**, *21*, 1120–1126. [CrossRef] [PubMed]
17. Pan, M.H.; Maresz, K.; Lee, P.S.; Wu, J.C.; Ho, C.T.; Popko, J.; Mehta, D.S.; Stohs, S.J.; Badmaev, V. Inhibition of TNF-alpha, IL-1alpha, and IL-1beta by Pretreatment of Human Monocyte-Derived Macrophages with Menaquinone-7 and Cell Activation with TLR Agonists In Vitro. *J. Med. Food* **2016**, *19*, 663–669. [CrossRef]
18. Budoff, M.J.; Nasir, K.; Katz, R.; Takasu, J.; Carr, J.J.; Wong, N.D.; Allison, M.; Lima, J.A.; Detrano, R.; Blumenthal, R.S.; et al. Thoracic aortic calcification and coronary heart disease events: The multi-ethnic study of atherosclerosis (MESA). *Atherosclerosis* **2011**, *215*, 196–202. [CrossRef]
19. Chen, J.; Budoff, M.J.; Reilly, M.P.; Yang, W.; Rosas, S.E.; Rahman, M.; Zhang, X.; Roy, J.A.; Lustigova, E.; Nessel, L.; et al. Coronary Artery Calcification and Risk of Cardiovascular Disease and Death Among Patients with Chronic Kidney Disease. *JAMA Cardiol.* **2017**, *2*, 635–643. [CrossRef]
20. Santos, R.D.; Rumberger, J.A.; Budoff, M.J.; Shaw, L.J.; Orakzai, S.H.; Berman, D.; Raggi, P.; Blumenthal, R.S.; Nasir, K. Thoracic aorta calcification detected by electron beam tomography predicts all-cause mortality. *Atherosclerosis* **2010**, *209*, 131–135. [CrossRef]
21. Wilson, P.W.; Kauppila, L.I.; O'Donnell, C.J.; Kiel, D.P.; Hannan, M.; Polak, J.M.; Cupples, L.A. Abdominal aortic calcific deposits are an important predictor of vascular morbidity and mortality. *Circulation* **2001**, *103*, 1529–1534. [CrossRef] [PubMed]
22. Berkner, K.L.; Runge, K.W. The physiology of vitamin K nutriture and vitamin K-dependent protein function in atherosclerosis. *J. Thromb. Haemost.* **2004**, *2*, 2118–2132. [CrossRef] [PubMed]
23. Harshman, S.G.; Shea, M.K. The Role of Vitamin K in Chronic Aging Diseases: Inflammation, Cardiovascular Disease, and Osteoarthritis. *Curr. Nutr. Rep.* **2016**, *5*, 90–98. [CrossRef] [PubMed]
24. Kramer, C.K.; Zinman, B.; Gross, J.L.; Canani, L.H.; Rodrigues, T.C.; Azevedo, M.J.; Retnakaran, R. Coronary artery calcium score prediction of all cause mortality and cardiovascular events in people with type 2 diabetes: Systematic review and meta-analysis. *BMJ* **2013**, *346*, f1654. [CrossRef]
25. Henaut, L.; Chillon, J.M.; Kamel, S.; Massy, Z.A. Updates on the Mechanisms and the Care of Cardiovascular Calcification in Chronic Kidney Disease. *Semin. Nephrol.* **2018**, *38*, 233–250. [CrossRef]
26. Leopold, J.A. Vascular calcification: Mechanisms of vascular smooth muscle cell calcification. *Trends Cardiovasc. Med.* **2015**, *25*, 267–274. [CrossRef]
27. Ceneri, N.; Zhao, L.; Young, B.D.; Healy, A.; Coskun, S.; Vasavada, H.; Yarovinsky, T.O.; Ike, K.; Pardi, R.; Qin, L.; et al. Rac2 Modulates Atherosclerotic Calcification by Regulating Macrophage Interleukin-1beta Production. *Arterioscler. Thromb. Vasc. Biol.* **2017**, *37*, 328–340. [CrossRef]
28. Parhami, F.; Basseri, B.; Hwang, J.; Tintut, Y.; Demer, L.L. High-density lipoprotein regulates calcification of vascular cells. *Circ. Res.* **2002**, *91*, 570–576. [CrossRef]

29. Tintut, Y.; Patel, J.; Territo, M.; Saini, T.; Parhami, F.; Demer, L.L. Monocyte/macrophage regulation of vascular calcification in vitro. *Circulation* **2002**, *105*, 650–655. [CrossRef]
30. Kakutani, Y.; Shioi, A.; Shoji, T.; Okazaki, H.; Koyama, H.; Emoto, M.; Inaba, M. Oncostatin M Promotes Osteoblastic Differentiation of Human Vascular Smooth Muscle Cells Through JAK3-STAT3 Pathway. *J. Cell. Biochem.* **2015**, *116*, 1325–1333. [CrossRef]
31. Aikawa, E.; Nahrendorf, M.; Figueiredo, J.L.; Swirski, F.K.; Shtatland, T.; Kohler, R.H.; Jaffer, F.A.; Aikawa, M.; Weissleder, R. Osteogenesis associates with inflammation in early-stage atherosclerosis evaluated by molecular imaging in vivo. *Circulation* **2007**, *116*, 2841–2850. [CrossRef] [PubMed]
32. Dweck, M.R.; Aikawa, E.; Newby, D.E.; Tarkin, J.M.; Rudd, J.H.; Narula, J.; Fayad, Z.A. Noninvasive Molecular Imaging of Disease Activity in Atherosclerosis. *Circ. Res.* **2016**, *119*, 330–340. [CrossRef] [PubMed]
33. Lariviere, R.; Gauthier-Bastien, A.; Ung, R.V.; St-Hilaire, J.; Mac-Way, F.; Richard, D.E.; Agharazii, M. Endothelin type A receptor blockade reduces vascular calcification and inflammation in rats with chronic kidney disease. *J. Hypertens.* **2017**, *35*, 376–384. [CrossRef] [PubMed]
34. Benz, K.; Hilgers, K.F.; Daniel, C.; Amann, K. Vascular Calcification in Chronic Kidney Disease: The Role of Inflammation. *Int. J. Nephrol.* **2018**, *2018*, 4310379. [CrossRef] [PubMed]
35. Al-Aly, Z. Medial vascular calcification in diabetes mellitus and chronic kidney disease: The role of inflammation. *Cardiovasc. Hematol. Disord. Drug Targets* **2007**, *7*, 1–6. [CrossRef]
36. Cho, H.H.; Shin, K.K.; Kim, Y.J.; Song, J.S.; Kim, J.M.; Bae, Y.C.; Kim, C.D.; Jung, J.S. NF-kappaB activation stimulates osteogenic differentiation of mesenchymal stem cells derived from human adipose tissue by increasing TAZ expression. *J. Cell. Physiol.* **2010**, *223*, 168–177.
37. Herzmann, N.; Salamon, A.; Fiedler, T.; Peters, K. Lipopolysaccharide induces proliferation and osteogenic differentiation of adipose-derived mesenchymal stromal cells in vitro via TLR4 activation. *Exp. Cell Res.* **2017**, *350*, 115–122. [CrossRef]
38. Feng, X.; Feng, G.; Xing, J.; Shen, B.; Li, L.; Tan, W.; Xu, Y.; Liu, S.; Liu, H.; Jiang, J.; et al. TNF-alpha triggers osteogenic differentiation of human dental pulp stem cells via the NF-kappaB signalling pathway. *Cell Biol. Int.* **2013**, *37*, 1267–1275. [CrossRef]
39. Hess, K.; Ushmorov, A.; Fiedler, J.; Brenner, R.E.; Wirth, T. TNFalpha promotes osteogenic differentiation of human mesenchymal stem cells by triggering the NF-kappaB signaling pathway. *Bone* **2009**, *45*, 367–376. [CrossRef]
40. Ye, Y.; Bian, W.; Fu, F.; Hu, J.; Liu, H. Selenoprotein S inhibits inflammation-induced vascular smooth muscle cell calcification. *J. Biol. Inorg. Chem.* **2018**, *23*, 739–751. [CrossRef]
41. He, X.; Jiang, H.; Gao, F.; Liang, S.; Wei, M.; Chen, L. Indoxyl sulfate-induced calcification of vascular smooth muscle cells via the PI3K/Akt/NF-kappaB signaling pathway. *Microsc. Res. Tech.* **2019**, *82*, 2000–2006. [CrossRef] [PubMed]
42. Voelkl, J.; Luong, T.T.; Tuffaha, R.; Musculus, K.; Auer, T.; Lian, X.; Daniel, C.; Zickler, D.; Boehme, B.; Sacherer, M.; et al. SGK1 induces vascular smooth muscle cell calcification through NF-kappaB signaling. *J. Clin. Investig.* **2018**, *128*, 3024–3040. [CrossRef] [PubMed]
43. Zhao, M.M.; Xu, M.J.; Cai, Y.; Zhao, G.; Guan, Y.; Kong, W.; Tang, C.; Wang, X. Mitochondrial reactive oxygen species promote p65 nuclear translocation mediating high-phosphate-induced vascular calcification in vitro and in vivo. *Kidney Int.* **2011**, *79*, 1071–1079. [CrossRef] [PubMed]
44. Voelkl, J.; Lang, F.; Eckardt, K.U.; Amann, K.; Kuro, O.M.; Pasch, A.; Pieske, B.; Alesutan, I. Signaling pathways involved in vascular smooth muscle cell calcification during hyperphosphatemia. *Cell. Mol. Life Sci.* **2019**, *76*, 2077–2091. [CrossRef] [PubMed]
45. Saputra, W.D.; Aoyama, N.; Komai, M.; Shirakawa, H. Menaquinone-4 Suppresses Lipopolysaccharide-Induced Inflammation in MG6 Mouse Microglia-Derived Cells by Inhibiting the NF-kappaB Signaling Pathway. *Int. J. Mol. Sci.* **2019**, *20*, 2317. [CrossRef] [PubMed]
46. Reddi, K.; Henderson, B.; Meghji, S.; Wilson, M.; Poole, S.; Hopper, C.; Harris, M.; Hodges, S.J. Interleukin 6 production by lipopolysaccharide-stimulated human fibroblasts is potently inhibited by naphthoquinone (vitamin K) compounds. *Cytokine* **1995**, *7*, 287–290. [CrossRef]
47. Varsha, M.K.; Thiagarajan, R.; Manikandan, R.; Dhanasekaran, G. Vitamin K1 alleviates streptozotocin-induced type 1 diabetes by mitigating free radical stress, as well as inhibiting NF-kappaB activation and iNOS expression in rat pancreas. *Nutrition* **2015**, *31*, 214–222. [CrossRef]

48. Shea, M.K.; Dallal, G.E.; Dawson-Hughes, B.; Ordovas, J.M.; O'Donnell, C.J.; Gundberg, C.M.; Peterson, J.W.; Booth, S.L. Vitamin K, circulating cytokines, and bone mineral density in older men and women. *Am. J. Clin. Nutr.* **2008**, *88*, 356–363. [CrossRef]
49. Shea, M.K.; Cushman, M.; Booth, S.L.; Burke, G.L.; Chen, H.; Kritchevsky, S.B. Associations between vitamin K status and haemostatic and inflammatory biomarkers in community-dwelling adults. The Multi-Ethnic Study of Atherosclerosis. *Thromb. Haemost.* **2014**, *112*, 438–444.
50. Wei, F.F.; Trenson, S.; Verhamme, P.; Vermeer, C.; Staessen, J.A. Vitamin K-Dependent Matrix Gla Protein as Multifaceted Protector of Vascular and Tissue Integrity. *Hypertension* **2019**, *73*, 1160–1169. [CrossRef]
51. Luo, G.; Ducy, P.; McKee, M.D.; Pinero, G.J.; Loyer, E.; Behringer, R.R.; Karsenty, G. Spontaneous calcification of arteries and cartilage in mice lacking matrix GLA protein. *Nature* **1997**, *386*, 78–81. [CrossRef] [PubMed]
52. Murshed, M.; Schinke, T.; McKee, M.D.; Karsenty, G. Extracellular matrix mineralization is regulated locally; different roles of two gla-containing proteins. *J. Cell Biol.* **2004**, *165*, 625–630. [CrossRef] [PubMed]
53. Mori, K.; Shioi, A.; Jono, S.; Nishizawa, Y.; Morii, H. Expression of matrix Gla protein (MGP) in an in vitro model of vascular calcification. *FEBS Lett.* **1998**, *433*, 19–22. [CrossRef]
54. Munroe, P.B.; Olgunturk, R.O.; Fryns, J.P.; Van Maldergem, L.; Ziereisen, F.; Yuksel, B.; Gardiner, R.M.; Chung, E. Mutations in the gene encoding the human matrix Gla protein cause Keutel syndrome. *Nat. Genet.* **1999**, *21*, 142–144. [CrossRef]
55. Hur, D.J.; Raymond, G.V.; Kahler, S.G.; Riegert-Johnson, D.L.; Cohen, B.A.; Boyadjiev, S.A. A novel MGP mutation in a consanguineous family: Review of the clinical and molecular characteristics of Keutel syndrome. *Am. J. Med. Genet. A* **2005**, *135*, 36–40. [CrossRef]
56. O'Young, J.; Liao, Y.; Xiao, Y.; Jalkanen, J.; Lajoie, G.; Karttunen, M.; Goldberg, H.A.; Hunter, G.K. Matrix Gla protein inhibits ectopic calcification by a direct interaction with hydroxyapatite crystals. *J. Am. Chem. Soc.* **2011**, *133*, 18406–18412. [CrossRef]
57. Wallin, R.; Cain, D.; Hutson, S.M.; Sane, D.C.; Loeser, R. Modulation of the binding of matrix Gla protein (MGP) to bone morphogenetic protein-2 (BMP-2). *Thromb. Haemost.* **2000**, *84*, 1039–1044.
58. Zebboudj, A.F.; Imura, M.; Bostrom, K. Matrix GLA protein, a regulatory protein for bone morphogenetic protein-2. *J. Biol. Chem.* **2002**, *277*, 4388–4394. [CrossRef]
59. Shanahan, C.M.; Cary, N.R.; Metcalfe, J.C.; Weissberg, P.L. High expression of genes for calcification-regulating proteins in human atherosclerotic plaques. *J. Clin. Investig.* **1994**, *93*, 2393–2402. [CrossRef]
60. Tyson, K.L.; Reynolds, J.L.; McNair, R.; Zhang, Q.; Weissberg, P.L.; Shanahan, C.M. Osteo/chondrocytic transcription factors and their target genes exhibit distinct patterns of expression in human arterial calcification. *Arterioscler. Thromb. Vasc. Biol.* **2003**, *23*, 489–494. [CrossRef]
61. Spronk, H.M.; Soute, B.A.; Schurgers, L.J.; Cleutjens, J.P.; Thijssen, H.H.; De Mey, J.G.; Vermeer, C. Matrix Gla protein accumulates at the border of regions of calcification and normal tissue in the media of the arterial vessel wall. *Biochem. Biophys. Res. Commun.* **2001**, *289*, 485–490. [CrossRef] [PubMed]
62. Engelse, M.A.; Neele, J.M.; Bronckers, A.L.; Pannekoek, H.; de Vries, C.J. Vascular calcification: Expression patterns of the osteoblast-specific gene core binding factor alpha-1 and the protective factor matrix gla protein in human atherogenesis. *Cardiovasc. Res.* **2001**, *52*, 281–289. [CrossRef]
63. Shioi, A.; Taniwaki, H.; Jono, S.; Okuno, Y.; Koyama, H.; Mori, K.; Nishizawa, Y. Monckeberg's medial sclerosis and inorganic phosphate in uremia. *Am. J. Kidney Dis.* **2001**, *38*, S47–S49. [CrossRef] [PubMed]
64. Wu, G.; Ma, Z.; Hu, W.; Wang, D.; Gong, B.; Fan, C.; Jiang, S.; Li, T.; Gao, J.; Yang, Y. Molecular insights of Gas6/TAM in cancer development and therapy. *Cell Death Dis.* **2017**, *8*, e2700. [CrossRef] [PubMed]
65. Son, B.K.; Kozaki, K.; Iijima, K.; Eto, M.; Nakano, T.; Akishita, M.; Ouchi, Y. Gas6/Axl-PI3K/Akt pathway plays a central role in the effect of statins on inorganic phosphate-induced calcification of vascular smooth muscle cells. *Eur. J. Pharmacol.* **2007**, *556*, 1–8. [CrossRef] [PubMed]
66. Qiu, C.; Zheng, H.; Tao, H.; Yu, W.; Jiang, X.; Li, A.; Jin, H.; Lv, A.; Li, H. Vitamin K2 inhibits rat vascular smooth muscle cell calcification by restoring the Gas6/Axl/Akt anti-apoptotic pathway. *Mol. Cell. Biochem.* **2017**, *433*, 149–159. [CrossRef]
67. Viegas, C.S.; Rafael, M.S.; Enriquez, J.L.; Teixeira, A.; Vitorino, R.; Luis, I.M.; Costa, R.M.; Santos, S.; Cavaco, S.; Neves, J.; et al. Gla-rich protein acts as a calcification inhibitor in the human cardiovascular system. *Arterioscler. Thromb. Vasc. Biol.* **2015**, *35*, 399–408. [CrossRef]

68. Willems, B.A.; Furmanik, M.; Caron, M.M.J.; Chatrou, M.L.L.; Kusters, D.H.M.; Welting, T.J.M.; Stock, M.; Rafael, M.S.; Viegas, C.S.B.; Simes, D.C.; et al. Ucma/GRP inhibits phosphate-induced vascular smooth muscle cell calcification via SMAD-dependent BMP signalling. *Sci. Rep.* **2018**, *8*, 4961. [CrossRef]
69. Wilmer, W.A.; Magro, C.M. Calciphylaxis: Emerging concepts in prevention, diagnosis, and treatment. *Semin. Dial.* **2002**, *15*, 172–186. [CrossRef]
70. Polonsky, T.S.; McClelland, R.L.; Jorgensen, N.W.; Bild, D.E.; Burke, G.L.; Guerci, A.D.; Greenland, P. Coronary artery calcium score and risk classification for coronary heart disease prediction. *JAMA* **2010**, *303*, 1610–1616. [CrossRef]
71. Greenland, P.; LaBree, L.; Azen, S.P.; Doherty, T.M.; Detrano, R.C. Coronary artery calcium score combined with Framingham score for risk prediction in asymptomatic individuals. *JAMA* **2004**, *291*, 210–215. [CrossRef] [PubMed]
72. Detrano, R.; Guerci, A.D.; Carr, J.J.; Bild, D.E.; Burke, G.; Folsom, A.R.; Liu, K.; Shea, S.; Szklo, M.; Bluemke, D.A.; et al. Coronary calcium as a predictor of coronary events in four racial or ethnic groups. *N. Engl. J. Med.* **2008**, *358*, 1336–1345. [CrossRef] [PubMed]
73. Shea, M.K.; Booth, S.L.; Weiner, D.E.; Brinkley, T.E.; Kanaya, A.M.; Murphy, R.A.; Simonsick, E.M.; Wassel, C.L.; Vermeer, C.; Kritchevsky, S.B. Circulating Vitamin K Is Inversely Associated with Incident Cardiovascular Disease Risk among Those Treated for Hypertension in the Health, Aging, and Body Composition Study (Health ABC). *J. Nutr.* **2017**, *147*, 888–895. [CrossRef] [PubMed]
74. Shea, M.K.; Holden, R.M. Vitamin K status and vascular calcification: Evidence from observational and clinical studies. *Adv. Nutr.* **2012**, *3*, 158–165. [CrossRef] [PubMed]
75. Villines, T.C.; Hatzigeorgiou, C.; Feuerstein, I.M.; O'Malley, P.G.; Taylor, A.J. Vitamin K1 intake and coronary calcification. *Coron. Artery Dis.* **2005**, *16*, 199–203. [CrossRef] [PubMed]
76. Shea, M.K.; Booth, S.L.; Miller, M.E.; Burke, G.L.; Chen, H.; Cushman, M.; Tracy, R.P.; Kritchevsky, S.B. Association between circulating vitamin K1 and coronary calcium progression in community-dwelling adults: The Multi-Ethnic Study of Atherosclerosis. *Am. J. Clin. Nutr.* **2013**, *98*, 197–208. [CrossRef] [PubMed]
77. Beulens, J.W.; Bots, M.L.; Atsma, F.; Bartelink, M.L.; Prokop, M.; Geleijnse, J.M.; Witteman, J.C.; Grobbee, D.E.; van der Schouw, Y.T. High dietary menaquinone intake is associated with reduced coronary calcification. *Atherosclerosis* **2009**, *203*, 489–493. [CrossRef]
78. Torii, S.; Ikari, Y.; Tanabe, K.; Kakuta, T.; Hatori, M.; Shioi, A.; Okano, T. Plasma phylloquinone, menaquinone-4 and menaquinone-7 levels and coronary artery calcification. *J. Nutr. Sci.* **2016**, *5*, e48. [CrossRef]
79. Cranenburg, E.C.; Brandenburg, V.M.; Vermeer, C.; Stenger, M.; Muhlenbruch, G.; Mahnken, A.H.; Gladziwa, U.; Ketteler, M.; Schurgers, L.J. Uncarboxylated matrix Gla protein (ucMGP) is associated with coronary artery calcification in haemodialysis patients. *Thromb. Haemost.* **2009**, *101*, 359–366.
80. Shea, M.K.; O'Donnell, C.J.; Hoffmann, U.; Dallal, G.E.; Dawson-Hughes, B.; Ordovas, J.M.; Price, P.A.; Williamson, M.K.; Booth, S.L. Vitamin K supplementation and progression of coronary artery calcium in older men and women. *Am. J. Clin. Nutr.* **2009**, *89*, 1799–1807. [CrossRef]
81. Kurnatowska, I.; Grzelak, P.; Masajtis-Zagajewska, A.; Kaczmarska, M.; Stefanczyk, L.; Vermeer, C.; Maresz, K.; Nowicki, M. Effect of vitamin K2 on progression of atherosclerosis and vascular calcification in nondialyzed patients with chronic kidney disease stages 3–5. *Pol. Arch. Med. Wewn.* **2015**, *125*, 631–640. [CrossRef] [PubMed]
82. Ikari, Y.; Torii, S.; Shioi, A.; Okano, T. Impact of menaquinone-4 supplementation on coronary artery calcification and arterial stiffness: An open label single arm study. *Nutr. J.* **2016**, *15*, 53. [CrossRef] [PubMed]
83. Zwakenberg, S.R.; de Jong, P.A.; Bartstra, J.W.; van Asperen, R.; Westerink, J.; de Valk, H.; Slart, R.; Luurtsema, G.; Wolterink, J.M.; de Borst, G.J.; et al. The effect of menaquinone-7 supplementation on vascular calcification in patients with diabetes: A randomized, double-blind, placebo-controlled trial. *Am. J. Clin. Nutr.* **2019**, *110*, 883–890. [CrossRef] [PubMed]
84. Krueger, T.; Schlieper, G.; Schurgers, L.; Cornelis, T.; Cozzolino, M.; Jacobi, J.; Jadoul, M.; Ketteler, M.; Rump, L.C.; Stenvinkel, P.; et al. Vitamin K1 to slow vascular calcification in haemodialysis patients (VitaVasK trial): A rationale and study protocol. *Nephrol. Dial. Transplant.* **2014**, *29*, 1633–1638. [CrossRef] [PubMed]
85. Holden, R.M.; Booth, S.L.; Day, A.G.; Clase, C.M.; Zimmerman, D.; Moist, L.; Shea, M.K.; McCabe, K.M.; Jamal, S.A.; Tobe, S.; et al. Inhibiting the progression of arterial calcification with vitamin K in HemoDialysis patients (iPACK-HD) trial: Rationale and study design for a randomized trial of vitamin K in patients with end stage kidney disease. *Can. J. Kidney Health Dis.* **2015**, *2*, 17. [CrossRef] [PubMed]

86. Vossen, L.M.; Schurgers, L.J.; van Varik, B.J.; Kietselaer, B.L.; Vermeer, C.; Meeder, J.G.; Rahel, B.M.; van Cauteren, Y.J.; Hoffland, G.A.; Rennenberg, R.J.; et al. Menaquinone-7 Supplementation to Reduce Vascular Calcification in Patients with Coronary Artery Disease: Rationale and Study Protocol (VitaK-CAC Trial). *Nutrients* **2015**, *7*, 8905–8915. [CrossRef]
87. Chen, X.; Jin, D.Y.; Stafford, D.W.; Tie, J.K. Evaluation of oral anticoagulants with vitamin K epoxide reductase in its native milieu. *Blood* **2018**, *132*, 1974–1984. [CrossRef]
88. Palaniswamy, C.; Sekhri, A.; Aronow, W.S.; Kalra, A.; Peterson, S.J. Association of warfarin use with valvular and vascular calcification: A review. *Clin. Cardiol.* **2011**, *34*, 74–81. [CrossRef]
89. Schurgers, L.J.; Spronk, H.M.; Skepper, J.N.; Hackeng, T.M.; Shanahan, C.M.; Vermeer, C.; Weissberg, P.L.; Proudfoot, D. Post-translational modifications regulate matrix Gla protein function: Importance for inhibition of vascular smooth muscle cell calcification. *J. Thromb. Haemost.* **2007**, *5*, 2503–2511. [CrossRef]
90. Price, P.A.; Faus, S.A.; Williamson, M.K. Warfarin causes rapid calcification of the elastic lamellae in rat arteries and heart valves. *Arterioscler. Thromb. Vasc. Biol.* **1998**, *18*, 1400–1407. [CrossRef]
91. Schurgers, L.J.; Joosen, I.A.; Laufer, E.M.; Chatrou, M.L.; Herfs, M.; Winkens, M.H.; Westenfeld, R.; Veulemans, V.; Krueger, T.; Shanahan, C.M.; et al. Vitamin K-antagonists accelerate atherosclerotic calcification and induce a vulnerable plaque phenotype. *PLoS ONE* **2012**, *7*, e43229. [CrossRef] [PubMed]
92. Schurgers, L.J.; Spronk, H.M.; Soute, B.A.; Schiffers, P.M.; DeMey, J.G.; Vermeer, C. Regression of warfarin-induced medial elastocalcinosis by high intake of vitamin K in rats. *Blood* **2007**, *109*, 2823–2831. [CrossRef] [PubMed]
93. Peeters, F.; Dudink, E.; Kimenai, D.M.; Weijs, B.; Altintas, S.; Heckman, L.I.B.; Mihl, C.; Schurgers, L.J.; Wildberger, J.E.; Meex, S.J.R.; et al. Vitamin K Antagonists, Non-Vitamin K Antagonist Oral Anticoagulants, and Vascular Calcification in Patients with Atrial Fibrillation. *TH Open* **2018**, *2*, e391–e398. [CrossRef] [PubMed]
94. Han, K.H.; O'Neill, W.C. Increased Peripheral Arterial Calcification in Patients Receiving Warfarin. *J. Am. Heart Assoc.* **2016**, *5*, e002665. [CrossRef]
95. Tantisattamo, E.; Han, K.H.; O'Neill, W.C. Increased vascular calcification in patients receiving warfarin. *Arterioscler. Thromb. Vasc. Biol.* **2015**, *35*, 237–242. [CrossRef]
96. Unlu, S.; Sahinarslan, A.; Kilic, H.K.; Gokalp, G.; Sezenoz, B.; Erbas, G.; Yalcin, R.M.; Arac, M. Long-term vitamin-K antagonist use and coronary artery calcification. *Herz* **2018**. [CrossRef]
97. Andrews, J.; Psaltis, P.J.; Bayturan, O.; Shao, M.; Stegman, B.; Elshazly, M.; Kapadia, S.R.; Tuzcu, E.M.; Nissen, S.E.; Nicholls, S.J.; et al. Warfarin Use Is Associated with Progressive Coronary Arterial Calcification: Insights From Serial Intravascular Ultrasound. *JACC Cardiovasc. Imaging.* **2018**, *11*, 1315–1323. [CrossRef]
98. Cranenburg, E.C.; Koos, R.; Schurgers, L.J.; Magdeleyns, E.J.; Schoonbrood, T.H.; Landewe, R.B.; Brandenburg, V.M.; Bekers, O.; Vermeer, C. Characterisation and potential diagnostic value of circulating matrix Gla protein (MGP) species. *Thromb. Haemost.* **2010**, *104*, 811–822. [CrossRef]
99. Dalmeijer, G.W.; van der Schouw, Y.T.; Magdeleyns, E.; Ahmed, N.; Vermeer, C.; Beulens, J.W. The effect of menaquinone-7 supplementation on circulating species of matrix Gla protein. *Atherosclerosis* **2012**, *225*, 397–402. [CrossRef]
100. Knapen, M.H.; Braam, L.A.; Drummen, N.E.; Bekers, O.; Hoeks, A.P.; Vermeer, C. Menaquinone-7 supplementation improves arterial stiffness in healthy postmenopausal women. A double-blind randomised clinical trial. *Thromb. Haemost.* **2015**, *113*, 1135–1144. [CrossRef]
101. Caluwe, R.; Vandecasteele, S.; Van Vlem, B.; Vermeer, C.; De Vriese, A.S. Vitamin K2 supplementation in haemodialysis patients: A randomized dose-finding study. *Nephrol. Dial. Transplant.* **2014**, *29*, 1385–1390. [CrossRef] [PubMed]
102. Shea, M.K.; O'Donnell, C.J.; Vermeer, C.; Magdeleyns, E.J.; Crosier, M.D.; Gundberg, C.M.; Ordovas, J.M.; Kritchevsky, S.B.; Booth, S.L. Circulating uncarboxylated matrix gla protein is associated with vitamin K nutritional status, but not coronary artery calcium, in older adults. *J. Nutr.* **2011**, *141*, 1529–1534. [CrossRef] [PubMed]
103. Jono, S.; Ikari, Y.; Vermeer, C.; Dissel, P.; Hasegawa, K.; Shioi, A.; Taniwaki, H.; Kizu, A.; Nishizawa, Y.; Saito, S. Matrix Gla protein is associated with coronary artery calcification as assessed by electron-beam computed tomography. *Thromb. Haemost.* **2004**, *91*, 790–794. [PubMed]

104. Dalmeijer, G.W.; van der Schouw, Y.T.; Vermeer, C.; Magdeleyns, E.J.; Schurgers, L.J.; Beulens, J.W. Circulating matrix Gla protein is associated with coronary artery calcification and vitamin K status in healthy women. *J. Nutr. Biochem.* **2013**, *24*, 624–628. [CrossRef]
105. Meuwese, C.L.; Olauson, H.; Qureshi, A.R.; Ripsweden, J.; Barany, P.; Vermeer, C.; Drummen, N.; Stenvinkel, P. Associations between Thyroid Hormones, Calcification Inhibitor Levels and Vascular Calcification in End-Stage Renal Disease. *PLoS ONE* **2015**, *10*, e0132353. [CrossRef]
106. Dalmeijer, G.W.; van der Schouw, Y.T.; Magdeleyns, E.J.; Vermeer, C.; Elias, S.G.; Velthuis, B.K.; de Jong, P.A.; Beulens, J.W. Circulating species of matrix Gla protein and the risk of vascular calcification in healthy women. *Int. J. Cardiol.* **2013**, *168*, e168–e170. [CrossRef]
107. Liabeuf, S.; Bourron, O.; Olivier, B.; Vemeer, C.; Theuwissen, E.; Magdeleyns, E.; Aubert, C.E.; Brazier, M.; Mentaverri, R.; Hartemann, A.; et al. Vascular calcification in patients with type 2 diabetes: The involvement of matrix Gla protein. *Cardiovasc. Diabetol.* **2014**, *13*, 85. [CrossRef]
108. Schurgers, L.J.; Barreto, D.V.; Barreto, F.C.; Liabeuf, S.; Renard, C.; Magdeleyns, E.J.; Vermeer, C.; Choukroun, G.; Massy, Z.A. The circulating inactive form of matrix gla protein is a surrogate marker for vascular calcification in chronic kidney disease: A preliminary report. *Clin. J. Am. Soc. Nephrol.* **2010**, *5*, 568–575. [CrossRef]
109. Delanaye, P.; Krzesinski, J.M.; Warling, X.; Moonen, M.; Smelten, N.; Medart, L.; Pottel, H.; Cavalier, E. Dephosphorylated-uncarboxylated Matrix Gla protein concentration is predictive of vitamin K status and is correlated with vascular calcification in a cohort of hemodialysis patients. *BMC Nephrol.* **2014**, *15*, 145. [CrossRef]
110. Dalmeijer, G.W.; van der Schouw, Y.T.; Magdeleyns, E.J.; Vermeer, C.; Verschuren, W.M.; Boer, J.M.; Beulens, J.W. Matrix Gla protein species and risk of cardiovascular events in type 2 diabetic patients. *Diabetes Care* **2013**, *36*, 3766–3771. [CrossRef]
111. van den Heuvel, E.G.; van Schoor, N.M.; Lips, P.; Magdeleyns, E.J.; Deeg, D.J.; Vermeer, C.; den Heijer, M. Circulating uncarboxylated matrix Gla protein, a marker of vitamin K status, as a risk factor of cardiovascular disease. *Maturitas* **2014**, *77*, 137–141. [CrossRef] [PubMed]
112. Dalmeijer, G.W.; van der Schouw, Y.T.; Magdeleyns, E.J.; Vermeer, C.; Verschuren, W.M.; Boer, J.M.; Beulens, J.W. Circulating desphospho-uncarboxylated matrix gamma-carboxyglutamate protein and the risk of coronary heart disease and stroke. *J. Thromb. Haemost.* **2014**, *12*, 1028–1034. [CrossRef] [PubMed]
113. Keyzer, C.A.; Vermeer, C.; Joosten, M.M.; Knapen, M.H.; Drummen, N.E.; Navis, G.; Bakker, S.J.; de Borst, M.H. Vitamin K status and mortality after kidney transplantation: A cohort study. *Am. J. Kidney Dis.* **2015**, *65*, 474–483. [CrossRef] [PubMed]
114. Mayer, O., Jr.; Seidlerova, J.; Vanek, J.; Karnosova, P.; Bruthans, J.; Filipovsky, J.; Wohlfahrt, P.; Cifkova, R.; Windrichova, J.; Knapen, M.H.; et al. The abnormal status of uncarboxylated matrix Gla protein species represents an additional mortality risk in heart failure patients with vascular disease. *Int. J. Cardiol.* **2016**, *203*, 916–922. [CrossRef]
115. Liu, Y.P.; Gu, Y.M.; Thijs, L.; Knapen, M.H.; Salvi, E.; Citterio, L.; Petit, T.; Carpini, S.D.; Zhang, Z.; Jacobs, L.; et al. Inactive matrix Gla protein is causally related to adverse health outcomes: A Mendelian randomization study in a Flemish population. *Hypertension* **2015**, *65*, 463–470. [CrossRef]
116. Mayer, O., Jr.; Seidlerova, J.; Bruthans, J.; Filipovsky, J.; Timoracka, K.; Vanek, J.; Cerna, L.; Wohlfahrt, P.; Cifkova, R.; Theuwissen, E.; et al. Desphospho-uncarboxylated matrix Gla-protein is associated with mortality risk in patients with chronic stable vascular disease. *Atherosclerosis* **2014**, *235*, 162–168. [CrossRef]

6

Drug Delivery Systems for Vitamin D Supplementation and Therapy

Eliza Glowka *, Joanna Stasiak and Janina Lulek

Department of Pharmaceutical Technology, Poznan University of Medical Sciences, 6 Grunwaldzka Street, 60-780 Poznan, Poland
* Correspondence: eglowka@ump.edu.pl

Abstract: Vitamin D (VD) is a fat-soluble prohormone well known for its role in regulating calcium and phosphate metabolism. It has been clinically used for many years to prevent rickets in children, osteomalacia, and osteoporosis in adults. VD insufficiency is a common medical condition, and many supplements are available in the market in order to increase serum 25-hydroxy VD levels to recommended amounts. Over the course of the last decades, it has become increasingly clear that calcitriol, an active form of VD, regulates multiple cellular processes with effects on normal and malignant cell growth and differentiation, and on the immune and cardiovascular function. Increasing evidence supports the role of the VD system in cancer prevention and therapy. Due to many pleiotropic and beneficial effects in extra-skeletal disorders, VD has gained potential and become an interesting active for encapsulation into drug delivery systems. The purpose of this review is to present the diversity of drug delivery systems that have been reported for VD or VD derivatives in an orderly manner across the following categories: Oral administration, application on the skin, cancer prevention/therapy, and other diseases or routes of administration.

Keywords: vitamin D; cholecalciferol; drug delivery systems; targeted delivery; nanoparticles; food fortification; cancer

---

1. Introduction

Vitamin D (VD) is one of the lipophilic vitamins. The most important forms of VD are cholecalciferol (vitamin D3, VD3) and ergocalciferol (vitamin D2, VD2) (Figure 1). VD3 is the main form and is available in some natural dietary products (egg yolk, flesh of fatty fish, and fish liver oils), food fortified with VD, and many forms of dietary supplements. VD2 is of plant origin and present in low amounts, e.g., in some mushrooms. VD2, being less potent than VD3, is rarely present in commercial preparations and fortified food. Despite that, it is a good alternative for vegans and vegetarians. However, the main source of VD is endogenous synthesis from 7-dehydrocholesterol in the human skin after sun exposure. Part of VD is stored in adipose and muscle tissue, and part of it gets hydroxylated. Independent of the source, VD3 and VD2 act as hormone precursors since they require two stages of metabolism: First to 25-hydroxy VD (25(OH)D, calcidiol) in the liver; then to 1α,25-dihydroxy VD (1,25(OH)D, calcitriol) in the kidney [1]. 25(OH)D3 is significantly less active than calcitriol and is transported in the circulation by binding to VD binding proteins. The amount of circulating 25(OH)D3 is the most reliable measurement and is thought to reflect body VD status best. The chemical structures of the vitamin and its active derivatives are presented in Figure 1, whereas the fate of VD in the body is presented in Figure 2.

It is considered that most people are insufficient or deficient in VD due to a lack of sun exposure, extensive use of sunscreens, which block VD synthesis, and poor dietary intake. Maintaining recommended serum levels, i.e., 30–60 ng/mL of 25(OH)D3, can be achieved through vitamin supplementation or food fortification without changing lifestyle to avoid impaired skeletal and overall health [2].

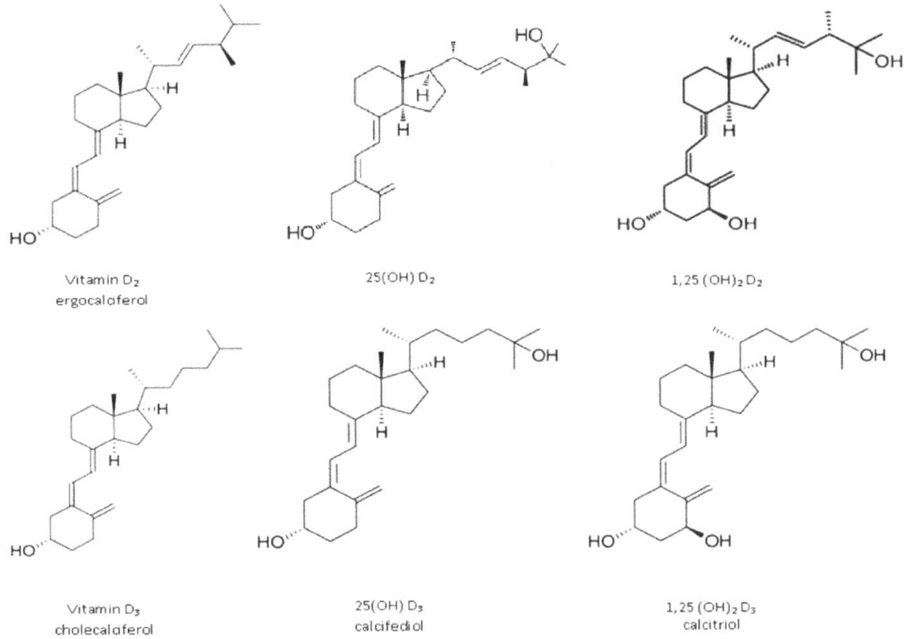

Figure 1. The chemical structure of ergocalciferol, cholecalciferol, and their active derivatives.

Nowadays, a lot is known and written about the mechanism of action and the beneficial effects of VD on the human body [1,3,4]. Similar to other steroid hormones, the active form of VD binds to a nuclear receptor (VDR, vitamin D receptor) and modulates gene expression. As the VDR is present in most cells in the body and calcitriol directly or indirectly regulates as much as 3–5% of the human genome, VD activity is widespread, and it exerts actions that can limit the progression of multiple diseases [5]. One of the most important functions of VD is to maintain skeletal calcium and phosphate balance, and VD deficiency can result in lower mineral density. For this reason, VD has been used in order to prevent or treat rickets in children, osteomalacia, osteoporosis, bone fractures, and secondary hyperparathyroidism in adults. There is also evidence that VD can prevent or has beneficial effects in many other diseases such as malignancies, diabetes, and cardiovascular or autoimmune diseases [3]. A few drugs with VD-like activity (VD analogues), with more or less pronounced calcemic action (e.g., calcifediol, alfacalcidiol, paricalcitol, calcitriol, eldecalcitol), are also clinically available and used topically to treat psoriasis due to the regulation of keratinocytes proliferation, differentiation, and apoptosis [6].

Nowadays, the use of VD or VD analogues in prophylaxis or in the therapy of many beyond-skeletal diseases seems to be very interesting, especially for possible use in cancer treatment [7–9]. In such a case, the calcemic activity becomes undesirable and targeting delivery to cancer cells could be expected. However, anti-proliferative activity is associated with high concentrations of calcitriol at which hypercalcemia may be induced due to the action of calcitriol in stimulating intestinal calcium absorption. Additionally, the activity of the hormone is self-regulated as it simultaneously induces its inactivation [5]. To overcome these barriers, several analogues of calcitriol with lower calcemic activities that activate the target receptor have been synthesised [10–12]. The analogues should be selective and should have increased pro-differentiating and anti-proliferative properties. Therefore, it is necessary to characterize new VD analogues fully. Some of the analogues have undergone evaluation in preclinical or clinical trials for potential anticancer activity [11]. It is worth paying attention to seocalcitol (EB 1089), which is one of the potential analogues. Seocalcitol is 50–200 times more potent than calcitriol concerning regulation of cell growth and differentiation in vitro as well as in vivo. It has reduced calcemic activity in vivo compared to that of calcitriol, but a lower binding affinity for the VDR [13].

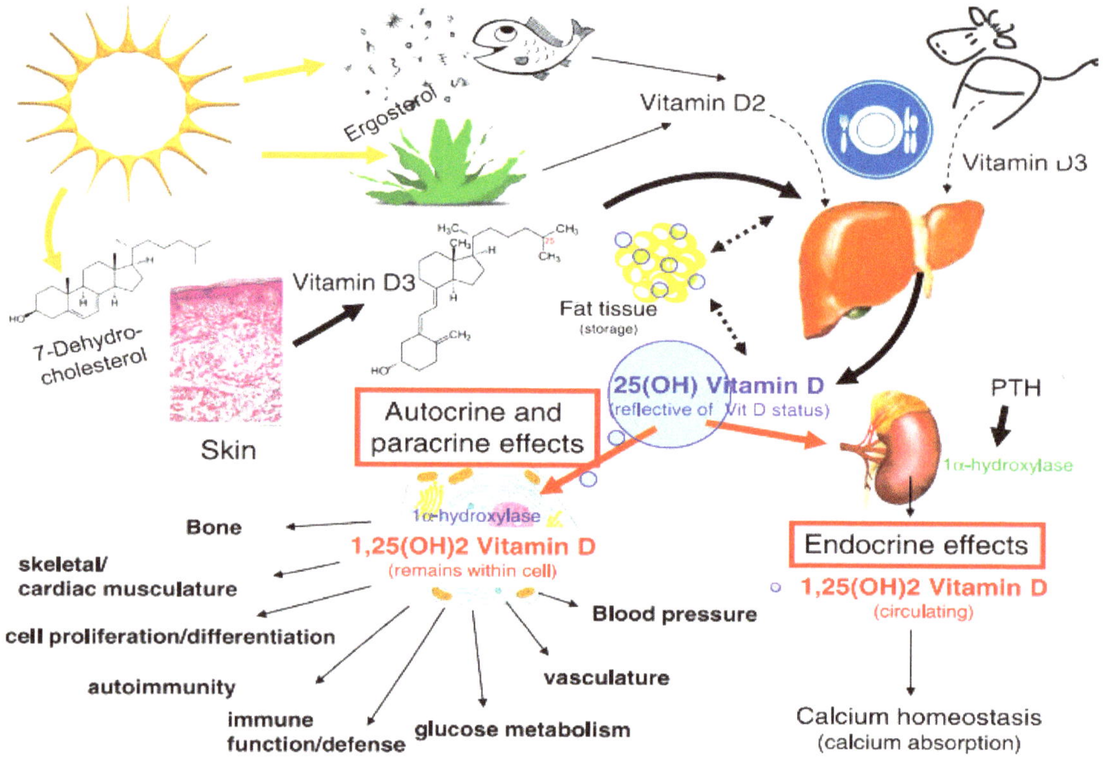

Figure 2. Scheme of vitamin D sources, fate in the body, and pleiotropic actions of 1,25-dihydroxy vitamin D (calcitriol), the active form of vitamin D. Reproduced with permission from [14]; published by Elsevier, 2011.

Many attempts have been made to harness some drug delivery systems (DDS) to deliver VD or VD analogues for skeletal or non-skeletal effects. A drug delivery system is defined as a formulation or a device that enables the introduction of a therapeutic substance into the body and improves its efficacy and safety by controlling the rate, time, and place of drug release. Ideal DDS should increase the bioavailability of the drug, provide for controlled or sustained drug delivery, and transport the drug intact to the site of action, while avoiding the non-diseased host tissues. The product should be safe and reliable, cost effective, stable, easy to administer to the patients, and drug delivery should be maintained under various physiological variables [15]. Meeting all these requirements at the same time is often impossible and not always necessary. The development of DDS has been going on for a few decades (starting from the discovery of liposomes in the 1960s) and this advanced drug delivery is promising much in the treatment of disease, with superior control of delivery and action over conventional formulations. However, development of such a delivery system with zero-order release kinetics, suitable stability, and ease of scaling up is a difficult task. Therefore, the vast majority of potential applications of DDS remain at the initial research stage.

Nowadays, the diversity of DDS is enormous, including nano- and microparticulate DDS that may be composed of a range of materials such as polymers, lipids, surfactants, and inorganic or hybrid materials [15–17]. The structure of the selected DDS is shown in Figure 3.

The recent increase in VD interest by the general public has fuelled a big rise in sales of over-the-counter VD preparations. Additionally, products with progressively increasing content of VD have been introduced with similar rapidity. Many types of pharmaceutical preparations for VD supplementation are commercially available, including oily drops, capsules, and tablets. At the same time, considering the potential use of VD and its analogues in the therapy of various diseases, they have become interesting candidates for encapsulation into DDS. This review of the published literature was conducted to present various types of delivery systems loaded with VD or VD-related compounds across the following categories: Oral administration (food fortification), application on the skin, cancer prevention/treatment, and finally other diseases or routes of administration.

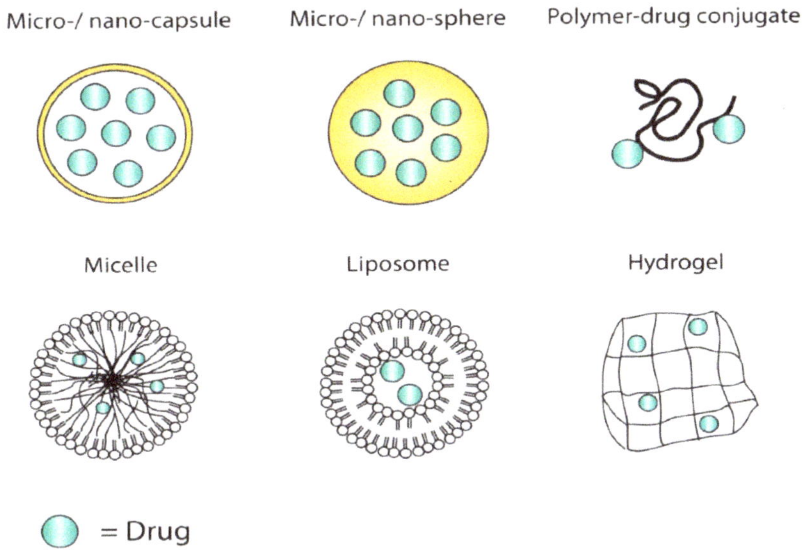

Figure 3. Different structures of drug delivery systems (not-exhaustive). Each structure has its advantages and disadvantages to incorporate and release different types of drugs. Reproduced with permission from [18]; published by MDPI, 2014.

2. Drug Delivery Systems for Oral Administration (Food Fortification)

Most dietary products are a poor source of VD, including breast milk. VD is minimally found in fat-free and low-fat dairy products, which are in growing demand. VD intake is found to be very low in vegetarians and vegans. The high phytate and fiber content of vegetarian diets may also reduce VD absorption [19]. Since VD insufficiency is a widespread public health problem, functional food fortified with this vitamin during processing has received increasing attention in recent years. While the use of oral VD supplements is a low-cost and practical method to treat deficiency, clinical advancements in VD oral administration are limited by its lipophilic character, low solubility in gastrointestinal fluid, and, thus, low bioavailability. Moreover, the facile degradation of VD by light, air, and heat should also be considered during manufacturing, storage, and use. In a moderate climate, VD supplementation should take place every day for most of the year. Thus, patient compliance could be low. Thereby, there is a need to develop new formulations of VD, especially those with prolonged release. In this context, the everyday consumption of foods enriched with VD seems to be a simpler and cheaper alternative.

In the gastrointestinal tract, after release from the food matrix or supplements, VD is included in micelles made by bile acids and enters the enterocytes via passive diffusion through an unsaturable mechanism [20]. Oral VD absorption requires three trans-membrane proteins that primarily function as cholesterol transporters in the intestine. Afterwards, it is included in chylomicrons and is then activated by the liver and kidneys. The absorption is blocked when there are not enough lipids in the intestine [19]. To improve VD bioavailability, it is important to enhance the water solubility [21]. Grossmann and Tangpricha (2010) reviewed a few studies that examined the effect of oil, cellulose, lactose, and ethanol vehicles on VD bioavailability from supplements. It was identified that VD in an oil vehicle has better oral bioavailability and produces a greater 25(OH)D response than VD in a powder (lactose or cellulose based) or an ethanol vehicle in healthy subjects [22]. However, a recent clinical trial concluded that oily drops (peanut oil) and capsules in lactose excipient, both containing VD, were bioequivalent [23].

2.1. Delivery Systems from a Food Processing Point of View

While the encapsulation of bioactive compounds in food products using nano/microparticulate systems is not a new concept [24], fortification of foods or beverages with VD still represents a big challenge for several reasons, including (i) high hydrophobicity that prevents direct dispersion of the vitamin in an aqueous food matrix, (ii) chemical degradation of VD leading to the reduction of functionality and bioavailability, and (iii) variable oral bioavailability [19,25,26]. In the vitamin structure (Figure 1), there are double bonds sensitive to oxidation. As mentioned earlier, light, oxygen, and high temperature induce vitamin isomerization and degradation into its inactive forms [22]. All these obstacles should be overcome to develop an efficient and inexpensive technology. Encapsulation into colloidal delivery systems could be a good solution, as it can either protect the vitamin against harmful conditions or make the vitamin soluble in aqueous systems. Various submicron-sized delivery systems are in particular interest. Over past years the popularity of nanotechnology in the food sector is increasing.

On the basis of the literature search, it is evident that most delivery systems for VD have been developed for potential application in the food industry. In the field of food technology, VD is often considered as a model nutraceutical, as it has more than nutritional value on health. The term "nutraceutical" simply combines the words "nutrition" and "pharmaceutical"; however, up to today, there is no official definition distinct from, e.g., dietary supplements. The importance of nanotechnology in food processing can be evaluated by considering its role in the improvement of food product quality in terms of food texture, appearance, taste, nutritional value of the food, and food shelf-life [27]. Colloidal systems such as micelles, liposomes, nanoemulsions, and solid nanoparticles have found numerous applications as delivery vehicles for active pharmaceutical ingredients. Their use as vehicles for functional food ingredients is relatively new in the food industry, and it is especially promising to improve the bioavailability of poorly soluble substances such as functional lipids (e.g., carotenoids, phytosterols, polyunsaturated fatty acids, fat-soluble vitamins) and natural antioxidants [21].

One of the main aspects of nutraceutical encapsulation is the selection of safe material for encapsulation and procedure, preferably without using toxic solvents. Several new methods and materials that are safe to be used in the food industry have been developed from natural materials for nanoparticle production [28]. Delivery systems are commonly classified according to the main building blocks, which are necessarily GRAS (generally recognized as safe) food materials, preferably natural, and ideally-endogenous components of the product, thereby shortening the ingredient list and minimizing changes to the product sensory attributes, for higher consumer satisfaction.

There are four main groups of delivery systems in food: Protein-based, carbohydrate-based, lipid-based, and mixed systems. Due to the negative health implications of high-fat consumption, there is a need for enriching low-fat and non-fat food and drinks with health-promoting oil-soluble bioactives, preferably using non-lipid, amphiphilic delivery systems [29]. It is obvious that delivery systems for such food application must be fabricated entirely from food-grade ingredients using economically viable processing operations and should provide suitable release of the nutraceuticals and their physical and chemical stability over the range of environmental conditions (e.g., temperature fluctuations, light, oxygen, and mechanical forces) that food and beverage products are usually exposed to during their manufacture, storage, and utilization. Additionally, the delivery system should not adversely influence the physicochemical or sensory properties of the food or beverage product that it is incorporated into, e.g., appearance, texture, or flavor [30].

According to the recommendations, the average daily requirement for VD for an adult is 1000–2000 international units (IU) [4]. This vitamin is a good candidate for encapsulation into drug delivery systems due to high activity (1 IU is equal to 0.025 μg), the relatively low daily requirement (25–50 μg/day), and high lipophilicity. Besides, most carriers are lipophilic in nature and generally the more lipophilic the active, the better encapsulation efficiency, and the lower the undesirable release. While the encapsulation of VD has been reported since 1993 [31], many disadvantages still exist, inhibiting further application and industrialization of VD supplementation or food fortification.

For instance, encapsulation technology may involve the use of high temperature during the preparation, which would cause loss of VD activity, or the use of toxic solvents, which would pose potential side effects to final products due to residues of these solvents. Other disadvantages may include low loading capacity and incomplete encapsulation due to adsorption on the carrier surface resulting in little protection against UV exposure [32]. Lack of long-term stability of some delivery systems is also a serious technological problem. It should be mentioned that food and beverage products vary in their pH, ionic composition, ingredient interactions, storage conditions, and preparation procedures. Consequently, it will be important to test the stability of both the vitamin and the delivery system under the precise conditions under which they will be utilized in food products [26].

2.2. *Types of Vitamin D Delivery Systems for Food Fortification*

Various types of delivery systems developed mainly over the last ten years for VD food fortification are described below or presented in Table 1. It was noticed that emulsions/nanoemulsions and nanoparticles are predominant types of vehicles for VD encapsulation. One of the most convenient means to incorporate lipophilic active components into aqueous media, so that they are suitable for utilization within food and beverage products, is to encapsulate them within colloidal lipid-based delivery systems. Such carriers may enhance VD bioaccessibility by forming mixed micelles in the small intestine that can solubilize and transport it [33].

There is increasing interest in the utilization of nanoemulsions in the food industry. Nanoemulsions are colloidal dispersions comprising two immiscible liquids with droplet sizes of the internal phase between 20 and 200 nm and are expected to improve oral bioavailability of poorly water-soluble drugs. Reducing droplet size in emulsion-based delivery systems has several consequences that may be beneficial for certain food applications: (i) Greater stability to droplet aggregation, and gravitational separation; (ii) higher optical clarity; and (iii) increased oral bioavailability. In particular, nanoemulsions may be particularly useful for encapsulating lipophilic nutraceuticals into aqueous-based food products that should be optically clear, such as fortified waters, soft drinks, or juices [26]. Additionally, nanoemulsions can be produced with natural food ingredients using simple production methods. Studies have shown that nanoemulsion composition effects lipid digestion and bioavailability so that the nature of the carrier oil is of great importance [34].

The most common technique used for the production of emulsion-type delivery systems is high-pressure homogenization. However, Guttoff et al. (2015) [26] proposed a spontaneous emulsification method that is simple and inexpensive to carry out, and therefore has great potential for forming nanoemulsion-based delivery systems for food, personal care, and pharmaceutical applications. Nevertheless, the method needs a higher surfactant concentration and may be less applicable to large-scale industrial processes [26].

An interesting approach has been taken by Salvia-Trujillo et al. (2017) [33]. They produced three VD2-enriched O/W emulsions with different particle size distributions (D4,3 values of 0.112, 0.53, and 14.5 μm) using different homogenization methods. To assess VD2 bioaccessibility (the fraction that is solubilized within the mixed micelle phase after lipid digestion), both an in-vitro gastrointestinal tract model consisting of mouth, stomach, and small intestine phases and in-vivo studies in rats were conducted. The in-vitro studies showed that smaller lipid droplets were digested more rapidly than larger ones and highest VD2 bioaccessibility was observed for the emulsions containing the smallest droplets. In contrast, the in-vivo rat feeding studies demonstrated that the absorption of VD2 was the highest for the emulsions containing the largest droplets [33].

Another of the most studied types of delivery systems for VD encapsulation is nanoparticles. Nanoencapsulation of nutraceuticals may be primarily used for better absorption, better stability, or sustained or even targeted delivery without affecting color or taste of food. Nanoparticles can be dispersed homogeneously and uniformly in the food system. They have more suitable properties compared to microstructures and can provide better bioavailability. There is a great number of synthetic polymers, biopolymers, and lipids available for the pharmaceutical, cosmetic, and food industries that may be used for the production of nanoparticles. However, only inexpensive food materials and technologies have the potential for commercialization. Abbasi et al. (2015) proposed whey protein isolate, which is a by-product of the dairy industry produced vastly in the world. Whey protein isolates have good nutritional and functional properties and can entrap hydrophobic compounds successfully. Furthermore, they can be digested and release their contents easily. Nanoparticles of whey protein isolate could entrap VD3 and delay its degradation in the presence of oxygen [28].

It is worth mentioning studies reported by researchers who prepared nanoparticles from hydrophobic alginate derivative (oleoyl alginate ester, OAE) loaded with VD3. They proved that such nanoparticles released in a sustained way in simulated gastric and intestinal fluid [21]. Next, they visualized the internalization of fluorescent VD3-loaded OAE nanoparticles by Caco-2 cells. Incorporation into OAE nanoparticles resulted in increased absorption of VD3 in mice. In in-vivo studies in rats with nutritionally induced VD-deficiency rickets, encapsulated VD3 had better efficacy than that of the VD3-free drug. Their studies provided evidence that OAE nanoparticles were valuable as nutraceutical delivery vehicles to enhance the absorption of VD3 [35].

Table 1. Examples of various types of delivery systems reported for vitamin D encapsulation for potential use in food and beverage fortification (VD2—vitamin D2, VD3—vitamin D3, MCT—medium chain triglycerides).

Delivery System	Active	Main Components	Technique/Method	Reference
O/W emulsions and microemulsions	VD2 VD3	Oil phase: Soybean oil, olive oil, or MCT; water phase containing Tween 20 or sodium cholate	Microchannel emulsification	[19]
	VD2 VD3	Oil phase: Soybean oil, olive oil, or MCT; water phase containing Tween 20	Rotor-stator and high-pressure homogenization	[36]
	VD3	Oil phase: MCT; water phase containing Tween 20, 60, or 80	High-speed blender and high-pressure homogenization	[30]
	VD2	Oil phase: Soybean oil; water phase containing modified lecithin, sodium caseinate, or decaglycerol monooleate	Rotor-stator and high-pressure homogenization	[37]
O/W nanoemulsions	VD3	Oil phase: MCT, corn oil, fish oil, mineral oil, or orange oil; water phase containing a natural surfactant	High-speed blender and high-pressure homogenization	[34]
	VD3	Oil phase: Fish oil; water phase containing Tween 20	Ultrasonication	[38]
Biopolymer-based nanoparticles	VD3	Zein nanoparticles coated with carboxymethyl chitosan	Phase separation method and coating by cross-linking with calcium	[32]
	VD2	Beta-lactoglobulin–sodium alginate complex	Electrostatic interactions	[39]
	VD3	High amylose corn starch	Ultrasonication	[40]
	VD3	Carboxymethyl chitosan–soy protein complex	Ionic gelation method	[41]

Table 1. *Cont.*

Delivery System	Active	Main Components	Technique/Method	Reference
Lipid-based nanoparticles	VD2	Solid lipid nanoparticles (glyceryl tripalmitate) stabilized by Tween 20	Hot homogenization technique using a high-pressure homogenizer	[42]
	VD3	Nanostructured lipid carriers (solid lipids: Precirol or Compritol, liquid lipid: Miglyol or octyloctanoat, surfactants: Tween 80 or 20 or Poloxamer 407)	Hot homogenization method	[43]
	VD3	Nanostructured lipid carriers (glycerol monostearate as solid lipid, oleic acid as liquid lipid, and Tween 80)	Hot high-pressure homogenization	[44]
Micelles	VD3	Amphiphilic chitosan derivative of *N,N*-dimethylhexadecyl carboxymethyl chitosan	Synthesis	[45]
Liposomes	VD3	Soybean phosphatidylcholine, cholesterol	Thin film hydration-sonication technique	[46]
Microparticles	VD2	Medium molecular weight sodium alginate	Ultrasonic atomization and microwave stabilization	[47]

An interesting approach was also presented by Semo et al. (2007). They proposed the use of bovine casein micelles for encapsulation and stabilization of VD2 that could enrich non-fat or low-fat food products. The authors demonstrated that these re-assembled casein micelles could provide protection against photochemical VD2 degradation [48]. In the next step, the authors improved the previous encapsulation technique by introducing ultra-high pressure homogenization and proved the protection conferred by the micelles to incorporated VD3 against heat-induced degradation and during cold storage. Finally, the bioavailability of a single high dose of 50,000 IU VD3 encapsulated in casein micelles in 1%-fat milk was at least as high as that using an aqueous Tween 80-emulsified VD3 supplement [25]. In another study, the authors compared the VD3 bioavailability in casein micelles to that in Tween 80, both in fat-free yogurt (VD3 dose: 50,000 IU), measuring serum 25(OH)D increase in subjects. No significant differences in mean 25(OH)D levels were observed, evidencing the fact that VD3 bioavailability in casein micelles was as high as that in the synthetic emulsifier [49]. Another recent clinical study found that the bioavailability of VD in casein micelles in the absence of fat was found to be insignificantly different from its bioavailability within fat, suggesting that the bioavailability of lipophilic bioactives in protein nanovehicles is not lower than in fat [50].

In the studies of Mohammadi et al. (2017), VD was incorporated into nanostructured lipid carriers (mean diameter of approximately 88 nm), and then the effect of rising 25(OH)D in rat blood was assessed. Nanoparticles demonstrated the faster and prolonged increase of 25(OH)D in plasma than the oily solution formulation of VD [43]. A different approach was proposed by Diarrassouba et al. (2015). They used food proteins (β-lactoglobulin and egg white lysozyme) to entrap VD3 and obtained microspheres (mean diameter of approximately 7 μm) by electrostatic interactions with an encapsulation efficiency of about 91%. The authors suggested the use of food proteins as potential food-grade vehicles for bioactives in the formulation of food products and pharmaceuticals [51].

Finally, as presented in Table 1, many other attempts were also carried out to improve water solubility, stability, and bioavailability of VD using different encapsulation strategies, like protein-based delivery systems [32,39,41], solid lipid [42] and nanostructured lipid carriers [43,44], liposomes [46], and microparticle [47]. Interestingly, most researchers underline the fact that VD is a vitamin sensitive to external factors. However, only some of the authors reported results concerning VD chemical stability studies. In such studies, the chemical stability of the vitamin is measured either by HPLC [37] or spectrophotometrically [19] and expressed as encapsulation efficiency decrease during storage of the formulation. Both report that the chemical stability of VD2 or VD3 loaded in oil-in-water nanoemulsions was dependent on the type of emulsifier; however, in these studies, there was no comparison to the stability of non-encapsulated VD, and the effect was not sufficient for long-term storage.

3. Drug Delivery Systems for Application on the Skin

Alternatively to the oral administration of VD, which can have low efficiency because of many barriers and differences of conditions along the route, skin application may provide several advantages. Transdermal delivery gives a chance to avoid the first-pass effect of the liver, ensures the release for a long period, and could be for people with diseases that impair the oral absorption of VD3. On the other side, the topical application could provide a high concentration of the active substance in the upper skin layers that is essential for the treatment of several skin diseases typified by the disfunction of keratinocytes in the lower epidermis, mainly psoriasis [52]. Analyzing the research described in the literature in which VD/VD analogue was loaded in drug delivery systems, most potential applications were designed for topical administration on the skin. However, a few interesting studies on transdermal VD delivery were also conducted.

3.1. *Transdermal Delivery*

The transdermal route of permeation of vitamin D3 may be interesting for people with fat malabsorption in the intestine, due to Crohn's disease, gastric bypass, bile acid-binding medications, cystic fibrosis, and celiac disease. However, the transdermal route has little use, and there is little scientific literature on the subject. D'Angelo Costa and co-workers [53] investigated the feasibleness of VD3 skin retention and permeation with the presence of chemical penetration enhancers (soybean lecithin, isopropyl palmitate, propylene glycol, ethoxydiglycol, and cereal alcohol) at different pharmaceutical forms (gel and cream) through human skin from abdominal surgery. However, according to their results, gel formulation showed VD3 detection at stratum corneum in 4 h and epidermis and dermis in 24 h, whereas VD3 from the cream was detected only at the skin surface (no VD3 was found at receptor fluid for both formulations). They concluded that VD3 did not indicate feasibleness for transdermal use since it did not permeate through human skin, probably due to high lipophilicity and, thus, high affinity with the vehicle in the cream. Nevertheless, the transdermal route could be more effective with less lipophilic derivates of VD3 and with a different combination of penetration enhancers in the gel [53]. In the research of Alsaqr et al. [54], ointments with oleic acid and dodecylamine as penetration enhancers were used to evaluate the transdermal delivery of VD3 through porcine skin in 24 h. The results were retention at stratum corneum and epidermis for three formulations assessed (control, oleic acid, and dodecylamine), but VD was detected in the receptor medium only in the case of formulation with dodecylamine. They concluded that the transdermal route could be effective. However, it should be noted that porcine skin has a higher permeability due to the greater amount of hair follicles than human skin [54].

The above results obtained for transdermal VD delivery with conventional formulations (ointments and gels) suggest that drug delivery systems could be attractive to enhance such delivery. To our knowledge, the report of Bubshait et al. (2018) is the only research on humans in this area that so far has been published [55]. They did a prospective randomized controlled trial in which patients in the study group were given Top-D (VD3 gel made from proniosomal technology, 1 g contained 5000 IU of VD3) to apply daily on the skin, while the control group was given 1 g of *Aloe vera* gel to be applied every day. All the patients had VD deficiency (25OHD level ≤ 20 ng/mL). After four months, only in the study group, the serum 25OHD level was sufficient (25OHD level 37.17 ± 6.04 ng/mL). However, the proniosomal technology was not described in detail, and the only information is that the average particle size of VD carriers is about 3.8 μm. Hence, the absorption of vitamin D3 through the pores occurred without difficulty, as skin pores are approximately 50 μm in diameter [55]. Already in 2014, this group of researchers from the same center did a randomized controlled pilot study on the transdermal route of vitamin D3 and received similar results. One group of patients applied a topical formulation with *Aloe vera* and VD3, and another group applied formulation without VD3. After three months, an increase in the 25OHD level was observed [56]. In this study, aromatic oils and glycerin were used as penetration enhancers, and the results were comparable to those obtained for proniosomal technology.

Untypical studies were conducted by Kim et al. (2018) in which, first, VD was encapsulated into poly(lactic-*co*-glycolic acid) (PLGA) nanoparticles by a well-known emulsion solvent evaporation method; then, nanoparticles were immobilized onto the microneedles by a dip-coating method. The overall system was designed for transdermal VD delivery as an alternation for oral supplementation. It should be explained that microneedles easily pierce the skin layer with enough mechanical strength and allow the localization of drugs within the dermal region. Finally, layers of nanoparticles coated on solid microneedles were dissolved entirely into the intradermal region in the porcine skin model and revealed better performance for VD3 release into the receptor compartment compared to the ointment-based transdermal method [57].

Finally, an interesting study was done by Yamagishi et al., who evaluated the effects of a reservoir-type calcitriol transdermal patch on plasma calcitriol and calcium concentrations in dairy cattle. Interestingly, VD3, or its active form (calcitriol), is used as a prophylaxis for parturient hypocalcemia in dairy cows. The patches were applied to the skin of the tail for two days at intervals of at least three weeks. The data of this study describe evidence of measurable transdermal absorption of exogenous calcitriol from a patch and its sufficient biological action to elevate plasma calcium concentrations [58].

3.2. *Topical Delivery*

VD and its analogues have been proven to have anti-psoriatic activity by decreasing the proliferation of epidermal keratinocytes, by regulating the differentiation process and apoptosis of keratinocytes, by regulating the cutaneous immune system, and through their anti-inflammatory ability [6,59]. The effectiveness on psoriasis of VD and its derivatives (calcitriol, calcipotriol, calcipotriene, tacalcitol, hexafluoro-1,25(OH)D, and maxacalcitol) has been known since 1985, being confirmed in numerous trials. The therapy with VD is one of the most popularly prescribed topical medications for this disease as the first-line, singly or in combination with topical corticosteroids, and numerous studies have documented the efficacy of such treatment [6].

Such activity in the skin is due to the presence of VD3 receptors on keratinocytes and fibroblasts and an autonomous VD3 pathway in which VD3 is converted to calcitriol, the hormonally active form. Nevertheless, the VD3 derivatives show also some hypercalcemic activity, which can be a limitation. That is why a significant challenge is to increase the limited drug penetration and to minimize systemic exposure [60,61]. Another issue that should be taken into consideration when developing topical delivery systems is the high sensitivity of VD3 to external environmental factors such as light, heat, and oxygen [57]. The success of drug delivery depends, among other things, on the physicochemical properties of the active and its carriers in the formulation. Several studies have been focused on using nanoparticles for topical delivery of VD or VD analogues, including liposomes, solid lipid nanoparticles, polymeric nanospheres, or combinations of PLGA nanoparticles and microneedles [52]. Table 2 summarizes the delivery systems and methods of preparation described below.

The idea of liposomal encapsulation for topical administration of VD derivatives is not new. For keeping small the negative side effects of VD3 derivatives and for increasing the drug concentration in the skin, Merz et al. (1994) investigated their incorporation in liposomes to optimize their use for psoriasis treatment; however, no in-vitro or ex-vivo study was done. They prepared liposomes made of synthetic or naturally occurring lipids and evaluated the incorporation of VD and VD analogues into liposomes and their thermal properties. Their results showed that VD3 and its analogues incorporated into the lipid bilayer, altering the lipid–lipid interactions in the liposomes. The incorporation rates were generally found to be high, i.e., ≥80% [62]. It is crucial to consider that liposomes which have a phase transition temperature (T_m) above the temperature of the skin (32 °C) will be in a rigid gel state and these with a T_m below 32 °C will be in a fluid liquid state. Several studies have presented that liposomes in a liquid state have improved penetration into the skin. It was also proven that the liposome-mediated delivery of calcipotriol to the epidermis of diseased skin is also affected by the fluidity of the liposomal membrane [63].

Table 2. Examples of various types of delivery systems reported for encapsulation of vitamin D or its analogues for potential topical delivery (VD3—vitamin D3).

Delivery System	Active	Main Components	Technique/Method	Reference
Liposomes	Calcipotriol	Dipalmitoylphosphatidyl-choline (DPPC) and dilauroylphosphatidylcholine (DLPC)	Thin film method and extrusion	[63]
	Calcipotriol	Distearoylphosphatidylcholine (DSPC), poly(ethylene glycol)-distearoylphosphoethanolamine (PEG_{2000}-DSPE), sodium cholate	Thin film method and extrusion	[61]
	Calcitriol and tacalcitol	Phosphatidylcholine, phosphatidic acid, phospha-tidylethanolamine	Made from concentrate (commercial kit)	[64]
Solid lipid nanoparticles	Bethamethasone and calcipotriol	Precirol® ATO 5	Hot melt high shear homogenization technique and incorporation in Carbol gel matrix	[65]
Polymeric nanoparticles	VD3	Poly(lactic acid) nanoparticles with non-ionic poly(ethylene glycol) or zwitterionic poly(2-methacryloyloxyethyl phosphorylcholine) (PMPC) coating	Flash nanoprecipitation	[66]
	VD3	ABA triblock copolymers composed of hydrophilic A blocks and hydrophobic B blocks that form TyroSpheres®	TyroSpheres® preparation	[52]

The major problem related to the exploit of liposomes is their impaired colloidal stability, which can be overcome by coating them with hydrophilic polymers. The one proposed by Knudsen et al. (2012) was poly(ethylene glycol) (PEG). Liposomes loaded with calcipotriol were prepared by the thin film method, and in their bilayer membrane, different molar ratios of PEG_{2000}-DSPE were included. The colloidal stability of the liposomes was received as a result of the inclusion of 0.5, 1, and 5 mol % PGE-DSPE in the membrane. PEGylation has been shown as a promising approach for stabilising calcipotriol-containing liposomes and improving skin penetration [61].

Earlier studies demonstrated that there is no remarkable improvement in the action of liposomal-incorporated vitamin D3 analogues compared to the free analogues related either to their proliferation or their IL1 alpha-releasing effects on keratinocytes. However, the authors suggested that the influence of liposomal-incorporated VD3 analogues in keeping small their adverse side effects has to be investigated at a more relevant model [60]. Results presented by Körbel et al. (2001) definitely suggest that using liposomal calcitriol and tacalcitol allows receiving a better anti-psoriatic effect compared to non-liposomal phospholipid gel and conventional formulations that are clinically used, i.e., ointments based on petrolatum. The authors suggested that, by using a liposomal formulation, the concentration of the analogue could be reduced compared to that of currently available commercial preparations without sacrificing any therapeutic effect, and thus lead to a reduction both in local side effects (skin irritation) and systemic side effects (hypercalcemia). The advantage of using liposomes is their physicochemical similarity to the lipid bilayer [64].

Another interesting approach for effective delivery is using solid lipid nanoparticles. They have good biocompatibility, the ability to protect some labile compounds against degradation, and the ability to modulate drug release. The research conducted by Sonawane et al. (2014) was focused on preparing betamethasone and calcipotriol co-loaded solid lipid nanoparticles for the treatment of psoriasis. Nanoparticles were prepared by hot melt high shear homogenization technique and incorporated in Carbol gel matrix. The average particle size was 188 nm, and entrapment efficiency of betamethasone and calcipotriol was very high for both drugs, 85%, and 97%, respectively. The versatile in-vitro (rat skin permeation and dermal distribution, anti-proliferative effect in human hyperproliferative keratinocyte cell lines) and in-vivo analysis (anti-psoriatic mouse tail studies, transepidermal water loss, and Draize patch irritation) proved the high potential use for skin application and higher anti-psoriatic efficiency compared to the commercial preparation (gel containing non-encapsulated betamethasone and calcipotriol). It was demonstrated for solid lipid nanoparticles that the drugs penetrated to epidermal and dermal skin layers, but were detected only in negligible amounts in the receptor compartment. Additionally, in in-vivo studies, nanoparticle-loaded gel significantly decreased the epidermal thickness and increased melanocyte count in comparison to commercial gel [65]. The work of Sonawane and co-workers is proof that drug delivery systems can provide safer and more effective anti-psoriatic therapy than conventional formulations.

On the contrary, in the study of Lalloz et al. (2018), it was not possible to penetrate VD into the epidermis through the intact pigskin with the use of poly(lactic acid) nanoparticles, regardless of the surface chemistry, although, the average particle size of nanoparticles was about 100 nm [66].

Finally, a different type of polymeric nanoparticles for local VD delivery was presented by Ramezanli et al. (2017). ABA triblock copolymers composed of hydrophilic A blocks and hydrophobic B blocks were used for the preparation of TyroSpheres. The polymers self-assemble in an aqueous environment to form a core-shell structure with a hydrophobic core in which VD3 is incorporated with hydrophilic blocks, making the shell and stabilizing the system. The average diameter was approximately 70 nm, and the encapsulation efficiency was high. VD3 was released from TyroSpheres in a sustained manner and was delivered across the stratum corneum separated from human cadaver skin. An ex-vivo skin distribution study showed that TyroSphere formulations delivered significantly higher amounts of active into the epidermis compared to VD dissolved in Transcutol®. Additionally, TyroSpheres protected the vitamin against photodegradation and hydrolysis [52].

4. Drug Delivery Systems for the Prevention and Treatment of Cancer

Increasing evidence supports the role of VD systems in cancer prevention and therapy. Many scientific articles have reported the role of VD systems in the onset, progression, prognosis, and treatment of cancer. The mechanisms of the genomic action of VD systems seems to be multidirectional.

Since the first hypothesis linking VD with possible anticancer activity in the early 1980s, a vast number of preclinical and clinical studies have been carried out, and various mechanisms of VD system actions in carcinogenesis have been reported in thousands of articles [5,7–9,67,68]. Non-specific, transversal anticancer actions of VD systems are presented in Figure 4. However, the possible actions of VD systems implicated in cancer development may be exerted upon specific histologic subtypes of cancer, including mainly breast, prostate, and colorectal cancer cells. Accumulating results from preclinical and some clinical studies strongly suggest that VD deficiency increases the risk of developing cancer and that avoiding deficiency and adding VD supplements might be an economical and safe way to reduce cancer incidence and improve cancer prognosis and outcome [5,8].

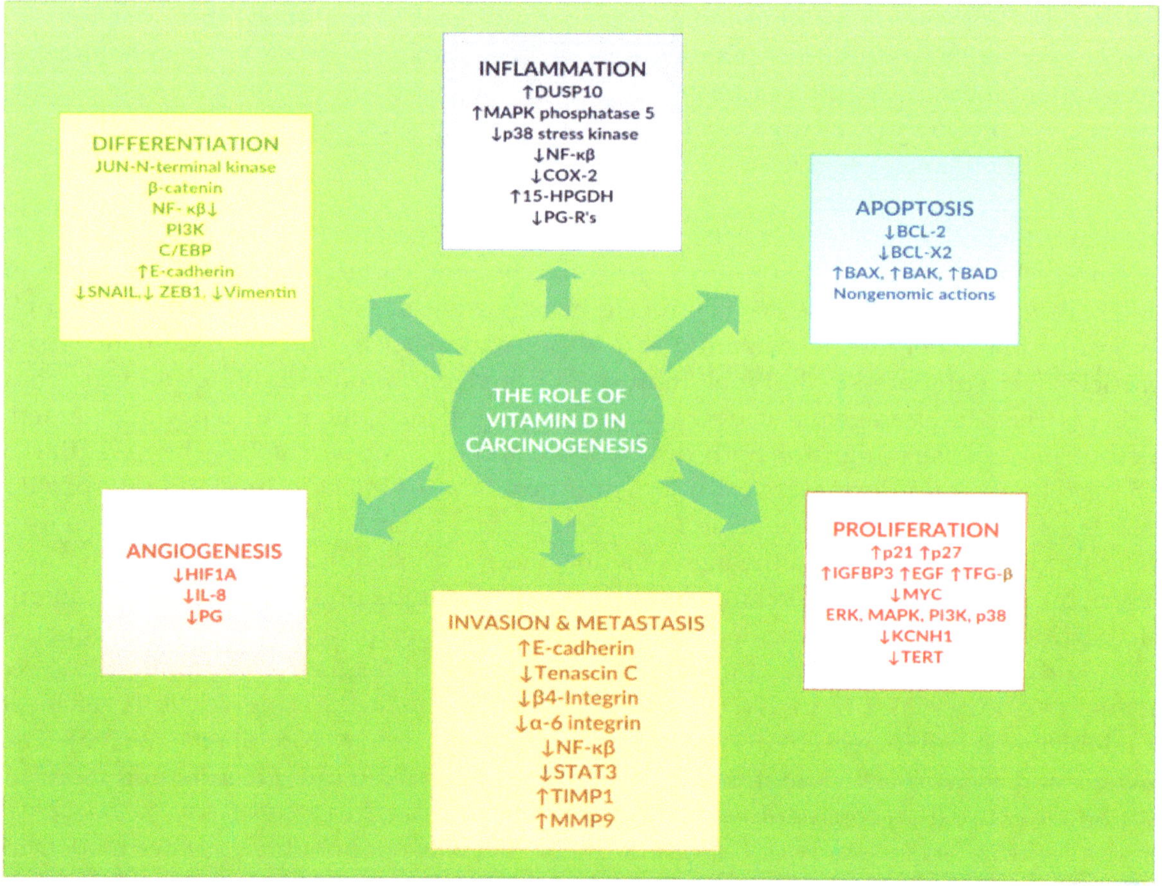

Figure 4. Preclinical basic-sciences studies show that the vitamin D system coordinates vital cellular processes such as cell differentiation, modulation of inflammation, apoptosis, cell proliferation, invasion, and metastatic processes, and angiogenesis. Reproduced with permission from [8], published by Elsevier, 2017.

In the review of Pandolfi et al. (2017), some forms of cancer are mentioned that benefit from a VD supplementation during treatment. For example, it has occurred that women with triple-negative breast cancer have lower cathelicidin antimicrobial peptide (CAMP), which is an essential cytotoxic and proapoptotic peptide. However, if the cells are stimulated with calcitriol, the level of CAMP rises, leading to potential advantages for treatment. Another positive effect and a new therapeutic avenue in breast cancer treatment may also be observed as a result of VD inhibition of the cluster of microRNA-199a/microRNA-214, a well-known tumor promoter. Aside from that, research in Norway has shown that patients who have prostate cancer had better outcomes during summer when sunlight exposure is higher as well as VD serum levels. A similar situation was observed in connection with the morbidity of colorectal cancer. Despite using different case populations, risk factors, and various techniques of VD measurement, the studies confirmed the inverse correlation between VD intake and colorectal cancer risk [9].

4.1. Vitamin D as an Adjuvant in Cancer Therapy

An interesting suggestion might also be a combination of VD with other active substances. Xu et al. (2018) investigated the synergistic effect of astemizole and VD in hepatocellular carcinoma cells in vitro and in vivo. Both actives were used as non-encapsulated. It has been proven in vitro that astemizole enhances VD-induced apoptosis and decreases cell proliferation and migration. However, the decrease of tumor number, mass, and incidence in hepatocellular carcinoma cells was demonstrated in vivo. Astemizole increased VDR expression both in cells in vitro and in tumor tissues in vivo. They also clarified that this combination inhibits the tumor suppressor miR-125a-5p and is responsible for subsequent upregulation of the VD receptor. These outcomes highlight the crucial role of combined treatment of astemizole and VD for the cure of hepatocellular carcinoma cells [69]. Similarly, in other studies, VD was encapsulated into nanostructured lipid carriers and was used as an adjuvant to elevate the efficacy of doxorubicin on concurrent administration in breast cancer treatment. The prepared lipid nanoparticles revealed a mean particle size of 87 nm and were in the range for passive targeting to cells. In-vitro cytotoxicity results exhibited that VD-loaded nanoparticles were more effective than free VD in the induction of breast cancer cell death after 24-h incubation. Indeed, cotreatment of the cells with VD-loaded nanoparticles and doxorubicin caused a twofold increase in the percentage of apoptosis [70]. An innovative approach was presented by Maayah et al. (2018). They synthesized doxorubicin-VD by conjugating VD to doxorubicin to increase the delivery of doxorubicin into human osteosarcoma cancer cells and mitigate the chemoresistance associated with doxorubicin. The results were very promising, as the conjugate doxorubicin-VD suppressed the growth of cancer cells by inducing apoptosis while inhibiting cell survival and proliferative signaling pathways. They proposed that VD may serve as a novel drug delivery approach to potentiate the delivery of anticancer drugs into cancer cells [71].

4.2. Vitamin D and Its Metabolites as Anticancer Drugs

Particularly in the case of anticancer application, drug delivery systems can be useful due to the possibility of selective drug delivery to tumor tissue either by passive targeting with the enhanced permeability and retention effect or by active targeting using functionalization. In this way, nanoparticles, when internalized by target cells, increase intracellular drug delivery, sustain drug release, increase therapeutic activity, and lower side effects. It is especially important knowing that calcitriol has anti-tumoral activity in supraphysiological doses which are associated with a high risk of hypercalcemia. Beyond very high toxicity, calcitriol has a very short half-life in bloodstream; this is why its administration is particularly problematic [72,73]. In the case of cancer therapy, parenteral administration of nanoparticles like intravenous injection/infusion or direct injection to the tumor are the most probable way of administration since the oral route requires additional resistance of drug and drug carriers to such factors as gastric juice and enzymes. From a variety of drug delivery systems, liposomes have been considered so far as the most successful drug delivery system as liposome-based drugs have been clinically used in cancer therapy (e.g., Doxil®, DaunoXome®, Depocyt®, Mepact®, Myocet®).

It is essential to mention studies prepared by Almouazen et al. (2013) where they encapsulated VD, calcidiol, or calcitriol into poly(lactic acid) (PLA) nanoparticles. As expected, encapsulation into PLA nanoparticles significantly improved the stability of VD, calcidiol, and calcitriol compared to non-encapsulated forms. Free or nanoencapsulated drugs were dispersed in cell culture medium (Dulbecco's Modified Eagle Medium with antibiotics) and incubated at 37 °C. After 24 h, more than 75% of the drugs remained in nanoparticles, whereas only about 25% of free VD and calcitriol remained in the medium, and free calcidiol was already totally degraded. In this study, loaded nanoparticles showed similar growth inhibition of human breast adenocarcinoma cells to non-encapsulated calcidiol and calcitriol [72]. This was not surprising, as calcidiol and calcitriol are lipophilic and readily cross the membranes to reach their nuclear receptors. A similar approach was presented by Ramalho et al. (2015). They prepared poly(lactic-*co*-glycolic-acid) (PLGA) nanoparticles as nanocarriers for calcitriol with a mean diameter of 186 nm. The in-vitro cytotoxic effects on three different human cell lines (two non-tumor pancreatic cell lines and one lung cancer cell line) after treatment with calcitriol-loaded nanoparticles were assessed relative to free calcitriol in terms of cell growth. Both free and encapsulated calcitriol exhibited a similar concentration-related decrease in cell growth and survival of the human non-tumor cells. However, calcitriol-loaded nanoparticles demonstrated an increased inhibitory effect on lung cancer cell line by inducing cell cycle arrest and morphological changes in the tumor cells [73].

A different approach was proposed by Vora et al. (2017), who created PLGA microspheres (28 µm) loaded with VD as an injectable controlled drug delivery system. The results showed that these microspheres could offer an interesting method for once-a-month delivery by the parenteral route (intramuscular injection), which was confirmed by in-vivo studies in rats [74]. However, such an approach could be an alternative for daily oral supplementation of this vitamin rather than a way to induce anticancer effects since such a system does not protect from hypercalcemia. On the other hand, Nguyen et al. (2007) reported a promising technique in liver cancer treatment by utilizing crosslinked microspheres (35 μm) prepared by polymerization as a carrier to control the release of calcitriol at the targeted site over a long period after direct injection of microspheres into the tumor. Local treatment through hepatic injection of calcitriol should prevent the development of hypercalcemia [75].

4.3. Active Targeting of Nanoparticles Loaded with Vitamin D to Cancer Cells

Very interesting studies were done by Liu et al. (2018). Calcitriol is also known as a promising agent for the treatment of non-small cell lung cancer with a developed resistance to inhibitors of EGFR (epidermal growth factor receptor) tyrosine kinase. However, calcitriol induces the expression of 24-hydroxylase, the enzyme that decreases calcitriol activity. That is why CTA091, a potent and selective 24-hydroxylase inhibitor, has been developed; however, CTA091 also suppresses renal 24-hydroxylase activity and so may promote hypercalcemia. To exploit the favorable effects of both calcitriol and CTA091 in tumor cells, tumor-targeted co-delivery of calcitriol and CTA091 was proposed by developing EGFR-targeted liposomes loaded with both drugs. Targeting of liposomes was achieved by conjugating human anti-EGFR monoclonal antibody to the liposomal surface. Liposomes were produced as uniformly distributed nanoparticles, with a mean diameter by volume of 157 nm and positive zeta potential. Compared with free calcitriol and CTA091, such targeted liposomes with co-loaded drugs have shown improved cellular uptake and effective inhibition of colony formation in lung cancer cells [76].

It should be mentioned that in some studies, conclusions suggest that VD is ineffective in cancer prevention/treatment and its role is overestimated. The research conducted by Maleklou et al. (2016) proved that targeted delivery of VD-loaded nanoparticles to C6 glioma cell lines reinforces the resistance to doxorubicin, epirubicin, and docetaxel and increases the cancerous characteristics in vitro [77]. It is also speculated that VD intake can be more significant in early carcinogenesis stages rather than advanced cancers [5]. Besides, many trials had some limitations, including being largely unable to observe a statistical relevant reduction in cancer occurrence or a lack of knowledge about the appropriate dose, the form of VD, and the length of time that it should be taken [10]. The large-scale and long-term human randomized controlled trials are not available so far, and there is no clear conclusion whether vitamin D can be beneficial during cancer treatment. Based on existing studies, it is crucial to avoid VD deficiency; VD might play a role in cancer risk reduction and treatment [5].

5. Drug Delivery Systems for Other Diseases or Routes of Administration

As mentioned earlier, VD was demonstrated to have multiple extra-skeletal effects on biological processes, such as immune regulation, neurogenesis, or genome stability, and the level of it can be associated with the therapy of other illnesses. Recent studies have focused on how VD can be exploited in the treatment of chronic, infectious, or autoimmune diseases. Some scientists also presume that we should consider VD as a hormone rather than a nutritional vitamin [78].

The immunomodulatory effects of VD through regulation and differentiation of lymphocytes, macrophages, and natural killer cells enhance opportunities to reinforce the treatment of arthritis. The research conducted by da Silveira et al. (2016) suggests that VD may inhibit the proinflammatory response. In the study, first arthritis was induced in rats, and then the groups were treated for 15 days with oral VD3 either in solution based on corn oil (120 IU/day) or VD3-loaded nanocapsules (15.84 IU/day). Lipid-core nanocapsules were made by interfacial deposition of preformed polymer technique using poly(ε-caprolactone) as a polymer making the shell. The versatile analysis was done before and after treatment for all the groups including chronic inflammation evaluation, histopathological observation, measurements of the activity of the inflammatory state enzymes in rat lymphocytes, and determination of many hematological and biochemical parameters in blood.

As a result, better anti-inflammatory activity was demonstrated for the oral oily solution of VD3. However, it should be mention that the dose of encapsulated VD3 was approximately more than 7.6-fold lower than the dose of non-encapsulated vitamin. While an increase in serum levels of 25OHD was observed only in groups receiving non-encapsulating VD3, histological analyses showed that both formulations were able to reduce the inflammatory changes [79].

Asthma is another immunologic disease characterized by chronic airway inflammation that is a promising target for VD. In the research done by Wei-hong et al. (2014), nanoemulsions were prepared for the delivery of VD in ovalbumin-induced asthmatic mice, and VD bioavailability and anti-inflammatory activity were evaluated. In the study, nanoemulsions were prepared from the established composition of solid self-emulsifying drug delivery systems (sSEDDS) by spray-drying technique. VD in the form of either the non-encapsulated one or nanoemulsion was administered to mice with induced asthma at a high dose of 2000 IU/kg. It was evident that nanoemulsions significantly increased oral VD absorption. This increase in bioavailability resulted in enhanced pharmacological activity. The anti-inflammatory and antioxidant assay revealed that the therapeutic efficiency of VD significantly enhanced upon nanoemulsion formation [80].

An interesting approach was presented by Goff et al. (2012). The purpose of this study was to evaluate whether β-glucuronides of 1,25(OH)D (calcitriol) could deliver free calcitriol to the colon to treat colitis while decreasing the risk of hypercalcemia. Several studies have demonstrated a direct therapeutic effect of VD and calcitriol in mouse models of inflammatory bowel disease, since VDRs are widely expressed in the epithelial cells and the immune cells in the colon. The authors conjugated glucuronic acid to the calcitriol molecule to form water-soluble 1,25-dihydroxy vitamin D-25-β-glucuronide that is inactive, and little of that glycosidic form can be absorbed across the intestine. Cleavage of the β-glucuronide of the calcitriol to free calcitriol upon hydrolysis by β-glucuronidase produced by bacteria in the lower intestinal tract would: (i) Reduce systemic absorption of the 1,25(OH)D, (ii) decrease hypercalcemic effects, and (iii) allow targeted delivery of 1,25(OH)D to the ileum/colon cells affected by the disease. As a result, the authors confirmed that β-glucuronides of vitamin D compounds delivered 1,25(OH)D to the lower intestine and reduced hypercalcemia and symptoms of acute colitis in this model [81].

The influence of VD on immune and anti-inflammatory regulation raises the question of potential benefit against bacterial infections. Therefore, the study presented by Castoldi et al. (2017) was focused on the encapsulation of calcifediol in liposomes to enable aerosolization. Prepared 25(OH)D-loaded liposomes were nanosized and monodisperse, with a negative surface charge and a 25(OH)D entrapment efficiency of approximately 23%. Jet nebulization of liposomes was seen to yield an aerosol suitable for tracheobronchial deposition. Calcifediol in either liposomes or ethanolic solution was tested for the capacity to prevent pulmonary infection by *Pseudomonas aeruginosa*. Interestingly, encapsulation into liposomes resulted in a significant reduction in bacterial survival. Besides, the formulation can be regarded as a means to achieve calcifediol lung deposition and as safe for pulmonary administration in humans [82].

In recent years it has been found that low serum 25-hydroxyvitamin D3 concentration is connected with periodontal destruction in periodontitis and likewise with osteoporosis in diabetes. Both studies conducted by Li et al. (2013, 2014) endeavoured to prove that 25OHD-loaded PLA microspheres may ensure a potential therapy for patients with periodontitis. These microspheres were prepared using an emulsion-solvent evaporation method and were evaluated due to the biological effect on both in-vitro and in-vivo models. As a result, drug release during these experiments remained almost steady, which is promising for long-term therapy. The 25OHD-loaded PLA microspheres upregulated VD receptor expression and impaired periodontal inflammatory infiltrate and bone loss in diabetic rats with periodontitis [83,84].

Furthermore, a growing body of evidence has pointed out that calcitriol, an active form of VD, takes a role in maintaining brain functions through stimulation of neurotrophic factors' expression, immune regulation, and prevention of neuronal damage. It is worth mentioning the approach made by Ślusarczyk et al. (2016), who prepared nanocapsules with calcitriol for neuroprotective targeted therapy to the brain and compared protective properties of calcitriol-loaded nanocapsules with those of non-encapsulated calcitriol in hippocampal organotypic cultures after treatment with lipopolysaccharide (LPS). The active substance was enclosed in a hydrophobic core coated with either PLL (poly(L-lysine hydrobromide)), PLL/PGA (poly(L-glutamic acid)), or PLL with pegylated PGA. The average size of nanocapsules ranged from 80 to 100 nm. The results demonstrated that carriers with PLL/PGA and PLL-PGA-PEG were recognized as non-toxic and as having a protective ability. Both forms of nanoparticles also exhibited a higher neuroprotective action than free calcitriol connected with the suppression of LPS-induced nitric oxide (NO) release. Since calcitriol can modulate the brain NO signalling, it may be used as a promising solution in neuroinflammation and neurodegenerative processes [85].

6. Conclusions

Due to its many beneficial effects, the interest in VD and its derivatives has increased, and they have become attractive as active substances for incorporation into DDS. In this review, we summarized and discussed the main directions of development of drug delivery technologies that have been reported in recent years for VD or VD analogues. Overall, although the number of works describing new technologies appears large at first glance, and they cover a wide range of strategies, they are all at an early stage of research. In this work, many types of DDS have been presented depending on the disease or route of administration. Oral administration is the most convenient route, and is cost-effective, to increasing 25(OH)D levels, especially since large proportions of the population have low VD levels. The implementation of DDS for food enrichment or VD therapy with dietary supplements seems to be justified and feasible in the near future. However, most interesting is the potential use of VD/VD analogues in anticancer therapy. The combination of both strategies, i.e., synthesis of low calcemic VD analogues and targeted delivery, seems to be most desirable. However, until now, no sophisticated technology with functionalization of DDS was introduced for VD or VD derivatives. Nevertheless, the delivery of VD-based drug payloads via tumor-targeted carriers seems to be a future direction.

Author Contributions: Conceptualization, E.G.; resources, E.G. and J.S.; writing—original draft preparation, E.G. and J.S; writing—review and editing, E.G. and J.L.; visualization, E.G and J.S.; funding acquisition, J.L.

References

1. Wimalawansa, S.J. Vitamin D in the New Millennium. *Curr. Osteoporos Rep.* **2012**, *10*, 4–15. [CrossRef] [PubMed]
2. Holick, M.F. The vitamin D deficiency pandemic: Approaches for diagnosis, treatment and prevention. *Rev. Endocr. Metab. Disord.* **2017**, *18*, 153–165. [CrossRef]
3. Christakos, S.; Dhawan, P.; Verstuyf, A.; Verlinden, L.; Carmeliet, G. Vitamin D: Metabolism, Molecular Mechanism of Action, and Pleiotropic Effects. *Physiol. Rev.* **2016**, *96*, 365–408. [CrossRef]
4. Cavalier, E.; Delanaye, P.; Chapelle, J.P.; Souberbielle, J.C. Vitamin D: Current status and perspectives. *Clin. Chem. Lab. Med.* **2009**, *47*, 120–127. [CrossRef] [PubMed]
5. Feldman, D.; Krishnan, A.V.; Swami, S.; Giovannucci, E.; Feldman, B.J. The role of vitamin D in reducing cancer risk and progression. *Nat. Rev. Cancer* **2014**, *14*, 342–357. Available online: http://www.nature.com/nrc/journal/v14/n5/abs/nrc3691.html#supplementary-information (accessed on 23 March 2019). [CrossRef] [PubMed]
6. Barrea, L.; Savanelli, M.C.; Di Somma, C.; Napolitano, M.; Megna, M.; Colao, A.; Savastano, S. Vitamin D and its role in psoriasis: An overview of the dermatologist and nutritionist. *Rev. Endocr. Metab. Disord.* **2017**, *18*, 195–205. [CrossRef] [PubMed]

7. Moukayed, M.; Grant, W.B. The roles of UVB and vitamin D in reducing risk of cancer incidence and mortality: A review of the epidemiology, clinical trials, and mechanisms. *Rev. Endocr. Metab. Disord.* **2017**, *18*, 167–182. [CrossRef] [PubMed]
8. Merchan, B.B.; Morcillo, S.; Martin-Nunez, G.; Tinahones, F.J.; Macias-Gonzalez, M. The role of vitamin D and VDR in carcinogenesis: Through epidemiology and basic sciences. *J. Steroid Biochem. Mol. Biol.* **2017**, *167*, 203–218. [CrossRef] [PubMed]
9. Pandolfi, F.; Franza, L.; Mandolini, C.; Conti, P. Immune Modulation by Vitamin D: Special Emphasis on Its Role in Prevention and Treatment of Cancer. *Clin. Ther.* **2017**, *39*, 884–893. [CrossRef] [PubMed]
10. Duffy, M.J.; Murray, A.; Synnott, N.C.; O'Donovan, N.; Crown, J. Vitamin D analogues: Potential use in cancer treatment. *Crit. Rev. Oncol. Hematol.* **2017**, *112*, 190–197. [CrossRef]
11. Corcoran, A.; Bermudez, M.A.; Seoane, S.; Perez-Fernandez, R.; Krupa, M.; Pietraszek, A.; Chodyński, M.; Kutner, A.; Brown, G.; Marcinkowska, E. Biological evaluation of new vitamin D2 analogues. *J. Steroid Biochem. Mol. Biol.* **2016**, *164*, 66–71. [CrossRef]
12. Maestro, M.A.; Molnár, F.; Mouriño, A.; Carlberg, C. Vitamin D receptor 2016: Novel ligands and structural insights. *Expert Opin. Ther. Pat.* **2016**, *26*, 1291–1306. [CrossRef]
13. Hansen, C.M.; Hamberg, K.J.; Binderup, E.; Binderup, L. Seocalcitol (EB 1089) A Vitamin D Analogue of Anti-cancer Potential. Background, Design, Synthesis, Pre-clinical and Clinical Evaluation. *Cur. Pharm. Des.* **2000**, *6*, 803–828. [CrossRef]
14. Dobnig, H. A review of the health consequences of the vitamin D deficiency pandemic. *J. Neurol. Sci.* **2011**, *311*, 15–18. [CrossRef]
15. Jain, K.K. Current status and future prospects of drug delivery systems. *Methods Mol. Biol.* **2014**, *1141*, 1–56. [CrossRef] [PubMed]
16. Banik, B.L.; Fattahi, P.; Brown, J.L. Polymeric nanoparticles: The future of nanomedicine. *Wiley Interdiscip Rev. Nanomed Nanobiotechnol* **2016**, *8*, 271–299. [CrossRef] [PubMed]
17. Crommelin, D.J.; Florence, A.T. Towards more effective advanced drug delivery systems. *Int. J. Pharm.* **2013**, *454*, 496–511. [CrossRef] [PubMed]
18. Janssen, M.; Mihov, G.; Welting, T.; Thies, J.; Emans, P. Drugs and Polymers for Delivery Systems in OA Joints: Clinical Needs and Opportunities. *Polymers* **2014**, *6*, 799–819. [CrossRef]
19. Khalid, N.; Kobayashi, I.; Wang, Z.; Neves, M.A.; Uemura, K.; Nakajima, M.; Nabetani, H. Formulation of monodisperse oil-in-water emulsions loaded with ergocalciferol and cholecalciferol by microchannel emulsification: Insights of production characteristics and stability. *Int. J. Food Sci. Technol.* **2015**, *50*, 1807–1814. [CrossRef]
20. Borel, P.; Caillaud, D.; Cano, N.J. Vitamin D Bioavailability: State of the Art. *Crit. Rev. Food Sci. Nutr.* **2015**, *55*, 1193–1205. [CrossRef] [PubMed]
21. Li, Q.; Liu, C.-G.; Huang, Z.-H.; Xue, F.-F. Preparation and Characterization of Nanoparticles Based on Hydrophobic Alginate Derivative as Carriers for Sustained Release of Vitamin D3. *J. Agric. Food Chem.* **2011**, *59*, 1962–1967. [CrossRef]
22. Grossmann, R.E.; Tangpricha, V. Evaluation of vehicle substances on vitamin D bioavailability: A systematic review. *Mol. Nutr. Food Res.* **2010**, *54*, 1055–1061. [CrossRef]
23. Coelho, I.M.G.; de Andrade, L.D.; Saldanha, L.; Diniz, E.T.; Griz, L.; Bandeira, F. Bioavailability of vitamin D3 in non-oily capsules: The role of formulated compounds and implications for intermittent replacement. *Arq. Bras. Endocrinol. Metab.* **2010**, *54*, 239–243. [CrossRef]
24. de Souza Simões, L.; Madalena, D.A.; Pinheiro, A.C.; Teixeira, J.A.; Vicente, A.A.; Ramos, Ó.L. Micro- and nano bio-based delivery systems for food applications: In vitro behavior. *Adv. Colloid Interface Sci.* **2017**, *243*, 23–45. [CrossRef]
25. Haham, M.; Ish-Shalom, S.; Nodelman, M.; Duek, I.; Segal, E.; Kustanovich, M.; Livney, Y.D. Stability and bioavailability of vitamin D nanoencapsulated in casein micelles. *Food Funct.* **2012**, *3*, 737–744. [CrossRef]
26. Guttoff, M.; Saberi, A.H.; McClements, D.J. Formation of vitamin D nanoemulsion-based delivery systems by spontaneous emulsification: Factors affecting particle size and stability. *Food Chem.* **2015**, *171*, 117–122. [CrossRef]
27. Singh, T.; Shukla, S.; Kumar, P.; Wahla, V.; Bajpai, V.K. Application of Nanotechnology in Food Science: Perception and Overview. *Front. Microbiol.* **2017**, *8*, 1501. [CrossRef]

28. Abbasi, A.; Emam-Djomeh, Z.; Mousavi, M.A.E.; Davoodi, D. Stability of vitamin D3 encapsulated in nanoparticles of whey protein isolate. *Food Chem.* **2014**, *143*, 379–383. [CrossRef]
29. Cohen, Y.; Levi, M.; Lesmes, U.; Margier, M.; Reboul, E.; Livney, Y.D. Re-assembled casein micelles improve in vitro bioavailability of vitamin D in a Caco-2 cell model. *Food Funct.* **2017**, *8*, 2133–2141. [CrossRef]
30. Ziani, K.; Fang, Y.; McClements, D.J. Encapsulation of functional lipophilic components in surfactant-based colloidal delivery systems: Vitamin E, vitamin D, and lemon oil. *Food Chem.* **2012**, *134*, 1106–1112. [CrossRef]
31. Kirilenko, V.; Gregoriadis, G. Fat Soluble Vitamins in Liposomes: Studies on Incorporation Efficiency and Bile Salt Induced Vesicle Disintegration. *J. Drug Target.* **1993**, *1*, 361–368. [CrossRef]
32. Luo, Y.; Teng, Z.; Wang, Q. Development of Zein Nanoparticles Coated with Carboxymethyl Chitosan for Encapsulation and Controlled Release of Vitamin D3. *J. Agric. Food Chem.* **2012**, *60*, 836–843. [CrossRef]
33. Salvia-Trujillo, L.; Fumiaki, B.; Park, Y.; McClements, D.J. The influence of lipid droplet size on the oral bioavailability of vitamin D2 encapsulated in emulsions: An in vitro and in vivo study. *Food Funct.* **2017**, *8*, 767–777. [CrossRef]
34. Ozturk, B.; Argin, S.; Ozilgen, M.; McClements, D.J. Nanoemulsion delivery systems for oil-soluble vitamins: Influence of carrier oil type on lipid digestion and vitamin D3 bioaccessibility. *Food Chem.* **2015**, *187*, 499–506. [CrossRef]
35. Sun, F.; Ju, C.; Chen, J.; Liu, S.; Liu, N.; Wang, K.; Liu, C. Nanoparticles Based on Hydrophobic Alginate Derivative as Nutraceutical Delivery Vehicle: Vitamin D3 Loading. *Artif. Cells Blood Substit. Biotechnol.* **2012**, *40*, 113–119. [CrossRef]
36. Khalid, N.; Kobayashi, I.; Neves, M.A.; Uemura, K.; Nakajima, M.; Nabetani, H. Encapsulation of cholecalciferol and ergocalciferol in oil-in-water emulsions by different homogenization techniques. *Eur. J. Lipid Sci. Technol.* **2017**, *119*, 1600247. [CrossRef]
37. Shu, G.F.; Khalid, N.; Zhao, Y.G.; Neves, M.A.; Kobayashi, I.; Nakajima, M. Formulation and stability assessment of ergocalciferol loaded oil-in-water nanoemulsions: Insights of emulsifiers effect on stabilization mechanism. *Food Res. Int.* **2016**, *90*, 320–327. [CrossRef] [PubMed]
38. Walia, N.; Dasgupta, N.; Ranjan, S.; Chen, L.; Ramalingam, C. Fish oil based vitamin D nanoencapsulation by ultrasonication and bioaccessibility analysis in simulated gastro-intestinal tract. *Ultrason. Sonochem* **2017**, *39*, 623–635. [CrossRef]
39. Hosseini, S.M.H.; Emam-Djomeh, Z.; Sabatino, P.; van der Meeren, P. Nanocomplexes arising from protein-polysaccharide electrostatic interaction as a promising carrier for nutraceutical compounds. *Food Hydrocoll.* **2015**, *50*, 16–26. [CrossRef]
40. Hassanvand, E.; Fathi, M.; Bassiri, A.; Javanmard, M.; Abbaszadeh, R. Novel starch based nanocarrier for Vitamin D fortification of milk: Production and characterization. *Food Bioprod. Process.* **2015**, *96*, 264–277. [CrossRef]
41. Teng, Z.; Luo, Y.; Wang, Q. Carboxymethyl chitosan–soy protein complex nanoparticles for the encapsulation and controlled release of vitamin D3. *Food Chem.* **2013**, *141*, 524–532. [CrossRef]
42. Patel, M.R.; Martin-Gonzalez, M.F.S. Characterization of Ergocalciferol Loaded Solid Lipid Nanoparticles. *J. Food Sci.* **2012**, *77*, N8–N13. [CrossRef]
43. Mohammadi, M.; Pezeshki, A.; Mesgari Abbasi, M.; Ghanbarzadeh, B.; Hamishehkar, H. Vitamin D (3)-Loaded Nanostructured Lipid Carriers as a Potential Approach for Fortifying Food Beverages; in Vitro and in Vivo Evaluation. *Adv. Pharm. Bull.* **2017**, *7*, 61–71. [CrossRef]
44. Park, S.J.; Garcia, C.V.; Shin, G.H.; Kim, J.T. Development of nanostructured lipid carriers for the encapsulation and controlled release of vitamin D3. *Food Chem.* **2017**, *225*, 213–219. [CrossRef]
45. Li, W.; Peng, H.; Ning, F.; Yao, L.; Luo, M.; Zhao, Q.; Zhu, X.; Xiong, H. Amphiphilic chitosan derivative-based core–shell micelles: Synthesis, characterisation and properties for sustained release of Vitamin D3. *Food Chem.* **2014**, *152*, 307–315. [CrossRef]
46. Mohammadi, M.; Ghanbarzadeh, B.; Hamishehkar, H. Formulation of nanoliposomal vitamin d3 for potential application in beverage fortification. *Adv. Pharm. Bull.* **2014**, *4*, 569–575. [CrossRef]
47. Barba, A.A.; Dalmoro, A.; d'Amore, M.; Lamberti, G. Liposoluble vitamin encapsulation in shell-core microparticles produced by ultrasonic atomization and microwave stabilization. *LWT-Food Sci. Technol.* **2015**, *64*, 149–156. [CrossRef]
48. Semo, E.; Kesselman, E.; Danino, D.; Livney, Y.D. Casein micelle as a natural nano-capsular vehicle for nutraceuticals. *Food Hydrocoll.* **2007**, *21*, 936–942. [CrossRef]

49. Levinson, Y.; Ish-Shalom, S.; Segal, E.; Livney, Y.D. Bioavailability, rheology and sensory evaluation of fat-free yogurt enriched with VD3 encapsulated in re-assembled casein micelles. *Food Funct.* **2016**, *7*, 1477–1482. [CrossRef]
50. Cohen, Y.; Ish-Shalom, S.; Segal, E.; Nudelman, O.; Shpigelman, A.; Livney, Y.D. The bioavailability of vitamin D3, a model hydrophobic nutraceutical, in casein micelles, as model protein nanoparticles: Human clinical trial results. *J. Funct. Food* **2017**, *30*, 321–325. [CrossRef]
51. Diarrassouba, F.; Remondetto, G.; Garrait, G.; Alvarez, P.; Beyssac, E.; Subirade, M. Self-assembly of β-lactoglobulin and egg white lysozyme as a potential carrier for nutraceuticals. *Food Chem.* **2015**, *173*, 203–209. [CrossRef] [PubMed]
52. Ramezanli, T.; Kilfoyle, B.E.; Zhang, Z.; Michniak-Kohn, B.B. Polymeric nanospheres for topical delivery of vitamin D3. *Int. J. Pharm.* **2017**, *516*, 196–203. [CrossRef]
53. D'Angelo Costa, G.M.; Sales de Oliveira Pinto, C.A.; Rodrigues Leite-Silva, V.; Rolim Baby, A.; Robles Velasco, M.V. Is Vitamin D3 Transdermal Formulation Feasible? An Ex Vivo Skin Retention and Permeation. *AAPS PharmSciTech* **2018**, *19*, 2418–2425. [CrossRef]
54. Alsaqr, A.; Rasoully, M.; Musteata, F.M. Investigating transdermal delivery of vitamin D3. *AAPS PharmSciTech* **2015**, *16*, 963–972. [CrossRef] [PubMed]
55. Bubshait, D.A.; Al-Dakheel, D.A.; Alanii, F.M. Topical vitamin D3: A randomized controlled trial (RCT). *Clin. Nutr. ESPEN* **2018**, *27*, 16–19. [CrossRef] [PubMed]
56. Sadat-Ali, M.; Bubshait, D.A.; Al-Turki, H.A.; Al-Dakheel, D.A.; Al-Olayani, W.S. Topical delivery of vitamin d3: A randomized controlled pilot study. *Int. J. Biomed. Sci.* **2014**, *10*, 21–24. [PubMed]
57. Kim, H.-G.; Gater, D.L.; Kim, Y.-C. Development of transdermal vitamin D3 (VD3) delivery system using combinations of PLGA nanoparticles and microneedles. *Drug Deliv. Transl. Res.* **2018**, *8*, 281–290. [CrossRef] [PubMed]
58. Yamagishi, N.; Namioka, T.; Okura, N.; Sato, S.; Kim, D.; Furuhama, K.; Naito, Y. Application of a Reservoir-Type Calcitriol Transdermal Patch in Dairy Cattle. *J. Vet. Med. Sci.* **2009**, *71*, 845–848. [CrossRef]
59. Prüfer, K.; Jirikowski, G.F. Liposomal incorporation changes the effect of 1.25-dihydroxyvitamin D3 on the phospholipase C signal transduction pathway and the eicosanoid cascade on keratinocytes in vitro. *Biochem. Pharmacol.* **1996**, *51*, 247–252. [CrossRef]
60. Prüfer, K.; Merz, K.; Barth, A.; Wollina, U.; Sternberg, B. Interaction of Liposomal Incorporated Vitamin D3-Analogues and Human Keratinocytes. *J. Drug Target.* **1994**, *2*, 419–429. [CrossRef]
61. Knudsen, N.O.; Ronholt, S.; Salte, R.D.; Jorgensen, L.; Thormann, T.; Basse, L.H.; Hansen, J.; Frokjaer, S.; Foged, C. Calcipotriol delivery into the skin with PEGylated liposomes. *Eur. J. Pharm. Biopharm.* **2012**, *81*, 532–539. [CrossRef]
62. Merz, K.; Sternberg, B. Incorporation of Vitamin D3-Derivatives in Liposomes of Different Lipid Types. *J. Drug Target.* **1994**, *2*, 411–417. [CrossRef]
63. Knudsen, N.Ø.; Jorgensen, L.; Hansen, J.; Vermehren, C.; Frokjaer, S.; Foged, C. Targeting of liposome-associated calcipotriol to the skin: Effect of liposomal membrane fluidity and skin barrier integrity. *Int. J. Pharm.* **2011**, *416*, 478–485. [CrossRef]
64. Körbel, J.N.; Sebök, B.; Kerényi, M.; Mahrle, G. Enhancement of the Antiparakeratotic Potency of Calcitriol and Tacalcitol in Liposomal Preparations in the Mouse Tail Test. *Skin Pharmacol. Physiol.* **2001**, *14*, 291–295. [CrossRef]
65. Sonawane, R.; Harde, H.; Katariya, M.; Agrawal, S.; Jain, S. Solid lipid nanoparticles-loaded topical gel containing combination drugs: An approach to offset psoriasis. *Expert Opin. Drug Deliv.* **2014**, *11*, 1833–1847. [CrossRef]
66. Lalloz, A.; Bolzinger, M.-A.; Faivre, J.; Latreille, P.-L.; Garcia Ac, A.; Rakotovao, C.; Rabanel, J.-M.; Hildgen, P.; Banquy, X.; Briançon, S. Effect of surface chemistry of polymeric nanoparticles on cutaneous penetration of cholecalciferol. *Int. J. Pharm.* **2018**, *553*, 120–131. [CrossRef]
67. Wu, X.Y.; Zhou, T.; Cao, N.; Ni, J.; Wang, X. Role of Vitamin D Metabolism and Activity on Carcinogenesis. *Oncol. Res.* **2015**, *22*, 129–137. [CrossRef]
68. Mondul, A.M.; Weinstein, S.J.; Layne, T.M.; Albanes, D. Vitamin D and Cancer Risk and Mortality: State of the Science, Gaps, and Challenges. *Epidemiol. Rev.* **2017**, *39*, 28–48. [CrossRef]
69. Xu, J.; Wang, Y.; Zhang, Y.; Dang, S.; He, S. Astemizole promotes the anti-tumor effect of vitamin D through inhibiting miR-125a-5p-meidated regulation of VDR in HCC. *Biomed. Pharm.* **2018**, *107*, 1682–1691. [CrossRef]

70. Sabzichi, M.; Mohammadian, J.; Mohammadi, M.; Jahanfar, F.; Movassagh Pour, A.; Hamishehkar, H.; Ostad-Rahimi, A. Vitamin D-Loaded Nanostructured Lipid Carrier (NLC): A New Strategy for Enhancing Efficacy of Doxorubicin in Breast Cancer Treatment. *Nutr. Cancer* **2017**, *69*, 840–848. [CrossRef]
71. Maayah, Z.H.; Zhang, T.; Forrest, M.L.; Alrushaid, S.; Doschak, M.R.; Davies, N.M.; El-Kadi, A.O.S. DOX-Vit D, a Novel Doxorubicin Delivery Approach, Inhibits Human Osteosarcoma Cell Proliferation by Inducing Apoptosis While Inhibiting Akt and mTOR Signaling Pathways. *Pharmaceutics* **2018**, *10*, 144. [CrossRef]
72. Almouazen, E.; Bourgeois, S.; Jordheim, L.P.; Fessi, H.; Briancon, S. Nano-encapsulation of Vitamin D-3 Active Metabolites for Application in Chemotherapy: Formulation Study and in Vitro Evaluation. *Pharm. Res.* **2013**, *30*, 1137–1146. [CrossRef] [PubMed]
73. Ramalho, M.J.; Loureiro, J.A.; Gomes, B.; Frasco, M.F.; Coelho, M.A.N.; Pereira, M.C. PLGA nanoparticles as a platform for vitamin D-based cancer therapy. *Beilstein J. Nanotechnol.* **2015**, *6*, 1306–1318. [CrossRef] [PubMed]
74. Vora, L.; Sita, V.G.; Vavia, P. Zero order controlled release delivery of cholecalciferol from injectable biodegradable microsphere: In-vitro characterization and in-vivo pharmacokinetic studies. *Eur. J. Pharm. Sci.* **2017**, *107*, 78–86. [CrossRef]
75. Nguyen, T.L.U.; Tey, S.Y.; Pourgholami, M.H.; Morris, D.L.; Davis, T.P.; Barner-Kowollik, C.; Stenzel, M.H. Synthesis of semi-biodegradable crosslinked microspheres for the delivery of 1,25 dihydroxyvitamin D3 for the treatment of hepatocellular carcinoma. *Eur. Polymer. J.* **2007**, *43*, 1754–1767. [CrossRef]
76. Liu, C.; Shaurova, T.; Shoemaker, S.; Petkovich, M.; Hershberger, P.A.; Wu, Y. Tumor-Targeted Nanoparticles Deliver a Vitamin D-Based Drug Payload for the Treatment of EGFR Tyrosine Kinase Inhibitor-Resistant Lung Cancer. *Mol. Pharm.* **2018**, *15*, 3216–3226. [CrossRef]
77. Maleklou, N.; Allameh, A.; Kazemi, B. Targeted delivery of vitamin D3-loaded nanoparticles to C6 glioma cell line increased resistance to doxorubicin, epirubicin, and docetaxel in vitro. *Vitro Cell. Dev. Biol. Anim.* **2016**, *52*, 989–1000. [CrossRef]
78. Wang, H.; Chen, W.; Li, D.; Yin, X.; Zhang, X.; Olsen, N.; Zheng, S.G. Vitamin D and Chronic Diseases. *Aging Dis.* **2017**, *8*, 346–353. [CrossRef]
79. Da Silveira, K.L.; da Silveira, L.L.; Thorstenberg, M.L.P.; Cabral, F.L.; Castilhos, L.G.; Rezer, J.F.P.; de Andrade, D.F.; Beck, R.C.R.; Einloft Palma, H.; de Andrade, C.M.; et al. Free and nanoencapsulated vitamin D3: Effects on E-NTPDase and E-ADA activities in an animal model with induced arthritis. *Cell Biochem. Function* **2016**, *34*, 262–273. [CrossRef]
80. Wei-hong, T.; Min-chang, G.; Zhen, X.; Jie, S. Pharmacological and Pharmacokinetic Studies with Vitamin D-loaded Nanoemulsions in Asthma Model. *Inflammation* **2014**, *37*, 723–728. [CrossRef]
81. Goff, J.P.; Koszewski, N.J.; Haynes, J.S.; Horst, R.L. Targeted delivery of vitamin D to the colon using β-glucuronides of vitamin D: Therapeutic effects in a murine model of inflammatory bowel disease. *Am. J. Physiol. Gastrointest. Liver Physiol.* **2012**, *302*, G460–G469. [CrossRef]
82. Castoldi, A.; Herr, C.; Niederstraßer, J.; Labouta, H.I.; Melero, A.; Gordon, S.; Schneider-Daum, N.; Bals, R.; Lehr, C.-M. Calcifediol-loaded liposomes for local treatment of pulmonary bacterial infections. *Eur. J. Pharm. Biopharm.* **2017**, *118*, 62–67. [CrossRef] [PubMed]
83. Li, H.; Wang, Q.; Xiao, Y.; Bao, C.; Li, W. 25-Hydroxyvitamin D(3)-Loaded PLA Microspheres: In Vitro Characterization and Application in Diabetic Periodontitis Models. *AAPS PharmSciTech* **2013**, *14*, 880–889. [CrossRef] [PubMed]
84. Li, H.; Li, B.; Wang, Q.; Xiao, Y.; Chen, X.M.; Li, W. Attenuation of Inflammatory Response by 25-hydroxyvitamin D3-loaded Polylactic Acid Microspheres in Treatment of Periodontitis in Diabetic Rats. *Chin. J. Dent. Res.* **2014**, *17*, 91–98. [PubMed]
85. Ślusarczyk, J.; Piotrowski, M.; Szczepanowicz, K.; Regulska, M.; Leśkiewicz, M.; Warszyński, P.; Budziszewska, B.; Lasoń, W.; Basta-Kaim, A. Nanocapsules with Polyelectrolyte Shell as a Platform for 1,25-dihydroxyvitamin D3 Neuroprotection: Study in Organotypic Hippocampal Slices. *Neurotox. Res.* **2016**, *30*, 581–592. [CrossRef] [PubMed]

7

Vitamin E Bioavailability: Mechanisms of Intestinal Absorption in the Spotlight

Emmanuelle Reboul

Aix Marseille University, INRA, INSERM, C2VN, 13005 Marseille, France; Emmanuelle.Reboul@univ-amu.fr

Abstract: Vitamin E is an essential fat-soluble micronutrient whose effects on human health can be attributed to both antioxidant and non-antioxidant properties. A growing number of studies aim to promote vitamin E bioavailability in foods. It is thus of major interest to gain deeper insight into the mechanisms of vitamin E absorption, which remain only partly understood. It was long assumed that vitamin E was absorbed by passive diffusion, but recent data has shown that this process is actually far more complex than previously thought. This review describes the fate of vitamin E in the human gastrointestinal lumen during digestion and focuses on the proteins involved in the intestinal membrane and cellular transport of vitamin E across the enterocyte. Special attention is also given to the factors modulating both vitamin E micellarization and absorption. Although these latest results significantly improve our understanding of vitamin E intestinal absorption, further studies are still needed to decipher the molecular mechanisms driving this multifaceted process.

Keywords: tocopherol; intestine; mixed micelles; dietary lipids; food matrix; membrane transporters; uptake; enterocytes; chylomicrons; HDL; fat-soluble vitamins

---

1. Introduction

Tocochromanols, a subset of isoprenoids better known as vitamin E, include four tocopherols and four tocotrienols (Figure 1). These lipophilic antioxidants are synthesized by plants and other photosynthetic organisms only [1]. The base of the molecule of tocopherol is a hydroxychromane nucleus upon which a phytyl saturated chain of 16 carbon atoms is fixed. Three of these carbons are asymmetric, which entails the possibility of the existence of eight stereoisomers. The different tocopherols are distinguished from each other by the number and the position of the methyl groups attached to the nucleus. RRR-α-tocopherol is the most common in nature and the tocopherol with the highest biological activity. In biological tests for vitamin evaluation (fetal resorption tests), β and γ-tocopherol display a reduced vitamin activity (from 15 to 30%), and δ-tocopherol is almost inactive. Tocotrienols are distinguished from tocopherols by the presence of three double bonds on the side chain. Only α and β-tocotrienol appear to have a significant vitamin activity [2].

The hydroxychromane nucleus of vitamin E can react with peroxyl radicals, generating a hydroperoxide (which can be inactivated by specific enzymes) and a tocopheryl radical (which can be regenerated by vitamin C or coenzyme Q10). This property places vitamin E at the forefront of anti-radical defense systems [2]. However, the beneficial effects of vitamin E in human health may also be due to the ability of its phosphorylated metabolite to modulate signal transduction and gene expression in numerous conditions, including inflammation and immune system disorders [3].

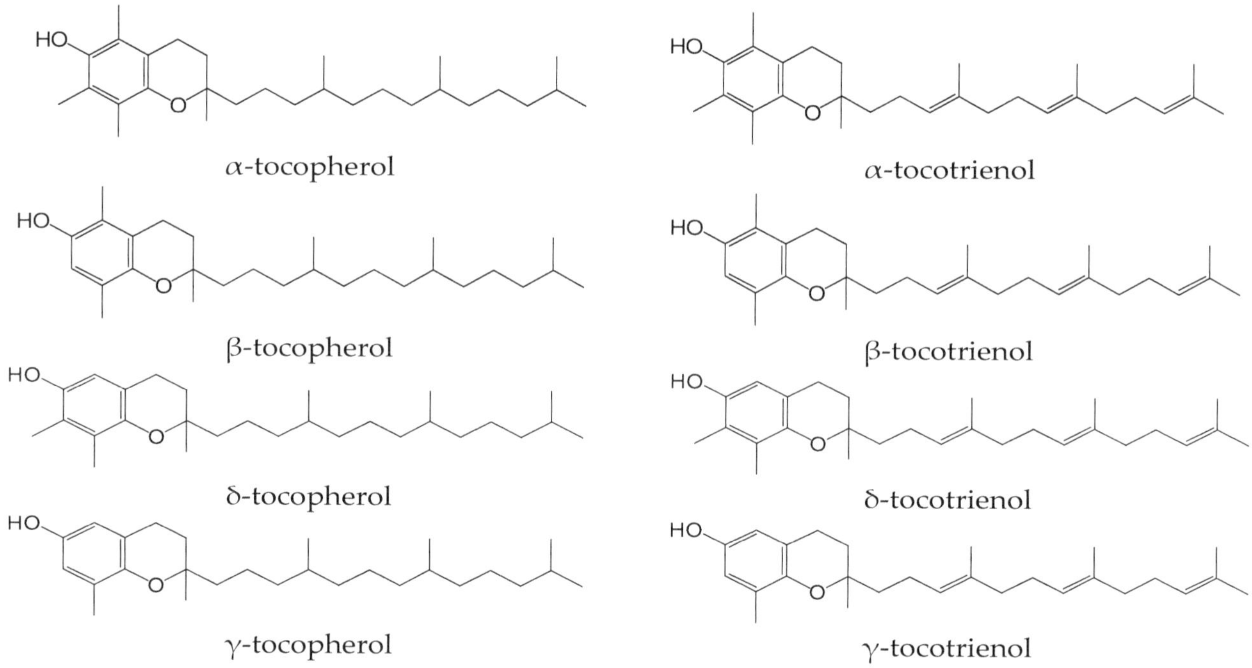

Figure 1. Vitamin E vitamers.

The main sources of vitamin E are vegetable oils and seeds. It can also be found in smaller quantities in some fruits and vegetables (Table 1). In France and Europe in general, α-tocopherol is the most consumed vitamin E vitamer [2], while in the US, it is γ-tocopherol [4].

Table 1. Vitamin E food content [2,5]. Average values in brackets.

Foods	Vitamin E Content (mg/100 g)
Sunflower oil	0.1–90 (58.3)
Sunflower seeds	0.01–57.6 (42.3)
Other vegetal oils	0.1–30
Almonds	0.01–24 (14.6)
Butter	1.5–2.3 (2.11)
Fatty fish	0.9–2
Fruits and vegetables (spinach, tomatoes, etc.)	0.8–2

In Europe, the Recommended Dietary Allowance (RDA) for vitamin E is 11 mg per day (as an α-tocopherol-equivalent) for women and 13 mg per day for men [6], while the RDA is 15 mg for all adults in the US [7]. Although there are no real vitamin E deficiencies in Western countries, three surveys carried out in France (Burgundy, ESVITAF, and Val-de-Marne surveys) showed that more than 30% of French people consumed less than 8 mg of vitamin E a day [8], which was recently confirmed in other European countries [9] as well as in the US, where over 90% of the population do not consume the estimated average requirements [10]. As recently shown, the low dietary intake of vitamin E may be worsened by the low stability of vitamin E in vegetable oils [11].

2. Vitamin E Digestion Process

2.1. The Fate of Vitamin E in the Gastrointestinal Tract

The first phase of the digestion–absorption process is the dissolution of vitamin E in the lipid phase of the meal. This phase is then emulsified into lipid droplets at both gastric and duodenal levels. No metabolism of vitamin E (i.e., degradation or absorption) appears to exist in the stomach.

In addition, the size of the droplets does not seem to have any effect on the efficiency of the subsequent absorption of the vitamin E in healthy humans [12].

In the duodenum, vitamin E is incorporated, along with lipid digestion products, in mixed micelles, structures that are theoretically essential for its absorption by the enterocyte. Indeed, mixed micelles can solubilize hydrophobic components and diffuse into the unstirred water layer (glycocalix) to approach the brush border membrane of the enterocytes.

2.2. Factors Affecting Vitamin E Transfer to Mixed Micelles

Numerous factors can affect vitamin E bioaccessibility (i.e., the fraction of vitamin E recovered in the mixed micelles compared to the initial amount of vitamin E provided by the meal) and thus in turn vitamin E bioavailability. The main factor is the food matrix in which vitamin E is embedded. For instance, it was shown that vitamin E bioaccessibility was low in apples but almost total in bananas, bread, or lettuce [13], and that vitamin E from durum wheat pasta was more bioaccessible than from pasta containing 10% eggs [14]. Unfortunately, it was not possible to identify the biochemical parameters of green leafy vegetables (cell-wall content, pectin, tannin, ...) governing α-tocopherol bioaccessibility [15]. However, as for other lipid micronutrients, matrix disruption can enhance vitamin E transfer to mixed micelles [16], while thermal or high pressure treatments have either no or negative effects [17].

Another important factor determining vitamin E bioaccessibility is the amount of fat provided in the meal, as fat likely facilitates vitamin E extraction from its food matrix, stimulates biliary secretion, and promotes micelle formation. It was first shown that various fats and oils, as well as long-chain triacylglycerols, did not significantly enhance vitamin E bioaccessibility. This was in contrast to more hydrophobic microconstituents such as β-carotene [18]. However, further data consistently showed that tocopherol acetate bioaccessibility was higher in long-chain rather than medium-chain triglyceride emulsions, probably due to a greater solubilization capacity of mixed micelles formed from long chain fatty acids and an enhanced conversion into tocopherol [19–21]. Vitamin E bioaccessibility was also increased by the presence of phospholipids [22].

2.3. Vitamin E Ester Hydrolysis

It is acknowledged that only the free forms of vitamin E are absorbed by the intestinal mucosa, suggesting that the esterified forms are hydrolyzed beforehand. This hydrolysis is probably carried out by cholesteryl ester hydrolase, also known as bile salt-dependent lipase [23]. Conversely to what we observed for retinyl esters [24], neither pancreatic lipase nor pancreatic lipase-related protein 2 were able to hydrolyze tocopheryl esters [25]. Surprisingly, it has been recently reported that α-tocopherol acetate absorption was equivalent to that of free α-tocopherol in the absence of both digestive enzymes and bile salts in healthy subjects [26]. This result signifies that enzymes originating from the enterocytes, such as endoplasmic reticulum esterases [27], are able to realize this hydrolysis in a very efficient manner.

3. Vitamin E Absorption Mechanisms by the Enterocyte

3.1. Apical Transport at the Brush Border Level

When approaching the brush border membrane, mixed micelles are supposed to dissociate due to the existing pH gradient. The released constituents can then be captured by different more or less specific systems to be absorbed by the enterocyte. For more than 30 years, due to the first results obtained in rat intestinal everted sacs [28,29], vitamin E absorption has been considered to occur by passive diffusion through enterocyte apical membrane. However, we showed for the first time in 2006 that α- and γ-tocopherol absorption was mediated, at least partly, by scavenger receptor class B type I (SR-BI) [30]. It was also shown that NPC1 like intracellular cholesterol transporter 1 (NPC1L1) was involved in α-tocopherol [31,32] and γ-tocotrienol [33] absorption. We finally highlighted the additional role of CD36 molecule (CD36) in the tocopherol absorption process [34].

These three membrane proteins have primarily been described as cholesterol transporters in the intestine [35,36]. However, they do display a relatively broad substrate specificity. Besides cholesterol, SRBI can mediate carotenoid [37,38], vitamin D [39], and K [40] transport; NPC1L1 is involved in phytosterols [41], vitamin D [39], K [42] and lutein [43] uptake; and CD36 is involved in very long chain fatty acid [44], vitamin D [39], K [40] and carotenoid [37] absorption. It is thus not surprising that they are involved in vitamin E uptake as well. Both SR-BI [45] and NPC1L1 [46] were showed to traffic in clathrin-coated lipid vesicles after a lipid load. The fact that these transporters seem to selectively mediate the transport of some molecules present in mixed micelles is an argument in favor of a direct interaction with their ligands. Interestingly, it was recently demonstrated that α-tocopherol competed with cholesterol to bind to the NPC1L1-N terminal domain, promoting NPC1L1 endocytosis [47].

CD36 [48] and SR-BI [49] have recently been described as intestinal lipid sensors, and they appear to be key modulators of chylomicron secretion [50,51]. These roles suggest that their impact on vitamin E transport may actually be a consequence of their role in other lipid absorption process. Indeed, by promoting lipid fluxes through the enterocyte, these receptors would create a driving force for absorption of minor lipids such as micronutrients, due to the lipid gradient.

We observed that the presence of tocopherol in structures mimicking mixed micelles (i.e., containing a biliary salt and at least oleic acid) was necessary for transporter-dependent absorption in Caco-2 cells [32]. This is in agreement with another study in which we showed that both SR-BI and CD36 extracellular loops were able to bind postprandial mixed micelles in a more efficient manner than interprandial micelles [52]. However, this does not indicate whether this interaction is the first step of either a sensing or an absorptive process—or if the two phenomena are coexisting.

Finally, it is worth mentioning that we observed that vitamin E could be effluxed back to the lumen after being absorbed in Caco-2 cells. This efflux was SR-BI-dependent and was increased in the presence of acceptors, e.g., mixed micelles that did not contain vitamin E [30]. The in vivo relevance of such observation should be further investigated.

3.2. Vitamin E Trafficking across the Enterocyte

Once absorbed, the fate of vitamin E across the enterocyte has been poorly described. Being hydrophobic, vitamin E likely localizes into organelle membranes, cytosolic lipid droplets, or traffic bound to binding proteins. Subcellular localization revealed that vitamin E could accumulate in microsomal membranes, i.e., the endoplasmic reticulum, Golgi, lysosomal and peroxisomal membranes [53]. However, it should be noted that in this study, vitamin E was delivered to cells with Tween 40, which may have influenced its targeting within the cells compared to a delivery in its physiological vehicles (i.e., mixed micelles).

Targeting to microsomal membranes may occur either via clathrin-coated vesicles as mentioned above, or thanks to the intervention of cytosolic carriers. A tocopherol-associated protein (TAP) expressed in the intestine has been shown to bind vitamin E in human tissues [54], but it actually displays a weak affinity towards tocopherols [55]. Sec14p-like proteins TAP1, 2 and 3, also expressed in the human intestine, are probably better candidates as they improved tocopherol transport to mitochondria as efficiently as the α-tocopherol transport protein (α-TTP) [56]. Additional research is needed to definitely confirm their role in the enterocyte.

3.3. Basolateral Secretion to the Lymph or to the Blood Circulation

Most of the vitamin E is incorporated into chylomicrons in its free form at the Golgi apparatus level before being released to the lymph.

In mice, it has been showed that in addition to this apolipoprotein-B (apoB)-dependent route, an non-apoB pathway could exist [57]. This non-apoB route involves ATB-binding cassette A1 (ABCA1) that allows the secretion of vitamin E via intestinal High Density Lipoproteins (HDL) [58], and maybe the ATP binding cassette sub-family G member 1 ABCG1 [59,60]. However, this pathway seems to remain minor in humans. Indeed, mutations in microsomal triglyceride transfer protein (MTP) or in secretion-associated Ras related GTPase 1B (SAR1B), lead to abetalipoproteinemia and chylomicron retention diseases, respectively [61]. These pathologies, characterized by a lack of chylomicrons, are associated with a massive impairment of vitamin E absorption that is not balanced by another pathway [62,63].

3.4. Vitamin E Absorption Site in the Intestine

It has long been assumed that vitamin E, as with other lipids and lipid micronutrients, is absorbed in the upper half of the small intestine [64]. However, recent work from our laboratory highlighted that vitamin E absorption was in fact mainly located in the distal part of mouse small intestine, i.e., in the distal jejunum and the ileum [32,65]. This data seems conflicting with the fact that identified vitamin E intestinal transporters, i.e., scavenger receptors and NPC1L1, have been described as mainly expressed in the duodenum and the jejunum, respectively [36,66,67]. However, this can be partly explained by the subcellular localization of these proteins. For instance, SR-BI is mostly expressed at the apical side of the duodenal enterocytes, but it is present on the basolateral surface of the distal intestine [68]. Besides, a postmortem study in humans showed that the expression of CD36, NPC1L1, and ABCA1 was highly variable and displayed a bell-shape pattern, with the highest levels in the ileum [69].

3.5. Factors Modulating Vitamin E Absorption by the Intestinal Cell

As for vitamin E transfer to mixed micelles, numerous factors can influence vitamin E transport across the intestinal cell, which likely explains the important variations observed regarding vitamin E absorption efficiency. Indeed, different studies report efficiency in ranges of 10–95% [70–72]. However when deuterium-labeled vitamin E was used to assess absorption, this range was reduced to 10–33% [73].

The intestine does not seem to specifically discriminate between vitamin E stereoisomers [74], or between α- and γ-tocopherol [30,75]. However, a study found a higher absorption of α-tocopherol compared to γ- and δ-tocopherol in lymph-cannulated rats [76], which is consistent with the existence of a ω-hydroxylase that preferentially metabolized these two last vitamers in $3'$ and $5'$ carboxychromanol metabolites that can be excreted in the urine [77].

The food matrix can also influence specifically this step of vitamin E absorption. The presence of fibers did not modify vitamin E absorption in humans [78,79]. Conversely, lipids can be classified as effectors of vitamin E absorption as they can promote chylomicron formation. It is interesting to note that a minimal quantity of fat of 3 g was required for an optimal tocopherol absorption, and that increasing further this amount did not led to a better vitamin E bioavailability [80]. This was partly confirmed in another trial where α-tocopherol-acetate was almost negligible when ingested with 2.7 g fat [81]. However, these data are conflicting with other studies showing that the higher the amount of fat, the better vitamin E absorption [73,82], or conversely that dairy fat from whole milk does not increase vitamin E absorption compared to low-fat milk [83]. Mono and polyunsaturated fatty acid seem to promote vitamin E absorption compared to saturated fatty acids in cockerels [84] and in Caco-2 cells [85]. Conversely, phosphatidylcholine decreased α-tocopherol absorption efficiency in rats [86,87], an effect that was reversed by the presence of lysophosphatidylcholine [86]. Authors suggested that vitamin E was associated with phospholipids, leading to a low uptake. As we showed that the presence of phosphatidylcholine in mixed micelles was associated with a decreased binding of mixed micelles on scavenger receptor extracellular loops [52], we suggest that neutral phospholipids can also impact vitamin E absorption by modifying micellar interaction with the membrane proteins responsible for its uptake.

We showed that α-tocopherol E could compete for absorption with other lipid micronutrients such as γ-tocopherol and carotenoids [30,88], as well as vitamin A, D, and K [65] in Caco-2 cells. Except for vitamin A, these competitions are presumably due to common uptake pathways involving cholesterol transporters. Vitamin A uptake mechanisms are still unknown. However, it has been hypothesized that vitamin E was protecting vitamin A against oxidation in the intestine, leading to vitamin E degradation and reduced absorption in chickens [89]. Polyphenols such as naringenin could also reduce vitamin E uptake in Caco-2 cells [88]. The underlying mechanisms still need to be resolved, but we can suggest that polyphenols can impair (micro) nutrient absorption by interfering with membrane protein functioning, as previously shown with digestive enzymes [90]. Although this is still debated [91], a study showed that phytosterols (2.2 g per day during 1 week) could inhibit vitamin E absorption in normocholesterolemic subjects [92].

Finally, it is noteworthy that genetic factors including polymorphisms in genes coding for vitamin E and lipid intestinal metabolism such as SR-BI, CD36, ABCA1, ABCG1, or apoB have been associated with a modulation of vitamin E bioavailability in humans [93].

4. Conclusions

Overall, this review highlights the fact that the molecular mechanisms of both intraluminal fate and intestinal absorption of vitamin E are only partly understood to date. The discovery of vitamin E intestinal transporters with broad substrate specificity has raised many questions with respect to the potential interactions with dietary lipids during the vitamin E absorption process. Besides, it is likely that other proteins involved in vitamin E absorption still remain to be identified. The modulation of the activity of these proteins, including the existence of functional polymorphisms in their encoding genes and the regulation of their expression levels by epigenetic to post-translational factors, may explain much of the observed large interindividual variation in postprandial responses to vitamin E. Further dedicated investigations are needed to address these presumptions in order to offer adequate vitamin E-tailored recommendations to individuals.

References

1. DellaPenna, D. A decade of progress in understanding vitamin E synthesis in plants. *J. Plant Physiol.* **2005**, *162*, 729–737. [CrossRef] [PubMed]
2. Martin, A. *Apports Nutritionnels Conseillés Pour la Population Française*, 3rd ed.; Tec & Doc. Lavoisier: Paris, France, 2001; p. 605.
3. Azzi, A.; Meydani, S.N.; Meydani, M.; Zingg, J.M. The rise, the fall and the renaissance of vitamin E. *Arch. Biochem. Biophys.* **2016**, *595*, 100–108. [CrossRef] [PubMed]
4. Jiang, Q.; Christen, S.; Shigenaga, M.K.; Ames, B.N. gamma-Tocopherol, the major form of vitamin E in the US diet, deserves more attention. *Am. J. Clin. Nutr.* **2001**, *74*, 714–722. [PubMed]
5. Table de Composition Nutritionnelle des Aliments Ciqual. 2016. Available online: https://www.anses.fr/fr/content/ciqual-la-table-de-composition-nutritionnelle-des-aliments (accessed on 31 October 2017).
6. EFSA Panel on Dietetic Products, Nutrition, and Allergies (NDA). Dietary Reference Values for vitamin E as α-tocopherol. *EFSA J.* **2015**, *13*. [CrossRef]
7. Medicine, I.O. *Dietary Reference Intakes for Vitamin C, Vitamin E, Selenium, and Carotenoids*; The National Academies Press: Washington, DC, USA, 2000; p. 529.
8. De Carvalho, M.J.; Guilland, J.C.; Moreau, D.; Boggio, V.; Fuchs, F. Vitamin status of healthy subjects in Burgundy (France). *Ann. Nutr. Metab.* **1996**, *40*, 24–51. [CrossRef] [PubMed]
9. Troesch, B.; Hoeft, B.; McBurney, M.; Eggersdorfer, M.; Weber, P. Dietary surveys indicate vitamin intakes below recommendations are common in representative western countries. *Br. J. Nutr.* **2012**, *108*, 692–698. [CrossRef] [PubMed]
10. Traber, M.G. Vitamin E inadequacy in humans: Causes and consequences. *Adv. Nutr.* **2014**, *5*, 503–514. [CrossRef] [PubMed]
11. Pignitter, M.; Stolze, K.; Gartner, S.; Dumhart, B.; Stoll, C.; Steiger, G.; Kraemer, K.; Somoza, V. Cold fluorescent light as major inducer of lipid oxidation in soybean oil stored at household conditions for eight weeks. *J. Agric. Food Chem.* **2014**, *62*, 2297–2305. [CrossRef] [PubMed]

12. Borel, P.; Pasquier, B.; Armand, M.; Tyssandier, V.; Grolier, P.; Alexandre-Gouabau, M.C.; Andre, M.; Senft, M.; Peyrot, J.; Jaussan, V.; et al. Processing of vitamin A and E in the human gastrointestinal tract. *Am. J. Physiol. Gastrointest. Liver Physiol.* **2001**, *280*, G95–G103. [PubMed]
13. Reboul, E.; Richelle, M.; Perrot, E.; Desmoulins-Malezet, C.; Pirisi, V.; Borel, P. Bioaccessibility of carotenoids and vitamin E from their main dietary sources. *J. Agric. Food Chem.* **2006**, *54*, 8749–8755. [CrossRef] [PubMed]
14. Werner, S.; Bohm, V. Bioaccessibility of carotenoids and vitamin e from pasta: Evaluation of an in vitro digestion model. *J. Agric. Food Chem.* **2011**, *59*, 1163–1170. [CrossRef] [PubMed]
15. Sriwichai, W.; Berger, J.; Picq, C.; Avallone, S. Determining Factors of Lipophilic Micronutrient Bioaccessibility in Several Leafy Vegetables. *J. Agric. Food Chem.* **2016**, *64*, 1695–1701. [CrossRef] [PubMed]
16. Mandalari, G.; Faulks, R.M.; Rich, G.T.; Lo Turco, V.; Picout, D.R.; Lo Curto, R.B.; Bisignano, G.; Dugo, P.; Dugo, G.; Waldron, K.W.; et al. Release of protein, lipid, and vitamin E from almond seeds during digestion. *J. Agric. Food Chem.* **2008**, *56*, 3409–3416. [CrossRef] [PubMed]
17. Cilla, A.; Alegria, A.; de Ancos, B.; Sanchez-Moreno, C.; Cano, M.P.; Plaza, L.; Clemente, G.; Lagarda, M.J.; Barbera, R. Bioaccessibility of tocopherols, carotenoids, and ascorbic acid from milk- and soy-based fruit beverages: Influence of food matrix and processing. *J. Agric. Food Chem.* **2012**, *60*, 7282–7290. [CrossRef] [PubMed]
18. Nagao, A.; Kotake-Nara, E.; Hase, M. Effects of fats and oils on the bioaccessibility of carotenoids and vitamin E in vegetables. *Biosci. Biotechnol. Biochem.* **2013**, *77*, 1055–1060. [CrossRef] [PubMed]
19. Yang, Y.; McClements, D.J. Vitamin E bioaccessibility: Influence of carrier oil type on digestion and release of emulsified alpha-tocopherol acetate. *Food Chem.* **2013**, *141*, 473–481. [CrossRef] [PubMed]
20. Yang, Y.; Decker, E.A.; Xiao, H.; McClements, D.J. Enhancing vitamin E bioaccessibility: Factors impacting solubilization and hydrolysis of alpha-tocopherol acetate encapsulated in emulsion-based delivery systems. *Food Funct.* **2015**, *6*, 84–97. [CrossRef] [PubMed]
21. Yang, Y.; Xiao, H.; McClements, D.J. Impact of Lipid Phase on the Bioavailability of Vitamin E in Emulsion-Based Delivery Systems: Relative Importance of Bioaccessibility, Absorption, and Transformation. *J. Agric. Food Chem.* **2017**, *65*, 3946–3955. [CrossRef] [PubMed]
22. Yang, Y.; McClements, D.J. Vitamin E and vitamin E acetate solubilization in mixed micelles: Physicochemical basis of bioaccessibility. *J. Colloid Interface Sci.* **2013**, *405*, 312–321. [CrossRef] [PubMed]
23. Lombardo, D.; Guy, O. Studies on the substrate specificity of a carboxyl ester hydrolase from human pancreatic juice. II. Action on cholesterol esters and lipid-soluble vitamin esters. *Biochim. Biophys. Acta* **1980**, *611*, 147–155. [CrossRef]
24. Reboul, E.; Berton, A.; Moussa, M.; Kreuzer, C.; Crenon, I.; Borel, P. Pancreatic lipase and pancreatic lipase-related protein 2, but not pancreatic lipase-related protein 1, hydrolyze retinyl palmitate in physiological conditions. *Biochim. Biophys. Acta* **2006**, *1761*, 4–10. [CrossRef] [PubMed]
25. Desmarchelier, C.; Tourniaire, F.; Preveraud, D.P.; Samson-Kremser, C.; Crenon, I.; Rosilio, V.; Borel, P. The distribution and relative hydrolysis of tocopheryl acetate in the different matrices coexisting in the lumen of the small intestine during digestion could explain its low bioavailability. *Mol. Nutr. Food Res.* **2013**, *57*, 1237–1245. [CrossRef] [PubMed]
26. Nagy, K.; Ramos, L.; Courtet-Compondu, M.C.; Braga-Lagache, S.; Redeuil, K.; Lobo, B.; Azpiroz, F.; Malagelada, J.R.; Beaumont, M.; Moulin, J.; et al. Double-balloon jejunal perfusion to compare absorption of vitamin E and vitamin E acetate in healthy volunteers under maldigestion conditions. *Eur. J. Clin. Nutr.* **2013**, *67*, 202–206. [CrossRef] [PubMed]
27. Mathias, P.M.; Harries, J.T.; Peters, T.J.; Muller, D.P. Studies on the in vivo absorption of micellar solutions of tocopherol and tocopheryl acetate in the rat: Demonstration and partial characterization of a mucosal esterase localized to the endoplasmic reticulum of the enterocyte. *J. Lipid Res.* **1981**, *22*, 829–837. [PubMed]
28. Muralidhara, K.S.; Hollander, D. Intestinal absorption of alpha-tocopherol in the unanesthetized rat. The influence of luminal constituents on the absorptive process. *J. Lab. Clin. Med.* **1977**, *90*, 85–91. [PubMed]
29. Hollander, D.; Rim, E.; Muralidhara, K.S. Mechanism and site of small intestinal absorption of alpha-tocopherol in the rat. *Gastroenterology* **1975**, *68*, 1492–1499. [PubMed]
30. Reboul, E.; Klein, A.; Bietrix, F.; Gleize, B.; Malezet-Desmoulins, C.; Schneider, M.; Margotat, A.; Lagrost, L.; Collet, X.; Borel, P. Scavenger receptor class B type I (SR-BI) is involved in vitamin E transport across the enterocyte. *J. Biol. Chem.* **2006**, *281*, 4739–4745. [CrossRef] [PubMed]

31. Narushima, K.; Takada, T.; Yamanashi, Y.; Suzuki, H. Niemann-pick C1-like 1 mediates alpha-tocopherol transport. *Mol. Pharmacol.* **2008**, *74*, 42–49. [CrossRef] [PubMed]
32. Reboul, E.; Soayfane, Z.; Goncalves, A.; Cantiello, M.; Bott, R.; Nauze, M.; Terce, F.; Collet, X.; Comera, C. Respective contributions of intestinal Niemann-Pick C1-like 1 and scavenger receptor class B type I to cholesterol and tocopherol uptake: In vivo v. in vitro studies. *Br. J. Nutr.* **2012**, *107*, 1296–1304. [CrossRef] [PubMed]
33. Abuasal, B.; Sylvester, P.W.; Kaddoumi, A. Intestinal absorption of gamma-tocotrienol is mediated by Niemann-Pick C1-like 1: In situ rat intestinal perfusion studies. *Drug Metab. Dispos.* **2010**, *38*, 939–945. [CrossRef] [PubMed]
34. Goncalves, A.; Roi, S.; Nowicki, M.; Niot, I.; Reboul, E. Cluster-determinant 36 (CD36) impacts on vitamin E postprandial response. *Mol. Nutr. Food Res.* **2014**, *58*, 2297–2306. [CrossRef] [PubMed]
35. Werder, M.; Han, C.H.; Wehrli, E.; Bimmler, D.; Schulthess, G.; Hauser, H. Role of scavenger receptors SR-BI and CD36 in selective sterol uptake in the small intestine. *Biochemistry* **2001**, *40*, 11643–11650. [CrossRef] [PubMed]
36. Altmann, S.W.; Davis, H.R., Jr.; Zhu, L.J.; Yao, X.; Hoos, L.M.; Tetzloff, G.; Iyer, S.P.; Maguire, M.; Golovko, A.; Zeng, M.; et al. Niemann-Pick C1 Like 1 protein is critical for intestinal cholesterol absorption. *Science* **2004**, *303*, 1201–1204. [CrossRef] [PubMed]
37. Borel, P.; Lietz, G.; Goncalves, A.; Szabo de Edelenyi, F.; Lecompte, S.; Curtis, P.; Goumidi, L.; Caslake, M.J.; Miles, E.A.; Packard, C.; et al. CD36 and SR-BI Are Involved in Cellular Uptake of Provitamin A Carotenoids by Caco-2 and HEK Cells, and Some of Their Genetic Variants Are Associated with Plasma Concentrations of These Micronutrients in Humans. *J. Nutr.* **2013**, *143*, 448–456. [CrossRef] [PubMed]
38. Reboul, E.; Abou, L.; Mikail, C.; Ghiringhelli, O.; Andre, M.; Portugal, H.; Jourdheuil-Rahmani, D.; Amiot, M.J.; Lairon, D.; Borel, P. Lutein transport by Caco-2 TC-7 cells occurs partly by a facilitated process involving the scavenger receptor class B type I (SR-BI). *Biochem. J.* **2005**, *387*, 455–461. [CrossRef] [PubMed]
39. Reboul, E.; Goncalves, A.; Comera, C.; Bott, R.; Nowicki, M.; Landrier, J.F.; Jourdheuil-Rahmani, D.; Dufour, C.; Collet, X.; Borel, P. Vitamin D intestinal absorption is not a simple passive diffusion: Evidences for involvement of cholesterol transporters. *Mol. Nutr. Food Res.* **2011**, *55*, 691–702. [CrossRef] [PubMed]
40. Goncalves, A.; Margier, M.; Roi, S.; Collet, X.; Niot, I.; Goupy, P.; Caris-Veyrat, C.; Reboul, E. Intestinal scavenger receptors are involved in vitamin K1 absorption. *J. Biol. Chem.* **2014**, *289*, 30743–30752. [CrossRef] [PubMed]
41. Davis, H.R., Jr.; Zhu, L.J.; Hoos, L.M.; Tetzloff, G.; Maguire, M.; Liu, J.; Yao, X.; Iyer, S.P.; Lam, M.H.; Lund, E.G.; et al. Niemann-Pick C1 Like 1 (NPC1L1) is the intestinal phytosterol and cholesterol transporter and a key modulator of whole-body cholesterol homeostasis. *J. Biol. Chem.* **2004**, *279*, 33586–33592. [CrossRef] [PubMed]
42. Takada, T.; Yamanashi, Y.; Konishi, K.; Yamamoto, T.; Toyoda, Y.; Masuo, Y.; Yamamoto, H.; Suzuki, H. NPC1L1 is a key regulator of intestinal vitamin K absorption and a modulator of warfarin therapy. *Sci. Transl. Med.* **2015**, *7*. [CrossRef] [PubMed]
43. Sato, Y.; Suzuki, R.; Kobayashi, M.; Itagaki, S.; Hirano, T.; Noda, T.; Mizuno, S.; Sugawara, M.; Iseki, K. Involvement of cholesterol membrane transporter Niemann-Pick C1-like 1 in the intestinal absorption of lutein. *J. Pharm. Pharm. Sci.* **2012**, *15*, 256–264. [CrossRef] [PubMed]
44. Drover, V.A.; Nguyen, D.V.; Bastie, C.C.; Darlington, Y.F.; Abumrad, N.A.; Pessin, J.E.; London, E.; Sahoo, D.; Phillips, M.C. CD36 mediates both cellular uptake of very long chain fatty acids and their intestinal absorption in mice. *J. Biol. Chem.* **2008**, *283*, 13108–13115. [CrossRef] [PubMed]
45. Hansen, G.H.; Niels-Christiansen, L.L.; Immerdal, L.; Danielsen, E.M. Scavenger receptor class B type I (SR-BI) in pig enterocytes: Trafficking from the brush border to lipid droplets during fat absorption. *Gut* **2003**, *52*, 1424–1431. [CrossRef] [PubMed]
46. Ge, L.; Wang, J.; Qi, W.; Miao, H.H.; Cao, J.; Qu, Y.X.; Li, B.L.; Song, B.L. The cholesterol absorption inhibitor ezetimibe acts by blocking the sterol-induced internalization of NPC1L1. *Cell Metab.* **2008**, *7*, 508–519. [CrossRef] [PubMed]
47. Kamishikiryo, J.; Haraguchi, M.; Nakashima, S.; Tasaka, Y.; Narahara, H.; Sugihara, N.; Nakamura, T.; Morita, T. N-terminal domain of the cholesterol transporter Niemann-Pick C1-like 1 (NPC1L1) is essential for alpha-tocopherol transport. *Biochem. Biophys. Res. Commun.* **2017**, *486*, 476–480. [CrossRef] [PubMed]

48. Tran, T.T.; Poirier, H.; Clement, L.; Nassir, F.; Pelsers, M.M.; Petit, V.; Degrace, P.; Monnot, M.C.; Glatz, J.F.; Abumrad, N.A.; et al. Luminal lipid regulates CD36 levels and downstream signaling to stimulate chylomicron synthesis. *J. Biol. Chem.* **2011**, *286*, 25201–25210. [CrossRef] [PubMed]
49. Beaslas, O.; Cueille, C.; Delers, F.; Chateau, D.; Chambaz, J.; Rousset, M.; Carriere, V. Sensing of dietary lipids by enterocytes: A new role for SR-BI/CLA-1. *PLoS ONE* **2009**, *4*, e4278. [CrossRef] [PubMed]
50. Buttet, M.; Traynard, V.; Tran, T.T.; Besnard, P.; Poirier, H.; Niot, I. From fatty-acid sensing to chylomicron synthesis: Role of intestinal lipid-binding proteins. *Biochimie* **2014**, *96*, 37–47. [CrossRef] [PubMed]
51. Briand, O.; Touche, V.; Colin, S.; Brufau, G.; Davalos, A.; Schonewille, M.; Bovenga, F.; Carriere, V.; de Boer, J.F.; Dugardin, C.; et al. Liver X Receptor Regulates Triglyceride Absorption Through Intestinal Down-regulation of Scavenger Receptor Class B, Type 1. *Gastroenterology* **2016**, *150*, 650–658. [CrossRef] [PubMed]
52. Goncalves, A.; Gontero, B.; Nowicki, M.; Margier, M.; Masset, G.; Amiot, M.J.; Reboul, E. Micellar lipid composition affects micelle interaction with class B scavenger receptor extracellular loops. *J. Lipid Res.* **2015**, *56*, 1123–1133. [CrossRef] [PubMed]
53. Anwar, K.; Kayden, H.J.; Hussain, M.M. Transport of vitamin E by differentiated Caco-2 cells. *J. Lipid Res.* **2006**, *47*, 1261–1273. [CrossRef] [PubMed]
54. Zimmer, S.; Stocker, A.; Sarbolouki, M.N.; Spycher, S.E.; Sassoon, J.; Azzi, A. A novel human tocopherol-associated protein—Cloning, in vitro expression, and characterization. *J. Biol. Chem.* **2000**, *275*, 25672–25680. [CrossRef] [PubMed]
55. Manor, D.; Atkinson, J. Is tocopherol associated protein a misnomer? *J. Nutr. Biochem* **2003**, *14*, 421–422. [CrossRef]
56. Zingg, J.M.; Kempna, P.; Paris, M.; Reiter, E.; Villacorta, L.; Cipollone, R.; Munteanu, A.; De Pascale, C.; Menini, S.; Cueff, A.; et al. Characterization of three human sec14p-like proteins: Alpha-tocopherol transport activity and expression pattern in tissues. *Biochimie* **2008**, *90*, 1703–1715. [CrossRef] [PubMed]
57. Anwar, K.; Iqbal, J.; Hussain, M.M. Mechanisms involved in vitamin E transport by primary enterocytes and in vivo absorption. *J. Lipid Res.* **2007**, *48*, 2028–2038. [CrossRef] [PubMed]
58. Reboul, E.; Trompier, D.; Moussa, M.; Klein, A.; Landrier, J.F.; Chimini, G.; Borel, P. ATP-binding cassette transporter A1 is significantly involved in the intestinal absorption of alpha- and gamma-tocopherol but not in that of retinyl palmitate in mice. *Am. J. Clin. Nutr.* **2009**, *89*, 177–184. [CrossRef] [PubMed]
59. Olivier, M.; Bott, G.R.; Frisdal, E.; Nowick, M.; Plengpanich, W.; Desmarchelier, C.; Roi, S.; Quinn, C.M.; Gelissen, I.; Jessup, W.; et al. ABCG1 is involved in vitamin E efflux. *Biochim. Biophys. Acta* **2014**, *1841*, 1741–1751. [CrossRef] [PubMed]
60. Nicod, N.; Parker, R.S. Vitamin E secretion by Caco-2 monolayers to APOA1, but not to HDL, is vitamer selective. *J. Nutr.* **2013**, *143*, 1565–1572. [CrossRef] [PubMed]
61. Ramasamy, I. Update on the molecular biology of dyslipidemias. *Clin. Chim. Acta* **2016**, *454*, 143–185. [CrossRef] [PubMed]
62. Cuerq, C.; Restier, L.; Drai, J.; Blond, E.; Roux, A.; Charriere, S.; Michalski, M.C.; Di Filippo, M.; Levy, E.; Lachaux, A.; et al. Establishment of reference values of alpha-tocopherol in plasma, red blood cells and adipose tissue in healthy children to improve the management of chylomicron retention disease, a rare genetic hypocholesterolemia. *Orphanet J. Rare Dis.* **2016**, *11*, 114. [CrossRef] [PubMed]
63. Burnett, J.R.; Hooper, A.J. Vitamin E and oxidative stress in abetalipoproteinemia and familial hypobetalipoproteinemia. *Free Radic. Biol. Med.* **2015**, *88*, 59–62. [CrossRef] [PubMed]
64. Reboul, E.; Borel, P. Proteins involved in uptake, intracellular transport and basolateral secretion of fat-soluble vitamins and carotenoids by mammalian enterocytes. *Prog. Lipid Res.* **2011**, *50*, 388–402. [CrossRef] [PubMed]
65. Goncalves, A.; Roi, S.; Nowicki, M.; Dhaussy, A.; Huertas, A.; Amiot, M.J.; Reboul, E. Fat-soluble vitamin intestinal absorption: Absorption sites in the intestine and interactions for absorption. *Food Chem.* **2015**, *172*, 155–160. [CrossRef] [PubMed]
66. Nassir, F.; Wilson, B.; Han, X.; Gross, R.W.; Abumrad, N.A. CD36 is important for fatty acid and cholesterol uptake by the proximal but not distal intestine. *J. Biol. Chem.* **2007**, *282*, 19493–19501. [CrossRef] [PubMed]
67. Bietrix, F.; Yan, D.; Nauze, M.; Rolland, C.; Bertrand-Michel, J.; Comera, C.; Schaak, S.; Barbaras, R.; Groen, A.K.; Perret, B.; et al. Accelerated lipid absorption in mice overexpressing intestinal SR-BI. *J. Biol. Chem.* **2006**, *281*, 7214–7219. [CrossRef] [PubMed]

68. Cai, S.F.; Kirby, R.J.; Howles, P.N.; Hui, D.Y. Differentiation-dependent expression and localization of the class B type I scavenger receptor in intestine. *J. Lipid Res.* **2001**, *42*, 902–909. [PubMed]
69. Masson, C.J.; Plat, J.; Mensink, R.P.; Namiot, A.; Kisielewski, W.; Namiot, Z.; Fullekrug, J.; Ehehalt, R.; Glatz, J.F.; Pelsers, M.M. Fatty acid- and cholesterol transporter protein expression along the human intestinal tract. *PLoS ONE* **2010**, *5*, e10380. [CrossRef] [PubMed]
70. Drevon, C.A. Absorption, transport and metabolism of vitamin E. *Free Radic. Res. Commun.* **1991**, *14*, 229–246. [CrossRef] [PubMed]
71. Traber, M.G.; Sies, H. Vitamin E in humans: Demand and delivery. *Annu. Rev. Nutr.* **1996**, *16*, 321–347. [CrossRef] [PubMed]
72. Cohn, W. Bioavailability of vitamin E. *Eur. J. Clin. Nutr.* **1997**, *51*, S80–S85. [PubMed]
73. Bruno, R.S.; Leonard, S.W.; Park, S.I.; Zhao, Y.; Traber, M.G. Human vitamin E requirements assessed with the use of apples fortified with deuterium-labeled alpha-tocopheryl acetate. *Am. J. Clin. Nutr.* **2006**, *83*, 299–304. [PubMed]
74. Traber, M.G.; Burton, G.W.; Ingold, K.U.; Kayden, H.J. RRR- and SRR-alpha-tocopherols are secreted without discrimination in human chylomicrons, but RRR-alpha-tocopherol is preferentially secreted in very low density lipoproteins. *J. Lipid Res.* **1990**, *31*, 675–685. [PubMed]
75. Traber, M.G.; Kayden, H.J. Preferential incorporation of alpha-tocopherol vs. gamma-tocopherol in human lipoproteins. *Am. J. Clin. Nutr.* **1989**, *49*, 517–526. [PubMed]
76. Porsgaard, T.; Hoy, C.E. Absorption by rats of tocopherols present in edible vegetable oils. *Lipids* **2000**, *35*, 1073–1078. [CrossRef] [PubMed]
77. Bardowell, S.A.; Ding, X.; Parker, R.S. Disruption of P450-mediated vitamin E hydroxylase activities alters vitamin E status in tocopherol supplemented mice and reveals extra-hepatic vitamin E metabolism. *J. Lipid Res.* **2012**, *53*, 2667–2676. [CrossRef] [PubMed]
78. Riedl, J.; Linseisen, J.; Hoffmann, J.; Wolfram, G. Some dietary fibers reduce the absorption of carotenoids in women. *J. Nutr.* **1999**, *129*, 2170–2176. [PubMed]
79. Greenwood, D.C.; Cade, J.E.; White, K.; Burley, V.J.; Schorah, C.J. The impact of high non-starch polysaccharide intake on serum micronutrient concentrations in a cohort of women. *Public Health Nutr.* **2004**, *7*, 543–548. [CrossRef] [PubMed]
80. Roodenburg, A.J.; Leenen, R.; van het Hof, K.H.; Weststrate, J.A.; Tijburg, L.B. Amount of fat in the diet affects bioavailability of lutein esters but not of alpha-carotene, beta-carotene, and vitamin E in humans. *Am. J. Clin. Nutr.* **2000**, *71*, 1187–1193. [PubMed]
81. Jeanes, Y.M.; Hall, W.L.; Ellard, S.; Lee, E.; Lodge, J.K. The absorption of vitamin E is influenced by the amount of fat in a meal and the food matrix. *Br. J. Nutr.* **2004**, *92*, 575–579. [CrossRef] [PubMed]
82. Kim, J.E.; Ferruzzi, M.G.; Campbell, W.W. Egg Consumption Increases Vitamin E Absorption from Co-Consumed Raw Mixed Vegetables in Healthy Young Men. *J. Nutr.* **2016**, *146*, 2199–2205. [CrossRef] [PubMed]
83. Mah, E.; Sapper, T.N.; Chitchumroonchokchai, C.; Failla, M.L.; Schill, K.E.; Clinton, S.K.; Bobe, G.; Traber, M.G.; Bruno, R.S. alpha-Tocopherol bioavailability is lower in adults with metabolic syndrome regardless of dairy fat co-ingestion: A randomized, double-blind, crossover trial. *Am. J. Clin. Nutr.* **2015**, *102*, 1070–1080. [CrossRef] [PubMed]
84. Preveraud, D.P.; Devillard, E.; Borel, P. Dietary fat modulates dl-alpha-tocopheryl acetate (vitamin E) bioavailability in adult cockerels. *Br. Poult. Sci.* **2015**, *56*, 94–102. [CrossRef] [PubMed]
85. Failla, M.L.; Chitchumronchokchai, C.; Ferruzzi, M.G.; Goltz, S.R.; Campbell, W.W. Unsaturated fatty acids promote bioaccessibility and basolateral secretion of carotenoids and alpha-tocopherol by Caco-2 cells. *Food Funct.* **2014**, *5*, 1101–1112. [CrossRef] [PubMed]
86. Koo, S.I.; Noh, S.K. Phosphatidylcholine inhibits and lysophosphatidylcholine enhances the lymphatic absorption of alpha-tocopherol in adult rats. *J. Nutr.* **2001**, *131*, 717–722. [PubMed]
87. Nishimukai, M.; Hara, H. Enteral administration of soybean phosphatidylcholine enhances the lymphatic absorption of lycopene, but reduces that of alpha-tocopherol in rats. *J. Nutr.* **2004**, *134*, 1862–1866. [PubMed]
88. Reboul, E.; Thap, S.; Perrot, E.; Amiot, M.J.; Lairon, D.; Borel, P. Effect of the main dietary antioxidants (carotenoids, gamma-tocopherol, polyphenols, and vitamin C) on alpha-tocopherol absorption. *Eur. J. Clin. Nutr.* **2007**, *61*, 1167–1173. [CrossRef] [PubMed]

89. Sklan, D.; Donoghue, S. Vitamin E response to high dietary vitamin A in the chick. *J. Nutr.* **1982**, *112*, 759–765. [PubMed]
90. Griffiths, D.W. The inhibition of digestive enzymes by polyphenolic compounds. *Adv. Exp. Med. Biol.* **1986**, *199*, 509–516. [PubMed]
91. Fardet, A.; Morise, A.; Kalonji, E.; Margaritis, I.; Mariotti, F. Influence of phytosterol and phytostanol food supplementation on plasma liposoluble vitamins and provitamin A carotenoid levels in humans: An updated review of the evidence. *Crit. Rev. Food Sci. Nutr.* **2017**, *57*, 1906–1921. [CrossRef] [PubMed]
92. Richelle, M.; Enslen, M.; Hager, C.; Groux, M.; Tavazzi, I.; Godin, J.P.; Berger, A.; Metairon, S.; Quaile, S.; Piguet-Welsch, C.; et al. Both free and esterified plant sterols reduce cholesterol absorption and the bioavailability of beta-carotene and alpha-tocopherol in normocholesterolemic humans. *Am. J. Clin. Nutr.* **2004**, *80*, 171–177. [PubMed]
93. Borel, P.; Desmarchelier, C. Genetic Variations Involved in Vitamin E Status. *Int. J. Mol. Sci.* **2016**, *17*. [CrossRef] [PubMed]

8

VKORC1 and VKORC1L1: Why do Vertebrates have Two Vitamin K 2,3-Epoxide Reductases?

Johannes Oldenburg [1,*], Matthias Watzka [1] and Carville G. Bevans [2]

[1] Institute of Experimental Haematology and Transfusion Medicine, University Clinic Bonn, Bonn 53105, Germany; E-Mail: matthias.watzka@ukb.uni-bonn.de

[2] Im Hermeshain 6, Frankfurt am Main 60388, Germany; E-Mail: bevans@jhu.edu

* Author to whom correspondence should be addressed; E-Mail: johannes.oldenburg@ukb.uni-bonn.de

Abstract: Among all cellular life on earth, with the exception of yeasts, fungi, and some prokaryotes, VKOR family homologs are ubiquitously encoded in nuclear genomes, suggesting ancient and important biological roles for these enzymes. Despite single gene and whole genome duplications on the largest evolutionary timescales, and the fact that most gene duplications eventually result in loss of one copy, it is surprising that all jawed vertebrates (gnathostomes) have retained two paralogous VKOR genes. Both VKOR paralogs function as entry points for nutritionally acquired and recycled K vitamers in the vitamin K cycle. Here we present phylogenetic evidence that the human paralogs likely arose earlier than gnathostomes, possibly in the ancestor of crown chordates. We ask why gnathostomes have maintained these paralogs throughout evolution and present a current summary of what we know. In particular, we look to published studies about tissue- and developmental stage-specific expression, enzymatic function, phylogeny, biological roles and associated pathways that together suggest subfunctionalization as a major influence in evolutionary fixation of both paralogs. Additionally, we investigate on what evolutionary timescale the paralogs arose and under what circumstances in order to gain insight into the biological *raison d'être* for both VKOR paralogs in gnathostomes.

Keywords: evolution; subfunctionalization; paralog; vitamin K; VKOR; VKORC1; VKORC1L1

---

1. Introduction

Genomes of higher vertebrates possess two paralog genes, *VKORC1* and *VKORC1L1* (see Note 1 [1]), that encode enzymes unique in catalyzing de-epoxidation of vitamin K 2,3-epoxide (K>O), a product of post-translational modification of vitamin K-dependent (VKD) proteins [2,3]. VKD proteins are known to be essential for diverse physiological functions including hemostasis and coagulation [4, 5]; bone development and homeostasis [6–8]; vascular homeostasis, remodeling and calcification [9–13]; cellular growth, survival, and signaling [14,15]; metabolic homeostasis [16,17]; and fertility [18]. While the respective VKORC1 and VKORC1L1 protein primary sequences share ~50% identity and highly homologous function (Figure 1), it is surprising that both genes have been maintained with high fidelity throughout over 400 million years of vertebrate evolution [3,19] (See also Bevans *et al.* [20] in this Special Issue). In the following review, we point out structural and functional similarities and differences between both paralog enzymes and explore phylogenetic relationships in order to construct a hypothesis that addresses the question "Why do vertebrates have two vitamin K 2,3-epoxide reductase (VKOR) enzymes?".

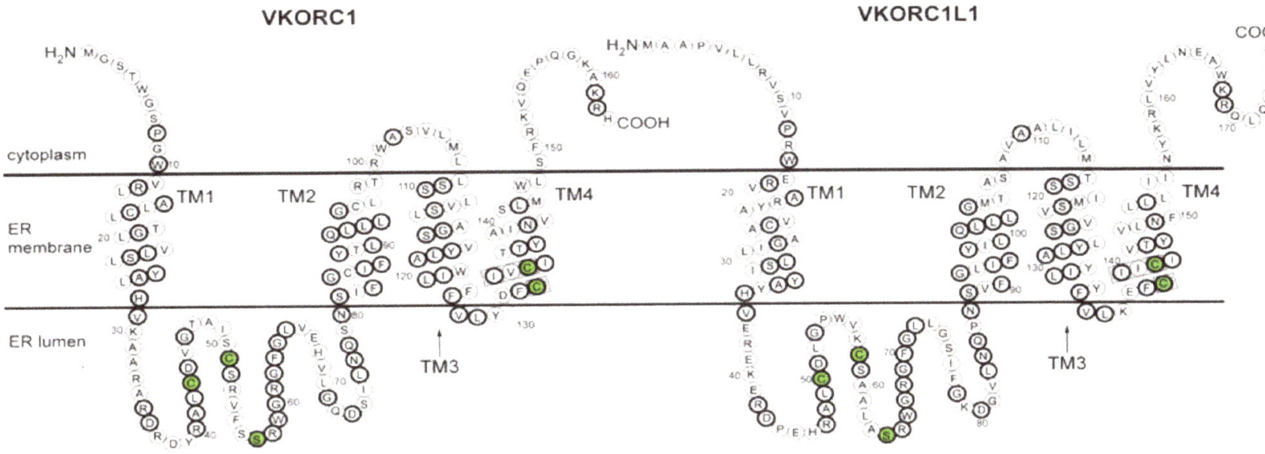

Figure 1. Primary protein sequence and predicted topology of human VKORC1 (left) and VKORC1L1 (right). Circles represent amino acid residues; bold circles indicate positions of sequence identity shared by both paralogs; green-filled circles, residues conserved among all VKOR family proteins; TM1–TM4, first through fourth transmembrane α-helices; gray-boxed regions, the catalytic CXXC active site motif.

1.1. *Catalytic Function and Biological Roles of VKOR Family Enzymes*

VKOR family homologs are expressed in the vast majority of the currently available sequenced genomes except those for all fungi and yeasts, and about half of the prokaryotic genomes available to-date, which almost always alternatively express DsbB oxidoreductases that function homologously to prokaryotic VKOR proteins [3,21–23] (See also Bevans *et al.* [20] in this Special Issue). Thus, VKOR homologs appear to have evolved very early in vertebrate evolutionary history and apparently carry out critical functions for most species, given their ubiquity and high degree of evolutionary conservation.

1.1.1. VKOR Enzymes Can Catalyze Multiple Reactions

Although the VKOR family is named for the first confirmed function of the human, rat and mouse orthologs [2,24], biochemical characterizations of non-vertebrate homologs reported to-date have indicated that they cannot catalyze VKOR activity, but alternatively catalyze vitamin K quinone reductase (VKR) or ubiquinone reductase activities [25–28]. To date, only one prokaryotic VKOR homolog from *Mycobacterium tuberculosis* has been demonstrated to possess VKOR activity *in vitro* when expressed in HEK 293 cells [27]. However, the native *M. tuberculosis* lipidome has been shown to possess only quinone and hydroquinone forms of menaquinones, but not menaquinone 2,3-epoxides [29], so it is not likely that the VKOR homolog of this bacterium catalyzes physiological VKOR activity *in vivo*. Subsequent to the initial reports identifying human VKORC1 by virtue of its VKOR de-epoxidase activity, the same enzyme was shown to additionally catalyze *in vitro* VKR activity that reduces vitamin K quinone (K) to vitamin K hydroquinone (KH_2) [30]. More recently, human VKORC1L1 was also confirmed to catalyze VKOR and VKR activities *in vitro* [31]. Thus, both vertebrate VKOR paralogs catalyze both VKOR and VKR enzymatic activities.

Four cysteine residues (human VKORC1 sequence numbering: Cys43, Cys51, Cys132, Cys135) are completely conserved among VKORC1 orthologs and are required for *in vivo* VKOR catalysis [27,32,33]. Only one *in vitro* study has investigated VKR enzymatic activity for VKORC1 and confirmed that Cys132 and Cys135 are required [30]. Additionally, a conserved serine or threonine (human VKORC1 sequence numbering: Ser57) has been shown to be essential for VKOR catalytic activity *in vitro* [32,34]. Based on sequence homology to the bacterial VKOR enzyme structure, the four redox-active cysteines are widely believed to be arranged in a double disulfide relay that shuttles reducing equivalents from ER-resident oxidoreductases, responsible for *de novo* oxidative protein folding (OPF), to membrane-soluble K>O [30,33–36]. Thus, VKORC1 accepts reducing equivalents from cysteine thiol groups of soluble oxidoreductase proteins in the ER lumen. Protein disulfide isomerase (PDI), TMX, TMX4 and ERp18, all with thioredoxin-like protein folds, have been implicated as physiological oxidoreductase partners by their ability to form intermolecular disulfide bonds with VKORC1 in cell culture experiments [36,37]. These ER-resident accessory oxidoreductases serve as the primary enzymes that interact with proteins and peptides undergoing oxidative folding by *de novo* disulfide formation [38]. Additionally, VKOR enzymes are the only OPF oxidoreductases that do not ultimately require molecular oxygen as the terminal electron acceptor by downstream enzymatic pathways, suggesting that the origin of these eukaryotic proteins may be very ancient, possibly having evolved before earth's atmosphere was substantially aerobic, and might predate the evolution of other enzymes involved in OPF in the ER including members of the Ero1, peroxiredoxin, and QSOX families [31,39].

1.1.2. Known Biological Roles for VKOR Family Enzymes

The first biological function attributed to VKORC1 was VKOR catalysis—the rate-limiting step in the classical vitamin K cycle [2,24,40,41]. In humans and other vertebrates, the vitamin K cycle drives post-translational modification of glutamic acid residues to form γ-carboxyglutamyl residues required for proper function of VKD proteins [42,43]. VKORC1 is the sole enzyme in vertebrates capable of sustaining sufficient VKOR activity to maintain hemostasis [42,44]. VKORC1L1 is apparently responsible for other functions as it cannot rescue VKORC1-specific production of VKD clotting factors in *vkorc1*$^{-/-}$ knock-out mice [44]. Newborn *vkorc1*$^{-/-}$ mice typically died within several days due to internal hemorrhage due to severe deficiency of γ-glutamyl carboxylated clotting factors. The lethal phenotype could be rescued by administration of large doses of vitamin K, similar to the rescue of the human VKCFD2 phenotype in patients homozygous for a VKORC1:Arg98Trp mutation [45]. Interestingly, with respect to hemostatic phenotype, heterozygous *vkorc1*$^{+/-}$ mice were indistinguishable from homozygous wild-type mice, suggesting that one wild-type *vkorc1* allele is sufficient for producing adequate levels of γ-glutamyl carboxylated VKD clotting factors to sustain normal development and growth. In contrast, with respect to bone morphology, eight-day old *vkorc1*$^{-/-}$ mice were found to have a pathological phenotype, whereby long bones were all found to be significantly shorter compared to those of homozygous wild-type *vkorc1* mice. In its fully γ-glutamyl carboxylated form, the VKD protein osteocalcin, secreted by osteoblast cells, has long been implicated in bone calcification and homeostasis [46]. Intriguingly, a recent study by Ferron *et al.* (2015) found that VKORC1L1 could not functionally substitute for VKORC1 in cultured osteoblast cells where VKORC1 expression level correlates with γ-glutamyl carboxylation of osteocalcin and modulation of its endocrine functions [47]. Thus, it appears that osteocalcin mediation of bone formation is a second example where VKORC1L1 cannot substitute for VKORC1-mediated biological function of a secreted VKD protein.

In addition to hemostatic functions of VKD clotting factors, other VKD proteins play crucial roles in bone growth and homeostasis [7,13], and recently were demonstrated to be necessary for inhibition of calcification in vasculature [9,10,12,48,49]. Vitamin K and VKD proteins have also been shown to protect oligodendrocytes and neurons from oxidative injury [50], function in cell signaling and growth [15,51], and support sphingomyelin synthesis and metabolism in nervous tissues [14].

A second important biological function was recently confirmed for VKORC1 as an acceptor of reducing equivalents from cysteines during oxidative protein folding in the ER [39]. This was independently confirmed by both siRNA silencing and warfarin knock-down of VKOR enzymatic activity in human hepatoma HepG2 cells after Ero1 α/β isoforms and peroxiredoxin IV (PRDX4) were first functionally silenced, demonstrating that VKORC1 alone can facilitate OPF.

That both vertebrate VKOR paralogs catalyze both VKOR and VKR reactions suggests that neofunctionalization of one of the evolved paralog enzymes, relative to the other retaining an ancestral function, has not occurred—at least with respect to catalytic reactions and substrates. Thus, further elucidation of biological functions for both enzymes may give clues to heretofore-unknown functional differences that might be the basis for selective pressure to conserve their otherwise redundant enzymatic activities in vertebrates. For example, there might be paralog-specific differences in which partner oxidoreductases pass reducing equivalents to each paralog or differences in tissue-specific or developmental stage-specific expression.

As a corollary to the above examples where VKORC1L1 cannot substitute for some of the biological functions of VKORC1 *in vivo*, we ask the question: Are there biological functions mediated by VKORC1L1 that VKORC1 cannot fulfill? Unfortunately, this question has not yet been experimentally addressed as it necessarily requires knock-down or knock-out of VKORC1L1 in cells or animal models that can be used to investigate its biological function. Recently, however, two lines of investigation have begun to focus on details of VKORC1L1 function.

First, a study by Westhofen *et al.* (2011) provided evidence from a number of different experimental perspectives. Expression of VKORC1L1 in HEK 293 T cells in the presence of vitamin K was found to promote vitamin K-dependent cell viability, elimination of intracellular reactive oxygen species and prevented oxidative damage to membrane proteins [31].

Second, a recent comprehensive study by Hammed *et al.* (2013) further measured and compared differential expression of vkorc1 and vkorc1l1 paralogs and tissue-specific VKOR activity of both paralogs in wild-type mice and the *vkorc1*$^{-/-}$ mouse line originally reported by Spohn *et al.* (2009) [44,52]. Expression levels of vkorc1l1 in all tissues investigated were not different in *vkorc1*$^{-/-}$ mice compared to mice with homozygous wild-type *vkorc1*. Thus, it appears that regulation of vkorc1l1 expression in mice is not sensitive to the level of vkorc1 expression, suggesting that the regulation of expression for both paralogs involves independent regulatory pathways. Furthermore, *in vitro* investigation of VKOR enzymatics for mouse and human VKOR paralog enzymes heterologously expressed in *Pichia pastoris* yielded surprising and unexpected results. While the Michaelis–Menton constants for $K_1 > O$ were determined to be similar for human VKORC1L1 and VKORC1 and for rat vkorc1l1 and vkorc1 (Table 1), the warfarin inhibition constants (K_i) for human VKORC1L1 and rat vkorc1l1 were found to be, respectively, 29-fold and 54-fold greater than for the respective VKORC1 and vkorc1 paralogs. Thus, it appears that both human and rat VKORC1L1 paralogs are ~1.5 orders of magnitude less warfarin sensitive than the respective VKORC1 paralogs. Based on these results, the study went on to show that tissue-specific expression of both paralogs contributes to overall level of VKOR activity (*i.e.*, tissue-specific VKOR activities of both paralogs are additive) and that the degree of warfarin sensitivity in various tissues is a function of the relative paralog expression ratio. Interestingly, by use of c-myc tagged expression constructs in *Pichia pastoris* cells, the authors were able to determine that the relative VKOR catalytic efficiency of rat vkorc1 is 30-fold greater than for rat vkorc1l1, while the VKOR catalytic efficiency of human VKORC1 is two-fold lower than that of human VKORC1L1. In summary, the study by Hammed *et al.* has demonstrated that VKORC1L1 is able to support VKOR activity and may constitute an alternative pathway that is able to substitute or partially complement for loss of VKORC1 function in various non-hepatic tissues of *vkorc1*$^{-/-}$ mice.

1.1.3. Evolutionary Origins of the VKORC1 and VKORC1L1 Paralogs

Robertson (2004) previously suggested that an ancestral VKOR gene duplication likely occurred in early vertebrates and resulted in the extant human and other gnathostome VKOR paralogs [3]. This would be in agreement with the divergence of the common ancestor of the jawed vertebrates (gnathostomes) from urochordates and cephalochordates, as has been suggested for many other vertebrate protein paralog pairs [53]. In the article by Bevans *et al.* [20] in this special issue, a broad phylogenetic study of VKOR family homologs yielded strong support for distinct monophyletic clades comprising vertebrate VKORC1 and VKORC1L1 homologs. Thus, it is likely that the paralogs arose one time and quickly became fixed in the genomes of subsequently diverged early (crown) vertebrate lineages. That all extant gnathostome genomes sequenced to date include both paralog genes suggests that the functions of both paralogs are indispensable to vertebrate life. In order to more accurately confirm the divergence point of the last common ancestor of modern vertebrates with two VKOR family paralogs, we chose a series of index genomes sampling various evolutionary groupings that diverged before, during and after the last universal common ancestor of gnathostomes, many only very recently sequenced in draft form, to reconstruct a likely metazoan VKOR phylogeny (Figure 2).

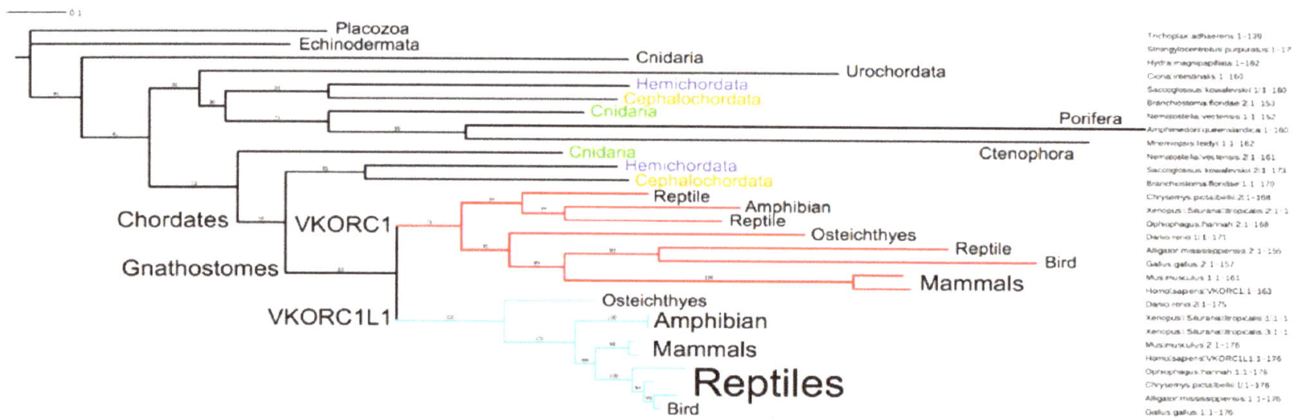

Figure 2. Reconstructed phylogeny (unrooted) for full-length sequences of index metazoans using PhyML with a WAG+I+G4 substitution model in the IQ-TREE ver1.2.3 server-based phylogenetics package with graphics generated using the iToL server (see Bevans *et al.* [20] in this Special Issue for details). Linnaean taxonomic names and primary sequence lengths are shown to the right; groupings shown on the left: Placozoa, basal invertebrate outgroup; Echinodermata and Hemichordata, basal deuterostomes belonging to the Ambulacaria; Cnidaria, basal metazoan invertebrates including jellyfish and sea anemonae; Urochordata, an invertebrate sister group to vertebrates; Porifera, basal non-metazoan animals including sponges; Ctenophora, basal non-bileterian metazoans including comb jellies; Cephalochordata, a basal chordate sister group to Olfactores which includes Urochordata and vertebrates; Chordates includes Cephalochordates, Tunicates (here represented by the Urochordate Ciona intestinalis) and Vertebrates; Gnathostomes are a subgroup of vertebrates with jaw bones that includes Chondrichthyes (sharks and rays—not included among the analyzed sequences; see Note 2 [54]) and Osteichthyes (bony fishes and tetrapods); VKORC1 and VKORC1L1 are paralog clades for Gnathostomes. Scale bar (upper left, labeled 0.1) represents single nucleotide substitution rate per million years; VKORC1 clade is represented by red lines, VKORC1L1 clade by cyan lines; numbers on branches are % support for 1000 bootstrap trees. VKOR paralogs encoded by non-gnathostome genomes are shown in blue (Hemichordata), orange (Cephalochordata) and green (Cnidaria) (see also Note 3 [55]).

As expected, we found high phylogenetic support for monophyletic VKORC1 and VKORC1L1 clades, which split uniformly for extant ganthostomes. Branch lengths for the VKORC1L1 clade (cyan) are relatively shorter than those for the VKORC1 clade (red), in agreement with earlier reports that primary sequences among VKORC1L1 orthologs are more highly conserved than for those among VKORC1 orthologs [2,3]. Reptilian VKORC1L1 orthologs appear on mixed branches with VKORC1L1 orthologs of amphibian, fish and bird as branch support for the VKORC1L1 clade is significantly weaker than for the VKORC1 clade. Surprisingly, for single genomes representing three non-gnathostome groups (Figure 2, indicated in blue, orange and green), we found pairs of VKOR paralogs where one paralog in each genome is inferred to be more similar to the gnathostome VKORs and the second paralogs for each genome are clustered together on a deeper-lying branch. However, inference support for the lower-lying branches (Figure 2, black lines) is considerably lower than the relatively high support for the gnathostome paralog clades. This is evident in the scrambled placement of representative non-gnathostome species in the tree that does not correlate well with the current consensus groupings on the Tree of Life (e.g., Echinodermata is placed on a low branch parallel to Placozoa, and chordate paralogs (Figure 2, blue and orange) are mixed with invertebrate

VKOR sequences on a single, deep branch (includes fourth through ninth sequences from the top). Notable results of our phylogenetic analysis include the VKOR paralog pairs of two invertebrate genomes (acorn worm, *Saccoglossus kowalevskii*; lancelet, *Branchiostoma floridae*) that are placed as basal deuterostomes, far deeper in the Tree of Life than vertebrates. This begs consideration that VKOR gene duplications may have occurred in these ancient invertebrate branches independent of the first whole genome duplication in gnathostomes, which, consistent with our inferred VKOR phylogeny, is the likeliest single event that resulted in the gnathostome paralogs. Similarly, the VKOR paralogs found in the Cnidarian sea anemone (*Nematostella vectensis*) may have arisen by a gene duplication unrelated to the gnathostome event. Whether these invertebrate genomes with VKOR paralog pairs represent isolated exceptions, or are evidence for deeper-rooted single gene duplication/loss events, will require more whole genome data from current and future sequencing efforts. In summary, our phylogenetic results suggest that the extant human VKOR paralogs VKORC1 and VKORC1L1 likely arose in an older common metazoan ancestor than the last universal common ancestor of gnathostomes, likely as early as the common ancestor of crown chordate groups.

2. Common Aspects of VKORC1 and VKORC1L1 Structure and Function

2.1. Gene and Protein Structural Organization

Parsing vertebrate *VKORC1* and *VKORC1L1* sequences in the NCBI Gene database confirmed both paralogs are organized into three exons of very similar lengths. Intron lengths vary considerably between the two paralogs with entire VKORC1L1 genes being typically 17–25 times longer than the respective VKORC1 paralogs (e.g., VKORC1: 2.3 kb mouse—human 3.5 kb; VKORC1L1: 40 kb mouse—86 kb human). In contrast, Robertson (2004) noted that three kinetoplast VKOR homologs, *Trypanosoma cruzi*, *T. brucei*, and *Leishmania major*, are encoded by single exon genes [3]. Pseudogenes found in the human, mouse and rat genomes have been previously reviewed in detail [3].

Inspection of vertebrate VKORC1 and VKORC1L1 full-length (isoform 1) protein sequences in the NCBI Proteins database revealed that most vertebrate VKORC1 orthologs are about 161–163 residues (Figure 3, yellow bars; range 160–163 residues), whereas VKORC1L1 sequences are predominantly 174–176 residues (Figure 3, cyan bars; range 161–190 residues). Most vertebrate VKORC1 ortholog primary sequences encompass a core domain of 153 residues (Figure 1, human VKORC1 residues Met1-Val153) with a *C*-terminus of variable length (7–14 residues). All VKORC1L1 sequences include an additional 3-residue insertion between corresponding human VKORC1 residues 10 and 11 (Figure 1, human VKORC1L1 residues Arg19-Tyr20-Ala21), effectively extending the length of the predicted 1st TMH by one α-helical turn and resulting in a core domain length of 152 residues (Figure 1, human VKORC1L1 residues Pro12-Leu163). The variable length *N*-termini of VKORC1L1 orthologs are 1–63 residues with the majority of orthologs having an *N*-terminal length of 11 residues. *C*-termini of VKORC1L1 orthologs are 8–13 residues with the majority having a length of 13 residues. Both VKORC1 and VKORC1L1 are localized to and retained in the ER [2,31], likely by a COP I-mediated mechanism of the *cis*-Golgi that recognizes known ER retention recognition sequences with adjacent pairs of positively charged amino acids in the *C*-termini of membrane-intrinsic proteins [56]. Recently, an additional ER retention motif in the short cytoplasmic loop connecting TMH2 and TMH3 of human VKORC1 has been identified [57].

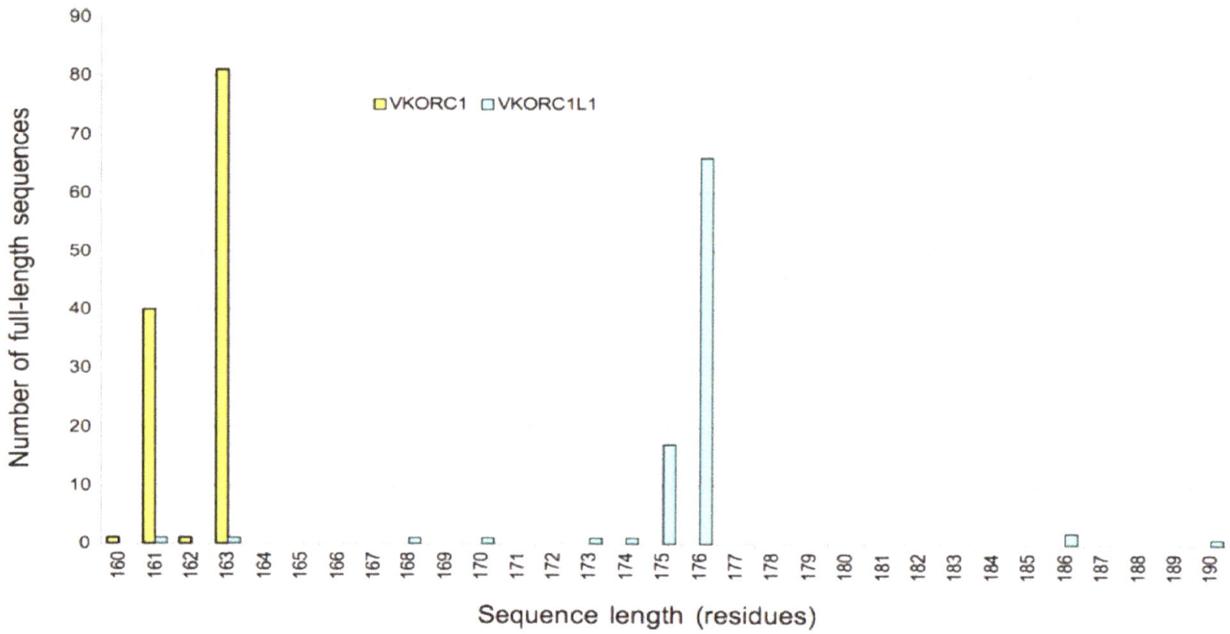

Figure 3. Histogram of vertebrate VKOR paralog sequence lengths in the NCBI Protein database. All sequences included were verified as full-length isoform 1 for VKORC1 (yellow bars) and VKORC1L1 (cyan bars).

Extramembraneous loops are of identical length among all sequenced vertebrate VKOR homologs. Thus, respective VKORC1 and VKORC1L1 proteins in vertebrates are expected to have highly homologous, evolutionarily conserved respective protein folds.

2.2. In Vitro VKOR Enzymatics—Substrates and Inhibitors

Although the first detailed enzymatic studies of VKOR activity in liver microsomes prepared from mice and rats commenced in 1984 [58–60], more recent studies, since 2011, characterizing the enzymatics of recombinantly produced human and rat VKORC1 and VKORC1L1 are just now gaining momentum among several active, independent research groups [31,52,61–68]. In order to form a comprehensive picture of our current understanding of VKOR enzymatics, we have summarized the basic results of these studies (Table 1). Of the dozen studies specifically addressing VKOR enzymatics, the initial three relied on rodent liver microsomal preparations as enzyme sources which, during preparation, substantially lose the ER lumenal oxidoreductases that are required for physiological VKOR activity *in vivo* [58]. In order to supply reducing equivalents to drive VKOR activity *in vitro*, DTT has been widely used since it was found to support VKOR activity (for a historical review of the DTT-driven *in vitro* VKOR assay, see [68]). Thus, in the DTT-driven VKOR assay, VKORC1 or VKORC1L1 catalyze reduction of K>O with concomitant oxidation of DTT. To achieve this, the enzymes function by a kinetic mechanism that alternates between two states where the active site CXXC motif cysteines are either oxidized (in the form of a disulfide bridge between them) or reduced [58,63,65,69]. Two different enzyme kinetic models have thus far been applied to VKOR studies—the "ping-pong" model takes enzymatic conversion of both substrates into account [58,63,65,68], while a simpler Michaelis–Menton single substrate kinetic model is based on enzymatic conversion of only the K>O substrate [31,52,59–62,64,66,67]. For the K>O single substrate model to be valid, the DTT substrate must be at saturating concentration in the VKOR assay a requisite condition for pseudo first-order kinetics [70]. Both kinetic models can yield valid enzymatic parameters (e.g., K_m, V_{max}, k_{cat}) from DTT-driven VKOR assay data. However, due to the fact that DTT competes with warfarin for binding to the enzymes, interpretation of warfarin dose-response data obtained using the DTT-driven VKOR assay has been extremely problematic [63,65,71,72]. For example, VKORC1 variants with single amino acid mutations that cause warfarin resistance in humans and rodents show dose-response data indicating warfarin susceptibility identical to wild-type VKORC1 [2,73]. This problem in *in vitro* assessment of resistance phenotypes for known VKORC1 warfarin-resistant variants has been recently overcome by use of alternative cell culture-based VKOR activity assays (see below) which yield warfarin resistance dose-response data in agreement with human and rodent resistance phenotypes. However, an advantage in continuing use of non-physiological reductant-driven VKOR assays lies in their ability to provide data suitable for detailed enzymatics and catalysis mechanism studies since, unlike in cell culture-based assays, the assay conditions can be strictly defined.

What we can generally conclude from VKOR enzymatics studies to-date includes (referring to Table 1): (1) wild-type VKORC1 and VKORC1L1 Michaelis-Menton constant (K_m) values determined for K>O substrates are in the low micromolar (~1–35 μM) range, while K_m for DTT and THPP reducing substrates are approximately millimolar (V_{max} values are not comparable between studies as they reflect a convolution of intrinsic enzyme turnover rate with the quantitative amount of enzyme used in the assay); (2) the enzymes to not appear to significantly discriminate between phylloquinone- and menaquinone-2,3-epoxide substrates; (3) for all warfarin resistance mutations studied, except for Tyr139 position mutations in rats, measured K_m values for K>O are considerably greater than for the respective wild-type enzymes, implying K>O substrate binding affinity is diminished by nearly all mutations; (4) the DTT-driven VKOR assay reveals warfarin-resistant *in vitro* phenotypes only for a very few mutations investigated (Table 1; last column, K_i values indicated in bold-face type are significantly increased with respect to the wild-type K_i in each study); and (5) both human and rat VKORC1L1 enzymes appear to be considerably less warfarin-sensitive than the respective VKORC1 enzymes. To-date, enzymatic studies of VKR catalytic function for VKORC1 and VKORC1L1 have not been reported. From enzymatic study of VKOR catalysis available so far for both VKORC1 and VKORC1L1, we are nudged towards the conclusion that there is no major difference in enzymatic function or substrate specificity between the vertebrate VKORC1 and VKORC1L1 paralogs.

Table 1. Summary of results from published VKORC1 and VKORC1L1 enzymatics studies.

Study	Enzyme	Species	K_m (K_1 > O) (μM)	K_m (K_2 > O) (μM)	K_m (DTT) (mM)	pH	K_m ($THPP_{Total}$) (μM)	K_i (warfarin) (μM)
Krettler *et al.* 2015 [65]	r VKORC1	human	**1.20**			7.4	431	
Goulois *et al.* 2015 [64]	r vkorc1	*R. rattus*	**15.9 ± 4.5**			7.4		0.32 ± 0.07
	r vkorc1	*R. norvegicus*				7.4		0.50 ± 0.01
	r vkorc1:Y25F	*R. rattus*	**15.9 ± 4.5**			7.4		**1.99**
Matagrin *et al.* 2014 [63]	r VKORC1	human				7.4		1.65
Hammed *et al.* 2013 [51]	r VKORC1	human	**21.5 ± 4.2**			7.4		1.8 ± 0.2
	r vkorc1	rat	**19.6 ± 1.6**			7.4		0.6 ± 0.04
	r VKORC1L1	human	**24.1 ± 3.0**			7.4		52.0 ± 3.0
	r vkorc1l11	rat	**35.0 ± 3.0**			7.4		32.6 ± 1.9
Matagrin *et al.* 2013 [61]	r vkorc1	rat	**7.2 ± 2.5**			7.4		
	r vkorc1:L120Q	rat	25.0 ± 4.0			7.4		
	r vkorc1:L128Q	rat	12.1 ± 1.0			7.4		
	r vkorc1:Y139C	rat	60.0 ± 6.0			7.4		
	r vkorc1:Y139F	rat	17.8 ± 4.5			7.4		
	r vkorc1:Y139S	rat	13.1 ± 1.3			7.4		
Bevans *et al.* 2013 [60]	r VKORC1	human	1.24		8.38	7.5		2.481
						7.5		2.633
						7.5		5.786
Hodroge *et al.* 2012 [59]	r VKORC1	human	**19.8 ± 4.5**			7.4		1.65 ± 0.79
	r VKORC1:A26P	human	57.4 ± 10.1			7.4		**18.43 ± 5.82**
	r VKORC1:A26T	human	18.7 ± 1.4			7.4		2.13 ± 0.56
	r VKORC1:L27V	human	22.8 ± 2.9			7.4		1.83 ± 0.62
	r VKORC1:H28Q	human	29.8 ± 4.6			7.4		0.65 ± 0.42
	r VKORC1:D36G	human	43.8 ± 0.2			7.4		0.74 ± 0.25
	r VKORC1:D36Y	human	23.6 ± 0.2			7.4		1.82 ± 0.70
	r VKORC1:A41S	human	65.9 ± 5.4			7.4		1.78 ± 0.02

Table 1. *Cont.*

Hodroge *et al.* 2012 [59]	r VKORC1:V45A	human	26.9 ± 2.3			7.4	1.10 ± 0.04
	r VKORC1V54L	human	102.5 ± 28.6			7.4	**7.95 ± 1.32**
	r VKORC1:S56F	human	23.2 ± 6.2			7.4	1.05 ± 0.82
	r VKORC1:R58G	human	71.0 ± 10.9			7.4	1.50 ± 0.36
	r VKORC1:W59C	human	179.7 ± 12.5			7.4	1.16 ± 0.20
	r VKORC1:H68Y	human	16.9 ± 2.8			7.4	**6.21 ± 0.85**
	r VKORC1:I123N	human	27.0 ± 2.1			7.4	**4.01 ± 1.01**
	r VKORC1:Y139H	human	9.2 ± 3.0			7.4	**5.91 ± 1.77**
Hodroge *et al.* 2011 [58]	r vkorc1	rat	**7.20 ± 2.50**			7.4	0.50 ± 0.05
	vkorc1$^{wt/wt}$	rat	**8.40 ± 0.90**			7.4	0.72 ± 0.01
	r vkorc1:L120Q	rat				7.4	**>100**
	r vkorc1:L128Q	rat				7.4	**4.0 ± 0.7**
	r vkorc1:Y139C	rat				7.4	**>100**
	r vkorc1:Y139F	rat	17.8 ± 4.5			7.4	**>100**
	vkorc1:Y139F$^{+/+}$	rat	19.5 ± 4.0			7.4	**29.0 ± 4.1**
	r vkorc1:Y139S	rat				7.4	**>100**
Westhofen *et al.* 2011 [30]	r VKORC1	human	**1.88 ± 0.13**	**1.55 ± 0.55**		7.6	
	r VKORC1L1	human	**4.15 ± 0.10**	**11.24 ± 0.23**		7.6	
Lasseur *et al.* 2006 [57]	vkorc1$^{wt/wt}$	mouse	**12.73 ± 0.93**			7.4	5.97 ± 0.38
	vkorc1$^{W59G/W59G}$	mouse	15.31 ± 4.92			7.4	3.5 ± 0.27
Lasseur *et al.* 2005 [56]	vkorc1$^{wt/wt}$	rat	**57.7 ± 12.5**			7.4	0.72 ± 0.06
	vkorc1$^{Y139F/Y139F}$	rat	19.5 ± 4			7.4	**29 ± 4.1**
Hildebrandt *et al.* 1984 [55]	vkorc1$^{wt/wt}$	rat	10.0 ± 0.7 *		0.60 ± 0.03	8.8	
	vkorc1$^{wt/wt}$	rat	9.1 ± 0.13 *		0.54 ± 0.04	8.8	
	vkorc1:$^{Y139S/Y139S}$	rat	4 *		0.16	8.8	
	vkorc1$^{wt/wt}$	rat	9		0.43	7.2	
	vkorc1:$^{Y139S/Y139S}$	rat	6		0.29	7.2	

Symbols: r, (Enzyme column) recombinantly produced enzyme; * (K_m ($K_1 > O$) column), sodium cholate-solubilized and partially purified enzyme. All enzymes are wild-type unless indicated by a colon followed by a specific mutation; samples prepared from liver microsomes are indicated with a superscript where individual *VKORC1* alleles (separated by a slash) are indicated as (wild-type) or a specific mutation. Bold-face type in columns for Michaelis–Menton constants (K_m values) indicates values for wild-type enzymes. Bold-face type in the column for warfarin inhibition constants (K_i) indicates warfarin resistance phenotypes confirmed by *in vitro* measurement.

2.3. *In Vitro Cell Culture-Based Assays of VKOR Activity*

Recent studies have confirmed *in vitro* warfarin resistance phenotypes for known human VKORC1 mutations that are in agreement with reported *in vivo* resistance phenotypes [74]. Compared to warfarin IC_{50} values for wild-type warfarin-sensitive and warfarin-resistant human VKORC1 variants determined by Fregin *et al.* (2013) [75] and Czogalla *et al.* (2013) [76], warfarin IC_{50} values determined in the study of Tie *et al.* (2013) are all about an order of magnitude lower, but all of these studies ranked *in vitro* phenotype severity, with respect to specific mutations, identically [77]. Although the purpose of the study by Haque *et al.* (2014) was to investigate dose-response for warfarin and its hydroxylated metabolites, and did not investigate warfarin-resistant VKORC1 variants, the warfarin IC_{50} value obtained for wild-type human VKORC1 is greater than the values obtained in all of the other studies [78]. Directly compared, warfarin IC_{50} values reported by Fregin *et al.* (2013) and Haque *et al.* (2014) are 6.9-fold and 18.3- to 35.4-fold greater than the value reported by Tie *et al.* (2013) [75,77,78]. Variations in assay conditions between the studies that could account for the differences in warfarin dose-response have not yet been identified. One important difference between the non-physiological reductant-driven VKOR assays and the more physiological cell culture-based assays is that the former directly assess enzyme function, while the latter are actually indirect assays of enzyme function in that they each rely on the rate-limiting function of VKOR enzymes in the vitamin K cycle to ultimately enable intracellular γ-gutamyl carboxylation of VKD proteins heterologously coexpressed by the cells and secreted into the culture medium. Thus, while the effects of warfarin inhibition on the read-out VKD protein status can be directly attributed to warfarin's localized interaction with VKORC1 or VKORC1L1, there are likely many other influences on the secreted VKD status (e.g., due to choices of cell line, specific VKD reporter protein, expression vector, and variability in culture medium constituents especially in amounts of warfarin-binding serum albumin, *etc.*) that could have profound influence on the correspondence between applied warfarin dosage and secreted VKD protein response. Balancing these possible uncertainties are the opportunities to use these cell culture-based assays to explore the nature of the enzymes' biological functions. Thus, identification of native partner oxidoreductases that provide the physiological reducing equivalents to drive VKOR activity and characterizing their interactions with VKORC1 and VKORC1L1 in the ER lumen could be experimentally addressed. Similarly, studies could be designed to elucidate regulation of the respective gene transcription and protein expression for VKOR paralogs in cell lines representative of various native tissues and developmental stages. Cultured cell assays would also be useful in identification and assessment of new pharmacological lead compounds based on vitamin K or intended for use as oral anticoagulants with desired qualities superior to currently available warfarin and other 4-hydroxycoumarin derivatives.

3. Differences between VKORC1 and VKORC1L1 Paralogs

3.1. *Tissue- and Developmental Stage-Specific Expression*

It has been known for a long time that liver is the primary location of VKOR enzymatic activity essential to the vitamin K cycle and production and secretion of VKD coagulation factors [35,71]. In 2000, before the identification of the *VKORC1* and *VKORC1L1* genes, a study by Itoh and Onishi investigated developmental changes in VKOR enzymatic activity of human liver sampled from autopsied samples representing individuals from 12 weeks post-fertilization to 18 years of age [79]. They found hepatic VKOR activity was low (mean 100 nmol/15 min/g_{liver}) and possibly declined through prenatal week 30, then increased abruptly by prenatal week 35 (mean 200 nmol/15 min/g_{liver}) and thereafter remained constant through age 18. With the identification of both VKOR paralogs in 2004, recent discoveries of biological roles for non-coagulation factor VKD proteins, and elucidation of what cells and tissues are their primary sites of expression, an increasing number of studies have been focused on assessing tissue-specific expression distributions for both VKORC1 and VKORC1L1

(Table 2). With respect to developmental expression of vkorc1 in mouse, two studies provided some early insight. Ko *et al.* (1998) constructed a cDNA library from total mRNA prepared from 7.5-day post-conception mouse embryonic and extraembryonic cells and found no evidence of vkorc1 expression by RT-PCR analysis [80]. A subsequent mouse tissue expression study by Diez-Roux *et al.* (2011) used *in situ* RNA hybridization on whole embryo sections and found diffuse, weak expression of vkorc1 by 14.5 day post-fertilization embryos [81].

Two recent studies determined mouse VKOR paralog expression profiles for mouse tissues by relative mRNA expression quantitation using qRT-PCR of cDNA prepared from tissue-specific mRNAs. Hammed *et al.* (2013) measured vkorc1l1 expression in liver, lung, and testis of both C57BL/6 wild-type and $vkorc1^{-/-}$ mice and in wild-type nine week-old OFA-Sprague Dawley rat brain, kidney, liver, lung and testis and rat osteosarcoma cell line ROS17/2.8 (Table 2) [52]. In mouse tissues, vkorc1l1 expression levels were highly similar between wild-type and $vkorc1^{-/-}$ strains, suggesting distinctly independent regulation of expression for both VKOR paralogs. For all tissues investigated, vkorc1 expression was also found, but most predominantly in liver (10-fold greater than for vkorc1l1), whereas brain had greater vkorc1l1 expression relative to that for vkorc1. Other tissues had intermediate expression levels for both paralogs. For expression levels in rat liver, lung, brain, kidney and testis assessed at three, six and nine weeks post-partum, both paralogs showed minor variations that were not statistically significant except for vkorc1 expression in liver which peaked significantly at six weeks before declining at nine weeks. Taken together, these results explain why some extrahepatic tissues may have near physiological VKOR activities and down-stream VKD protein function in the presence of warfarin concentrations that effectively inhibit VKD clotting factor production in the liver. Another study by Caspers *et al.* (2015) similarly investigated VKOR paralog expression levels in 29 different tissues of CD1 wild-type mouse [82]. Expression levels for vkorc1 were found to be greatest in liver, lung and exocrine tissues including mammary, salivary and prostate glands, whereas vkorc1l1 expression was greatest in brain (Table 2). Taken together, results of both studies investigating rodent tissue expression patterns for both VKOR paralogs strongly suggests an emerging picture of independent regulation of the vitamin K cycle by differential expression of both VKOR paralog enzymes.

In zebrafish, Fernández *et al.* (2015) have assessed Vkorc1 and Vkorc1l1 expression by qPCR analysis during larval development and in adult tissues [83]. Vkorc1l1 was expressed at highest levels overall at the post-fertilization 4-cell stage and diminished by Prim-5 stage, remaining stable at later stages. Vkorc1 expression was detectable at the 4-cell stage, but peaked at 72–96 h post-fertilization followed by lower, stable levels at later stages. In adults, Vkorc1l1 was ubiquitously expressed in all tissues investigated (Table 2) with greatest levels in brain, muscle and ovary, while Vkorc1 was only detectable in about half of the surveyed tissues with elevated levels in brain, muscle and vertebra. Interestingly, no Vkorc1 expression could be detected in adult intestine, kidney, ovary, spleen and stomach. Using the ZFB1 cell line developed in a previous study [84], the authors found Vkorc1 and Vkorc1l1 to be significantly overexpressed during differentiation, but not during induction of extracellular matrix (ECM) mineralization, in cells cultured for 1 week. In cells cultured for three weeks, there was no significant difference between differentiating cells or cells induced to mineralize ECM. Taken together with results reported for ROS 17/2.8 osteoblast-like cells by Hammed *et al.* (2013), and moderate expression levels of both VKOR paralogs in vertebral tissue, the authors suggest that osteoblast differentiation may require increased vitamin K cycle turnover [51].

Since the initial draft of the human, mouse and rat genomes completed in 2000, 2002 and 2004, respectively, whole genome and proteome investigations have enabled large-scale, high through-put investigation of gene and protein expression levels in various tissues and cells [85]. Less than a year after the identification of both VKOR paralogs in 2004, high-density nucleotide arrays including

VKORC1 and *VKORC1L1* sequences were already being used to explore gene expression on a genomics scale. CHiP-Seq mRNA quantification studies including data for *VKORC1* and *VKORC1L1* have been published for frog, fruitfly, human, rat, mouse, pig, and zebrafish [86–90].

We recently recovered human and mouse VKOR paralog mRNA expression profiles based on chromatin immunoprecipitation (ChIP-seq) technology from a large, high through-put transcriptomics study by Su *et al.* (2004) available through the BioGPS database portal [86,91]. Their data includes VKORC1 and VKORC1L1 expression levels for 79 human and 61 mouse tissues from pooled samples of typically 1–10 individuals. For simplification, in Table 2 we summarize only results including tissues with the 10 highest VKORC1 and VKORC1L1 expression levels above mean values for all tissues (for comprehensive tissue data, see Figure S1, online Supplemental Material). For human and mouse, VKORC1L1 is uniformly expressed at or near median value for most all tissues and cells surveyed. From among those surveyed, only adipocytes, CD34+ cell lines (including monocytic lines) and B lymphoblasts exhibit statistically significant higher levels of VKORC1L1 expression than the median. Westhofen *et al.* (2011) previously pointed out that all three tissues/cell types generate intensely and protractedly elevated levels of ROS under physiological conditions, suggesting a role for VKORC1L1 in redox homeostasis [31]. BioGPS tissue-specific expression levels for *VKORC1* mRNA exhibit more highly varied differences than for *VKORC1L1*. Among tissues with the highest expression levels are liver, where most of the vitamin K-dependent blood-clotting factors are produced, and adipocytes, smooth muscle, thyroid, lung and pineal body.

Data from the GTEx Portal [92], a large-scale, high through-put human genomics project published earlier this year, has recently been mined for a study by Melé *et al.* (2015) on RNA-seq deep-sequenced transcriptomes of 175 individuals that covers 29 solid organ tissues, 11 brain subregions, whole blood and two standard cell lines [93]. We summarize the top six expressing tissues for each VKOR paralog in this study (Figure S2, online Supplemental Material) for comparison with data from other studies. Tissues with highest levels of VKORC1 (ENSG#167397) expression from the GTEx project data included aorta and coronary artery, liver, pituitary and gland, while VKORC1L1 (ENSG#196715) expression was found to be greatest in adipose tissue, mammary gland, lung and tibial nerve (Table 2). Interestingly, the study results indicated that gene activity, in general, differed substantially more across tissues than across individuals and expression patterns for both *VKORC1* and *VKORC1L1* follow this trend. Genes that changed expression (FDR < 0.05) with age across all GTEx study tissues included *VKORC1L1*, but not *VKORC1* [94].

Table 2. Summary of results from expression studies of human, mouse and rat VKORC1 and VKORC1L1.

Study	Itoh & Onishi 2000 [76] *	Su *et al.* 2004 [83] *	Hammed *et al.* 2013 [51]	Kim *et al.* 2014 [93]	Wilhelm *et al.* 2014 [94]	Caspers *et al.* 2015 [79]	Melé *et al.* 2015 [90] *	Fernández *et al.* 2015 [80] *
Species	Human	Human, Mouse	Mouse, Rat	Human	Human	Mouse	Human	Zebrafish
Method	VKOR activity assay	CHiP-Seq	mRNA	Mass Spectroscopy	Mass Spectroscopy	mRNA	mRNA	mRNA
Tissue/cell types	**Liver (12 weeks post-fertilization to 18 years)**	**Adipocyte** **Brain (whole)** **Colon**	**Brain**	**Adrenal gland** Colon Esophagus	**Adipocyte** Adrenal gland Blood platelet Bone Brain Breast Cerebral cortex Colon Colonic epithelial cell	Adrenal gland Bone **Brain** Mammary gland Caecum Colon Diaphragm Duodenum Eye	**Adipose-visceral (omentum)** **Adipose-subcutaneous** **Aorta** **Breast-mammary** **Coronary artery**	Operculum **Brain** Eye

Table 2. *Cont.*

Tissue/cell types	**Liver (12 weeks post-fertilization to 18 years)**	**CD34+**		**Fetal Brain** Fetal Gut Fetal Heart Fetal Liver Fetal Ovary **Fetal Placenta** **Fetal Testis** Frontal cortex Gallbladder Heart Hematopoietic B cells Hematopoietic CD4+ T cells Hematopoietic CD8+ T cells **Hematopoietic Monocytes**	Gall bladder Gut Heart Helper T-lymphocyte **Monocyte**	Heart		Gills

Table 2. *Cont.*

Tissue/cell types	**Liver (12 weeks post-fertilization to 18 years)**	**Liver** **Lung** **721 B-ymphoblasts** **Mast-cells-IgE** **Mast-cells-IgE+antigen-1 h** **Mast-cells-IgE+antigen-6 h** **Mega-erythrocyte-progenitor**	**Kidney** **Liver** **Lung**	Hematopoietic NK cells **Hematopoietic Platelets** Kidney **Liver** **Lung**	Ileum epithelial cell Kidney Liver Lung Milk Myometrium Natural killer cell	Kidney **Liver** **Lung** Lymph node Masseter muscle Muscle Oesophagus	**Liver** **Lung** **EBV transformed lymphocytes** **Nerve-tibial**	Intestine Kidney Liver **Muscle**

Table 2. *Cont.*

Tissue/cell types	**Liver (12 weeks post-fertilization to 18 years)**	**Osteoblast-day 14** **Osteoblast-day 21** **Osteoblast-day 5** **Pineal body** **Pituitary** **Smooth-muscle** **Thyroid**	**Rat osteosarcoma cell line ROS 17/2.8** **Testis**	**Ovary** Pancreas Prostate Rectum Retina Spinal cord **Testis**	Osteosarcoma cell Ovary **Pancreas** **Pancreatic islet** Placenta Prefrontal cortex Prostate gland Rectum **Retina** Skin Spinal cord Stomach **Testis**	Ovary Pancreas **Prostate** **Salivary gland** Skin Soft tissue Stomach Spleen Testis	**Pituitary**	**Ovary** Skin Stomach Spleen

Table 2. *Cont.*

Tissue/cell types	**Liver (12 weeks post-fertilization to 18 years)**	**Umbilical-cord**		Urinary bladder	Urinary bladder	Tongue Uterus Vessels	**Transformed fibroblasts**	Vertebra

Symbols: * only cells and tissues shown with significantly greater expression than mean levels for all cells/tissues included in large-scale study; bold type indicates cells/tissues with expression levels significantly above means for each study; yellow, high VKORC1 expression level; blue, high VKORC1L1 expression, green high VKORC1 and VKORC1L1 coexpression.

Whole proteome studies using mass spectroscopic (MS) technologies have recently provided an opportunity to identify and quantitate intracellular pools of translated proteins across tissue types and populations of individuals [95]. Two recent MS proteomics studies include informative protein expression for human VKOR paralogs. Kim *et al.* (2014) systematically examined 30 different human tissues, including seven fetal tissues and six hematopoietic cell types from rapidly acquired postmortem samples from each of three donors [96]. Results for protein levels (~84% coverage of total predicted human proteome) of VKORC1 and VKORC1L1 from this study are available on the Human Proteome Map server [96]. VKORC1 proteolytic peptides (six 6–18 residue peptides representing 31% primary sequence coverage) were detected in six tissues including adrenal gland, monocytes, platelets, lung ovary and testes, while VKORC1L1 peptides (eleven 7–19 residue peptides representing 41% primary sequence coverage) were detected in fetal brain, placenta, testes and in adult lung (Table 2 lists all tissues in which VKOR paralog peptides were detected by MS). A similar MS proteomics study by Wilhelm *et al.* (2014) combined their own data from a similar number of tissues with >10,000 publicly available MS raw data files to generate a database encompassing 60 human tissues, 147 cell lines and 13 body fluids [97]. This study achieved a record 92% coverage of human proteome ORFs. VKORC1 (four 11–30 residue peptides representing 41.1% primary sequence coverage) was detected at higher than median expression levels only in monocytes, pancrease and retina, while VKORC1L1 (four 11–46 residue peptides representing 51.7% primary sequence coverage) was detected in higher than median expression levels only in brain. Compared to the results of Kim *et al.* (2014), this study had a very low detection efficiency for VKOR paralogs likely due to the much longer proteolytic fragments that were initially generated from tissue samples [96,97]. Comparing both MS studies to ChIP-seq method results (see above), it is clear that the MS-based techniques are still in their infancy as the number of tissues with detectable VKOR paralogs is low compared to the results from transcriptome studies. However, looking across all expression study results (Table 2), we find a general concurrence that VKORC1 is most highly expressed in liver, while VKORC1L1 is most highly expressed in brain.

3.2. Promoter Regions of VKORC1 and VKORC1L1 Genes

Since the coding regions of the *VKORC1* and *VKORC1L1* paralog genes are similarly organized and the respective expressed proteins are so highly conserved that their core domain sequence lengths, predicted folds, catalyzed reactions and substrate usage are essentially identical, we decided to survey existing published data for differences in non-coding regions of the genes for clues to why both paralogs have been preserved with complete fidelity in all extant (*i.e.*, sequenced to-date) vertebrate genomes. In a previously published study of human VKORC1L1 expression and function, we cited tissue-specific ChIP-seq gene expression data for both VKOR paralogs from the Functional ANnoTation Of the Mammalian genome phase 4 (FANTOM4) whole genome expression study [31,98]. For the purpose of exploring similarities and differences of the promoter regions for both human VKOR paralogs, we accessed deep-CAGE data using the FANTOM4 human genome viewer (Figure 4). FANTOM4 focused on the dynamics of transcription start site (TSS) usage in the myeloid cell line THP-1 [99]. We retrieved transcription start site (TSS) and predicted transcription factor binding site (TFBS) data for functionally expressed human *VKORC1* and *VKORC1L1* genes. In summary, *VKORC1* promoter organization is distinctly different from and relatively simpler than that for *VKORC1L1*. *VKORC1* uses four alternative TSSs spanning ~200 bp and 24 predicted TFBSs were identified around this region (Figure 4A, red arrows), while *VKORC1L1* uses seven alternative TSSs spanning ~150 bp with 53 predicted nearby TFBSs (Figure 4B, red arrows).

To predict putative binding sites for known TFBS motifs, a window of −300 to +100 bp flanking each promoter region was extracted, multiply aligned and the MotEvo algorithm applied [100]. Of the 52 predicted transcription regulators, 16 TFs were experimentally confirmed by systematic siRNA knock-down for the *VKORC1L1* promoter region, while only three TFs were found to bind the *VKORC1* promoter region (see Note 4 [101]) [98]. Taken together, these data support the notion that expression of each human VKOR paralog is apparently controlled by distinctly different transcriptional mechanisms, in agreement with previous study results for combined tissue expression levels and respective VKOR enzymatic activities in mice [52,82]. Furthermore, for *VKORC1*, there appear to be many predicted TFBSs in common with other hepatically expressed proteins, while predicted TFBSs for *VKORC1L1* are more similar to those from genes that express proteins with known house-keeping and homeostatic functions [31].

3.3. Human Coding Region Mutations

Naturally occurring coding region mutations for human, rat and mouse *VKORC1* genes mostly cause *in vivo* warfarin resistance phenotypes [73,74,102], and one human mutation causes VKCFD2, a severe deficiency in VKD clotting factors [2]. *VKORC1* mutations have been comprehensively reviewed elsewhere [103]. To gain insight into naturally occurring human *VKORC1L1* coding region mutations, we surveyed the NCBI dbVAR database, which includes combined whole genome sequence data for thousands of individuals, and found evidence for 21 total coding region SNPs in living adult humans of which seven are non-synonymous, one premature termination that shortens the *C*-terminus, and six synonymous variants that do not alter translated VKORC1L1 protein sequence. To date, no human *in vivo* phenotypes have been reported for VKORC1L1 non-wild type variants.

3.4. Commentary/Hypothesis: Why do Two VKOR Paralogs Persist in Vertebrates?

Here we summarize various conclusions drawn from the studies reviewed in this article and propose a novel hypothesis to explain why two VKOR paralogs with apparently identical enzymatic functions have persisted in vertebrates over ~400 million years of evolution. Rost *et al.* (2004) first noted that VKORC1L1 primary sequences are considerably more conserved among mammalian orthologs than the respective VKORC1 sequences [2]. Robertson (2004) suggested that the extant paralog genes likely arose in a common ancestor before the divergence of urochordates and vertebrates [3]. Phylogenetic analysis we present in this review suggests the last universal common ancestor (LUCA) of all extant metazoans with both VKOR paralogs was likely a crown chordate older than the LUCA of extant gnathostomes (Section 1.1.3. and Figure 2). Given aggregate evidence reviewed in this article that VKORC1 and VKORC1L1 enzymatic functions are virtually identical, but that regulation of developmental stage- and tissue-specific expression is the major notable difference between both paralogs, we further contemplate what other functional differences, at either the protein or biological pathway levels, could provide the required selection pressure to preserve both paralogs.

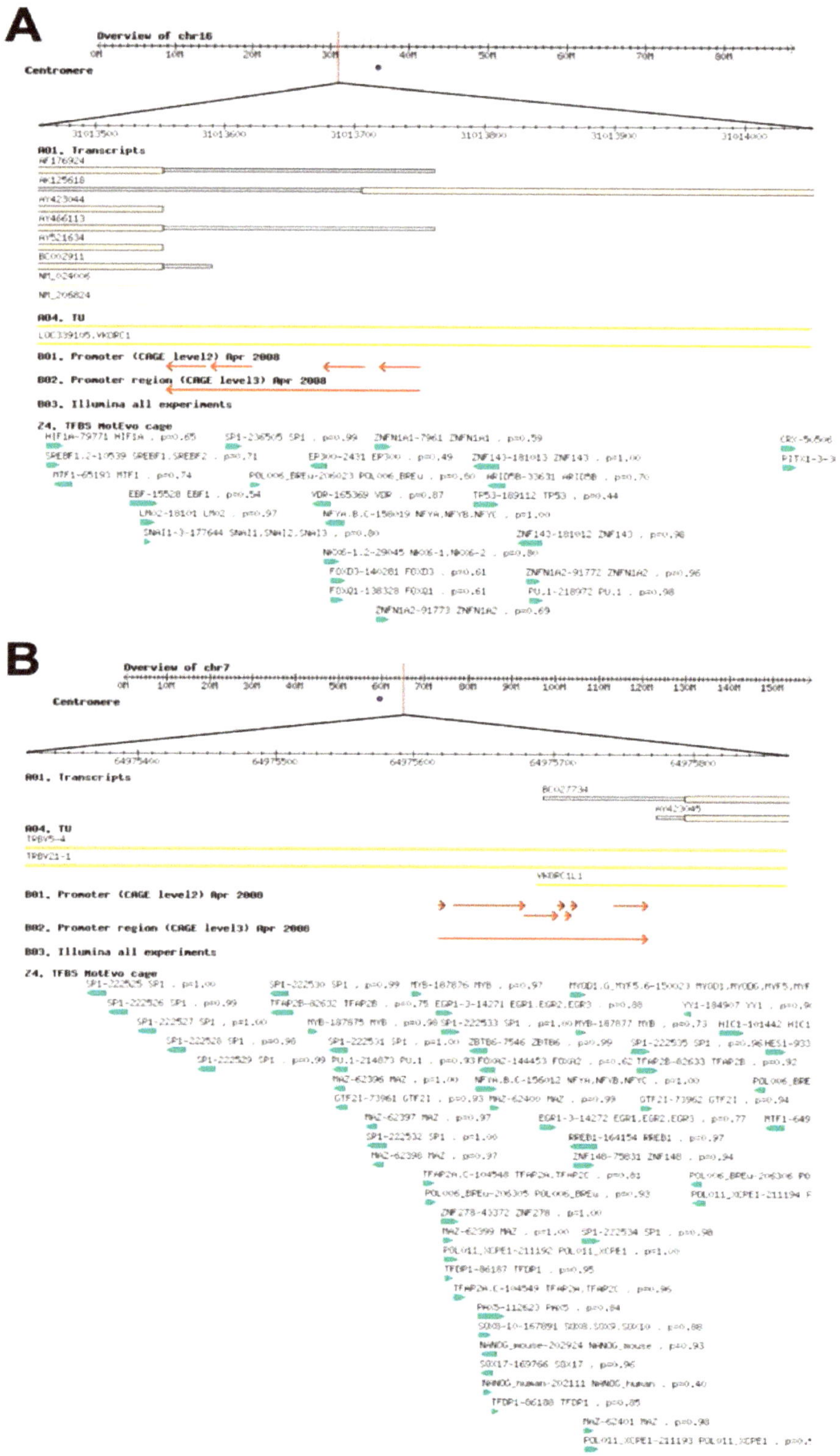

Figure 4. Overview of (top to bottom) chromosome maps (grey fields) showing genetic loci (vertical red lines), alternative mRNA transcripts (A01. Transcripts, tan bars), transcription start sequences (B01. Promoter (CAGE level 2, red arrows) and predicted transcription factor binding sites (24. TFBS MotEvo cage, blue arrows) for (**A**) human *VKORC1*; and (**B**) human *VKORC1L1*. Graphics are from the FANTOM4 Human (hg18) genome viewer (see Note 5 [104]).

Addressing this theme, Robertson (2004) commented, "...If this duplication follows the neofunctionalization model of gene duplication (Ohno, 1970) [105], then the rapid divergence of VKORC1 in vertebrates might suggest that its function related to vitamin K recycling might be the derived function, in which case the unknown VKORC1L1 function might better reflect the role of this protein in the other animals and trypanosomatids. Alternatively, if this duplication follows the subfunctionalization model of Lynch & Force (2000) [106], then both proteins might still be involved in vitamin K recycling; however, for some reason VKORC1 has been free to diverge more rapidly in vertebrates than has VKORC1L1..." It is clear from the evidence we review here that neofunctionalization cannot be the driving force for VKOR paralog maintenance, but that subfunctionalization, not of enzymatic function, but of developmental- and tissue-specific expression regulation, might be the basis for this unique preservation of paralogs. Furthermore, we can rationalize a biological need for this beginning with the evolution of aerobic heterotrophic organisms as the earth's atmosphere became increasingly oxygen-rich through photosynthesis. This led to evolution of multicellular animals and, eventually, vertebrates whose sizes increased over time [19,107]. Accordingly, closed circulatory systems of ever increasing volume and requiring increased cardiac capacity evolved leading to ever increasing circulatory pressure [108]. Parallel to these evolutionary developments in early metazoans, there arose the need for a robust hemostatic system and clotting capability to stem off bleeding through injury [109]. With all of this in mind, we propose that the regulatory mechanisms for VKOR paralog gene expression needed to keep pace with evolutionarily increasing circulatory volume and pressure, and so both VKOR paralogs were maintained in vertebrates due to selection pressure for distinct regulation of expression in non-coding regions of the genes. Thus, VKORC1L1 orthologs may have been maintained for more evolutionarily primitive housekeeping functions that might have included intracellular redox homeostasis and oxidative protein folding under anaerobic growth conditions [31,39]. In contrast, VKORC1 expression regulation has possibly evolved separately to sustain high systemic levels of secreted VKD proteins needed for maintaining large circulatory volume and pressure and also for development and homeostasis of a robust, calcified skeleton.

4. Conclusions and Future Perspectives

In this review, we have attempted to comprehensively summarize published results concerning structural and functional similarities and differences for VKORC1 and VKORC1L1 paralogs in extant metazoan genomes and to relate these to a rationale that explains why these proteins are evolutionarily maintained when their enzymatic functions are virtually identical. While it is presently clear that both enzymes are responsible for *de novo* reduction of K vitamins acquired from dietary sources, in addition to recycling oxidized forms of K vitamins to the respective reduced hydroquinone forms in the vitamin K cycle, evolutionary selection pressure has apparently maintained unique physiological functions for both paralogs by a tissue-specific "division of labor" under independent expression and regulatory controls.

In order to address important questions that remain about these paralogs, it will be necessary to more deeply investigate regulation of their expression with respect to cell and tissue type and developmental stage, to identify their functional intracellular protein partners, and to comprehensively identify and characterize new VKD proteins and the extent of the VKD proteome in individual species. We hope this review will stimulate discussion and cooperative investigation among researchers already engaged in vitamin K-related research areas as well as encourage researchers new to the field with expertise in complementary research methods.

Acknowledgments: This work was supported, in part, by funding from Baxter Germany GmbH (Johannes Oldenburg, Matthias Watzka), from Bayer AG for travel support and conference participation, and from the Deutsche Forschungsgemeinschaft (D.F.G.) grant Ol100 5-1 (Johannes Oldenburg, Matthias Watzka).

Author Contributions: Johannes Oldenburg, Matthias Watzka and Carville G. Bevans conceived and wrote the article. Carville G. Bevans provided literature and database analysis and figures.

References

1. Note 1: Official HUGO human gene designations are *VKORC1* and *VKORC1L1*; non-human orthologs are typically indicated using lower-case letters.
2. Rost, S.; Fregin, A.; Ivaskevicius, V.; Conzelmann, E.; Hörtnagel, K.; Pelz, H.J.; Lappegard, K.; Seifried, E.; Scharrer, I.; Tuddenham, E.G.D.; *et al.* Mutations in VKORC1 cause warfarin resistance and multiple coagulation factor deficiency type 2. *Nature* **2004**, *427*, 537–541. [CrossRef] [PubMed]
3. Robertson, H.M. Genes encoding vitamin-K epoxide reductase are present in Drosophila and trypanosomatid protists. *Genetics* **2004**, *168*, 1077–1080. [CrossRef] [PubMed]
4. Ferland, G. The vitamin K-dependent proteins: An update. *Nutr. Rev.* **1998**, *56*, 223–230. [CrossRef] [PubMed]
5. Willems, B.A.G.; Vermeer, C.; Reutelingsperger, C.P.M.; Schurgers, L.J. The realm of vitamin K dependent proteins: Shifting from coagulation toward calcification. *Mol. Nutr. Food Res.* **2014**, *58*, 1620–1635. [CrossRef] [PubMed]
6. Van Summeren, M.J.H.; van Coeverden, S.C.C.M.; Schurgers, L.J.; Braam, L.A.J.L.M.; Noirt, F.; Uiterwaal, C.S.P.M.; Kuis, W.; Vermeer, C. Vitamin K status is associated with childhood bone mineral content. *Br. J. Nutr.* **2008**, *100*, 852–858.
7. Gundberg, C.M.; Lian, J.B.; Booth, S.L. Vitamin K-dependent carboxylation of osteocalcin: Friend or foe? *Adv. Nutr. Bethesda Md.* **2012**, *3*, 149–157. [CrossRef] [PubMed]
8. Cancela, M.L.; Laizé, V.; Conceição, N. Matrix Gla protein and osteocalcin: From gene duplication to neofunctionalization. *Arch. Biochem. Biophys.* **2014**, *561*, 56–63. [CrossRef] [PubMed]
9. Laurance, S.; Lemarié, C.A.; Blostein, M.D. Growth arrest-specific gene 6 (gas6) and vascular hemostasis. *Adv. Nutr. Bethesda Md.* **2012**, *3*, 196–203. [CrossRef] [PubMed]
10. Shea, M.K.; Holden, R.M. Vitamin K status and vascular calcification: Evidence from observational and clinical studies. *Adv. Nutr. Bethesda Md.* **2012**, *3*, 158–165. [CrossRef] [PubMed]
11. Hegarty, J.M.; Yang, H.; Chi, N.C. UBIAD1-mediated vitamin K2 synthesis is required for vascular endothelial cell survival and development. *Dev. Camb. Engl.* **2013**, *140*, 1713–1719. [CrossRef] [PubMed]
12. Theuwissen, E.; Smit, E.; Vermeer, C. The role of vitamin K in soft-tissue calcification. *Adv. Nutr. Bethesda Md.* **2012**, *3*, 166–173. [CrossRef] [PubMed]
13. Cancela, M.L.; Conceicao, N.; Laize, V. Gla-rich protein, a new player in tissue calcification? *Adv. Nutr.* **2012**, *3*, 174–81. [CrossRef] [PubMed]
14. Ferland, G. Vitamin K and the nervous system: An overview of its actions. *Adv. Nutr. Bethesda Md.* **2012**, *3*, 204–212. [CrossRef] [PubMed]
15. Gely-Pernot, A.; Coronas, V.; Harnois, T.; Prestoz, L.; Mandairon, N.; Didier, A.; Berjeaud, J.M.; Monvoisin, A.; Bourmeyster, N.; de Frutos, P.G.; *et al.* An endogenous vitamin K-dependent mechanism regulates cell proliferation in the brain subventricular stem cell niche. *Stem Cells Dayt. Ohio* **2012**, *30*, 719–731. [CrossRef] [PubMed]
16. Lee, N.K.; Sowa, H.; Hinoi, E.; Ferron, M.; Ahn, J.D.; Confavreux, C.; Dacquin, R.; Mee, P.J.; McKee, M.D.; Jung, D.Y.; *et al.* Endocrine regulation of energy metabolism by the skeleton. *Cell* **2007**, *130*, 456–469. [CrossRef] [PubMed]
17. Ferron, M.; Hinoi, E.; Karsenty, G.; Ducy, P. Osteocalcin differentially regulates beta cell and adipocyte gene expression and affects the development of metabolic diseases in wild-type mice. *Proc. Natl. Acad. Sci. USA* **2008**, *105*, 5266–5270. [CrossRef] [PubMed]

18. Oury, F.; Sumara, G.; Sumara, O.; Ferron, M.; Chang, H.; Smith, C.E.; Hermo, L.; Suarez, S.; Roth, B.L.; Ducy, P.; *et al.* Endocrine regulation of male fertility by the skeleton. *Cell* **2011**, *144*, 796–809. [CrossRef] [PubMed]
19. Brazeau, M.D.; Friedman, M. The origin and early phylogenetic history of jawed vertebrates. *Nature* **2015**, *520*, 490–497. [CrossRef] [PubMed]
20. Bevans, C.G.; Krettler, C.; Reinhart, C.; Watzka, M.; Oldenburg, J. Phylogeny of the vitamin K 2,3-epoxide reductase (VKOR) family and evolutionary relationship to the disulfide bond formation protein B (DsbB) family. *Nutrients* **2015**, *7*, 6224–6249.
21. NCBI. Genome Information by Organism. Available online: http://www.ncbi.nlm.nih.gov/genome/browse/ (accessed on 30 April 2015).
22. NCBI. Bioproject Grid. Available online: http://www.ncbi.nlm.nih.gov/bioproject/browse/ (accessed on 30 April 2015).
23. Dutton, R.J.; Boyd, D.; Berkmen, M.; Beckwith, J. Bacterial species exhibit diversity in their mechanisms and capacity for protein disulfide bond formation. *Proc. Natl. Acad. Sci. USA* **2008**, *105*, 11933–11938. [CrossRef] [PubMed]
24. Li, T.; Chang, C.Y.; Jin, D.Y.; Lin, P.J.; Khvorova, A.; Stafford, D.W. Identification of the gene for vitamin K epoxide reductase. *Nature* **2004**, *427*, 541–544. [CrossRef] [PubMed]
25. Li, W.; Schulman, S.; Dutton, R.J.; Boyd, D.; Beckwith, J.; Rapoport, T.A. Structure of a bacterial homologue of vitamin K epoxide reductase. *Nature* **2010**, *463*, 507–512. [CrossRef] [PubMed]
26. Furt, F.; Oostende, C.; van Widhalm, J.R.; Dale, M.A.; Wertz, J.; Basset, G.J.C. A bimodular oxidoreductase mediates the specific reduction of phylloquinone (vitamin K_1) in chloroplasts. *Plant J. Cell Mol. Biol.* **2010**, *64*, 38–46. [CrossRef] [PubMed]
27. Tie, J.K.; Jin, D.Y.; Stafford, D.W. Mycobacterium tuberculosis vitamin K epoxide reductase homologue supports vitamin K-dependent carboxylation in mammalian cells. *Antioxid. Redox Signal.* **2012**, *16*, 329–338. [CrossRef] [PubMed]
28. Wan, C.M.; Yang, X.J.; Du, J.J.; Lu, Y.; Yu, Z.B.; Feng, Y.G.; Wang, X.Y. Identification and characterization of SlVKOR, a disulfide bond formation protein from Solanum lycopersicum, and bioinformatic analysis of plant VKORs. *Biochem. Biokhimiia* **2014**, *79*, 440–449. [CrossRef] [PubMed]
29. Collins, M.D.; Jones, D. Distribution of isoprenoid quinone structural types in bacteria and their taxonomic implication. *Microbiol. Rev.* **1981**, *45*, 316–354. [PubMed]
30. Jin, D.Y.; Tie, J.K.; Stafford, D.W. The conversion of vitamin K epoxide to vitamin K quinone and vitamin K quinone to vitamin K hydroquinone uses the same active site cysteines. *Biochemistry* **2007**, *46*, 7279–7283. [CrossRef] [PubMed]
31. Westhofen, P.; Watzka, M.; Marinova, M.; Hass, M.; Kirfel, G.; Müller, J.; Bevans, C.G.; Müller, C.R.; Oldenburg, J. Human vitamin K 2,3-epoxide reductase complex subunit 1-like 1 (VKORC1L1) mediates vitamin K-dependent intracellular antioxidant function. *J. Biol. Chem.* **2011**, *286*, 15085–15094. [CrossRef] [PubMed]
32. Goodstadt, L.; Ponting, C.P. Vitamin K epoxide reductase: Homology, active site and catalytic mechanism. *Trends Biochem. Sci.* **2004**, *29*, 289–292. [CrossRef] [PubMed]
33. Rishavy, M.A.; Usubalieva, A.; Hallgren, K.W.; Berkner, K.L. Novel insight into the mechanism of the vitamin K oxidoreductase (VKOR): Electron relay through Cys43 and Cys51 reduces VKOR to allow vitamin K reduction and facilitation of vitamin K-dependent protein carboxylation. *J. Biol. Chem.* **2011**, *286*, 7267–7278. [CrossRef] [PubMed]
34. Rost, S.; Fregin, A.; Hünerberg, M.; Bevans, C.G.; Müller, C.R.; Oldenburg, J. Site-directed mutagenesis of coumarin-type anticoagulant-sensitive VKORC1: Evidence that highly conserved amino acids define structural requirements for enzymatic activity and inhibition by warfarin. *Thromb. Haemost.* **2005**, *94*, 780–786. [PubMed]
35. Siegfried, C.M. Solubilization of vitamin K epoxide reductase and vitamin K-dependent carboxylase from rat liver microsomes. *Biochem. Biophys. Res. Commun.* **1978**, *83*, 1488–1495. [CrossRef]
36. Wajih, N.; Hutson, S.M.; Wallin, R. Disulfide-dependent protein folding is linked to operation of the vitamin K cycle in the endoplasmic reticulum. A protein disulfide isomerase-VKORC1 redox enzyme complex appears to be responsible for vitamin K1 2,3-epoxide reduction. *J. Biol. Chem.* **2007**, *282*, 2626–2635. [CrossRef] [PubMed]

37. Schulman, S.; Wang, B.; Li, W.; Rapoport, T.A. Vitamin K epoxide reductase prefers ER membrane-anchored thioredoxin-like redox partners. *Proc. Natl. Acad. Sci. USA* **2010**, *107*, 15027–15032. [CrossRef] [PubMed]
38. Depuydt, M.; Messens, J.; Collet, J.F. How proteins form disulfide bonds. *Antioxid. Redox Signal.* **2011**, *15*, 49–66. [CrossRef] [PubMed]
39. Rutkevich, L.A.; Williams, D.B. Vitamin K epoxide reductase contributes to protein disulfide formation and redox homeostasis within the endoplasmic reticulum. *Mol. Biol. Cell* **2012**, *23*, 2017–2027. [CrossRef] [PubMed]
40. Wajih, N.; Hutson, S.M.; Owen, J.; Wallin, R. Increased production of functional recombinant human clotting factor IX by baby hamster kidney cells engineered to overexpress VKORC1, the vitamin K 2,3-epoxide-reducing enzyme of the vitamin K cycle. *J. Biol. Chem.* **2005**, *280*, 31603–31607. [CrossRef] [PubMed]
41. Chu, P.H.; Huang, T.Y.; Williams, J.; Stafford, D.W. Purified vitamin K epoxide reductase alone is sufficient for conversion of vitamin K epoxide to vitamin K and vitamin K to vitamin KH_2. *Proc. Natl. Acad. Sci. USA* **2006**, *103*, 19308–19313. [CrossRef] [PubMed]
42. Oldenburg, J.; Bevans, C.G.; Müller, C.R.; Watzka, M. Vitamin K epoxide reductase complex subunit 1 (VKORC1): The key protein of the vitamin K cycle. *Antioxid. Redox Signal.* **2006**, *8*, 347–353. [CrossRef] [PubMed]
43. Oldenburg, J.; Marinova, M.; Müller-Reible, C.; Watzka, M. The vitamin K cycle. *Vitam. Horm.* **2008**, *78*, 35–62. [PubMed]
44. Spohn, G.; Kleinridders, A.; Wunderlich, F.T.; Watzka, M.; Zaucke, F.; Blumbach, K.; Geisen, C.; Seifried, E.; Müller, C.; Paulsson, M.; *et al.* VKORC1 deficiency in mice causes early postnatal lethality due to severe bleeding. *Thromb. Haemost.* **2009**, *101*, 1044–1050. [CrossRef] [PubMed]
45. Oldenburg, J.; von Brederlow, B.; Fregin, A.; Rost, S.; Wolz, W.; Eberl, W.; Eber, S.; Lenz, E.; Schwaab, R.; Brackmann, H.H.; *et al.* Congenital deficiency of vitamin K dependent coagulation factors in two families presents as a genetic defect of the vitamin K-epoxide-reductase-complex. *Thromb. Haemost.* **2000**, *84*, 937–941. [PubMed]
46. Price, P.A. Vitamin K-dependent formation of bone Gla protein (osteocalcin) and its function. *Vitam. Horm.* **1985**, *42*, 65–108. [PubMed]
47. Ferron, M.; Lacombe, J.; Germain, A.; Oury, F.; Karsenty, G. GGCX and VKORC1 inhibit osteocalcin endocrine functions. *J. Cell Biol.* **2015**, *208*, 761–776. [CrossRef] [PubMed]
48. Chatrou, M.L.L.; Reutelingsperger, C.P.; Schurgers, L.J. Role of vitamin K-dependent proteins in the arterial vessel wall. *Hämostaseologie* **2011**, *31*, 251–257. [CrossRef] [PubMed]
49. Chatrou, M.L.L.; Winckers, K.; Hackeng, T.M.; Reutelingsperger, C.P.; Schurgers, L.J. Vascular calcification: The price to pay for anticoagulation therapy with vitamin K-antagonists. *Blood Rev.* **2012**, *26*, 155–166. [CrossRef] [PubMed]
50. Li, J.; Lin, J.C.; Wang, H.; Peterson, J.W.; Furie, B.C.; Furie, B.; Booth, S.L.; Volpe, J.J.; Rosenberg, P.A. Novel role of vitamin K in preventing oxidative injury to developing oligodendrocytes and neurons. *J. Neurosci. Off. J. Soc. Neurosci.* **2003**, *23*, 5816–5826.
51. Varnum, B.C.; Young, C.; Elliott, G.; Garcia, A.; Bartley, T.D.; Fridell, Y.W.; Hunt, R.W.; Trail, G.; Clogston, C.; Toso, R.J. Axl receptor tyrosine kinase stimulated by the vitamin K-dependent protein encoded by growth-arrest-specific gene 6. *Nature* **1995**, *373*, 623–626. [CrossRef] [PubMed]
52. Hammed, A.; Matagrin, B.; Spohn, G.; Prouillac, C.; Benoit, E.; Lattard, V. VKORC1L1, an enzyme rescuing the vitamin K 2,3-epoxide reductase activity in some extrahepatic tissues during anticoagulation therapy. *J. Biol. Chem.* **2013**, *288*, 28733–28742. [CrossRef] [PubMed]
53. Holland, P.W.; Garcia-Fernàndez, J.; Williams, N.A.; Sidow, A. Gene duplications and the origins of vertebrate development. *Dev. Camb. Engl. Suppl.* **1994**, 125–133.
54. Note 2: The *Callorhinchus milii* (Australian ghostshark) genome, published in 2014, represents cartilagenous fishes among gnathostomes and includes entries of two VKOR family proteins. One apparently complete sequence (176 residues, NCBI genomic sequence entry XP_007894765.1, confirmed as transcriptome entry AFP01110.1) is homologous to vertebrate VKORC1L1 orthologs, while the second sequence (142 residues, NCBI genomic sequence entry XP_007894766.1) appears to be incomplete and possibly a concatenation of the 30 residue *N*-terminal sequence of a VKORC1 ortholog together with a *C*-terminal 112 residue sequence that

is identical to that of the putative VKORC1L1 paralog. Thus, the currently available data are inconclusive, but suggest that *Callorhinchus milii* possesses two VKOR paralogs.

55. Note 3: The genome of *Petromyzon marinus* (Japanese sea lamprey), published in 2011, represents the jawless vertebrates (Cyclostomata) and currently has no NCBI sequence entries. However, a BLAST search performed on the currently available lamprey genome (http://jlampreygenome.imcb.a-star.edu.sg, accessed 26 April 2015) using the human VKORC1 sequence returned only one partially homologous sequence (gene designation JL2487, 206 residues with no initial methionine, E-value 2e-22) with 57% identity to the human VKORC1 sequence from residue 11 through 95 and including the conserved loop cysteines and serine. However, the conserved active site CXXC motif is entirely absent from this sequence, suggesting an incorrect sequence assembly. Thus, no VKOR family homologs could be identified from the currently available lamprey genome data.
56. Vincent, M.J.; Martin, A.S.; Compans, R.W. Function of the KK*XX* Motif in Endoplasmic Reticulum Retrieval of a Transmembrane Protein Depends on the Length and Structure of the Cytoplasmic Domain. *J. Biol. Chem.* **1998**, *273*, 950–956. [CrossRef] [PubMed]
57. Czogalla, K.J.; Biswas, A.; Rost, S.; Watzka, M.; Oldenburg, J. The Arg98Trp mutation in human VKORC1 causing VKCFD2 disrupts a di-arginine-based ER retention motif. *Blood* **2014**, *124*, 1354–1362. [CrossRef] [PubMed]
58. Hildebrandt, E.F.; Preusch, P.C.; Patterson, J.L.; Suttie, J.W. Solubilization and characterization of vitamin K epoxide reductase from normal and warfarin-resistant rat liver microsomes. *Arch. Biochem. Biophys.* **1984**, *228*, 480–492. [CrossRef]
59. Lasseur, R.; Longin-Sauvageon, C.; Videmann, B.; Billeret, M.; Berny, P.; Benoit, E. Warfarin resistance in a French strain of rats. *J. Biochem. Mol. Toxicol.* **2005**, *19*, 379–385. [CrossRef] [PubMed]
60. Lasseur, R.; Grandemange, A.; Longin-Sauvageon, C.; Berny, P.; Benoit, E. Heterogeneity of the coumarin anticoagulant targeted vitamin K epoxide reduction system. Study of kinetic parameters in susceptible and resistant mice (Mus musculus domesticus). *J. Biochem. Mol. Toxicol.* **2006**, *20*, 221–229. [CrossRef] [PubMed]
61. Hodroge, A.; Longin-Sauvageon, C.; Fourel, I.; Benoit, E.; Lattard, V. Biochemical characterization of spontaneous mutants of rat VKORC1 involved in the resistance to antivitamin K anticoagulants. *Arch. Biochem. Biophys.* **2011**, *515*, 14–20. [CrossRef] [PubMed]
62. Hodroge, A.; Matagrin, B.; Moreau, C.; Fourel, I.; Hammed, A.; Benoit, E.; Lattard, V. VKORC1 mutations detected in patients resistant to vitamin K antagonists are not all associated with a resistant VKOR activity. *J. Thromb. Haemost. JTH* **2012**, *10*, 2535–2543. [CrossRef] [PubMed]
63. Bevans, C.G.; Krettler, C.; Reinhart, C.; Tran, H.; Koßmann, K.; Watzka, M.; Oldenburg, J. Determination of the warfarin inhibition constant K_i for vitamin K 2,3-epoxide reductase complex subunit-1 (VKORC1) using an *in vitro* DTT-driven assay. *Biochim. Biophys. Acta* **2013**, *1830*, 4202–4210. [CrossRef] [PubMed]
64. Matagrin, B.; Hodroge, A.; Montagut-Romans, A.; Andru, J.; Fourel, I.; Besse, S.; Benoit, E.; Lattard, V. New insights into the catalytic mechanism of vitamin K epoxide reductase (VKORC1)—The catalytic properties of the major mutations of rVKORC1 explain the biological cost associated to mutations. *FEBS Open Bio* **2013**, *3*, 144–150. [CrossRef] [PubMed]
65. Bevans, C.G.; Krettler, C.; Reinhart, C.; Tran, H.; Koßmann, K.; Watzka, M.; Oldenburg, J. Corrigendum to "Determination of the warfarin inhibition constant K_i for vitamin K 2,3-epoxide reductase complex subunit-1 (VKORC1) using an *in vitro* DTT-driven assay" [BBAGEN (2013) 4202–4210]. *Biochim. Biophys. Acta BBA—Gen. Subj.* **2014**, *1840*, 2382–2384. [CrossRef]
66. Matagrin, B.; Montagut-Romans, A.; Damin, M.; Lemaire, M.; Popowycz, F.; Benoit, E.; Lattard, V. Identification of VKORC1 genotype leading to resistance to tecarfarin. *J. Clin. Pharmacol.* **2014**, *54*, 896–900. [CrossRef] [PubMed]
67. Goulois, J.; Chapuzet, A.; Lambert, V.; Chatron, N.; Tchertanov, L.; Legros, L.; Benoît, E.; Lattard, V. Evidence of a target resistance to antivitamin K rodenticides in the roof rat Rattus rattus: Identification and characterization of a novel Y25F mutation in the Vkorc1 gene. *Pest Manag. Sci.* **2015**. [CrossRef]
68. Krettler, C.; Bevans, C.G.; Reinhart, C.; Watzka, M.; Oldenburg, J. Tris(3-hydroxypropyl)phosphine is superior to DTT for *in vitro* assessment of vitamin K 2,3-epoxide reductase activity. *Anal. Biochem.* **2015**, *474*, 89–94. [CrossRef] [PubMed]

69. Preusch, P.C.; Brummet, S.R. Steady-state kinetics of microsomal vitamin K epoxide reduction. In Current Advances in Vitamin K Research, Proceedings of the Seventeenth Steenbock Symposium, University of Wisconsin, Madison, WI, USA, 21–25 June 1987; Suttie, J.W., Ed.; Elsevier: New York, NY, USA, 1988; pp. 75–82.
70. Cornish-Bowden, A. *Fundamental of Enzyme Kinetics*; Butterworth & Co (Publishers) Ltd.: London, UK, 1979.
71. Whitlon, D.S.; Sadowski, J.A.; Suttie, J.W. Mechanism of coumarin action: Significance of vitamin K epoxide reductase inhibition. *Biochemistry* **1978**, *17*, 1371–1377. [CrossRef] [PubMed]
72. Silverman, R.B.; Oliver, J.S. 2-(Fluoromethyl)-3-phytyl-1,4-naphthoquinone and its 2,3-epoxide. Inhibition of vitamin K epoxide reductase. *J. Med. Chem.* **1989**, *32*, 2138–2141. [CrossRef] [PubMed]
73. Rost, S.; Pelz, H.J.; Menzel, S.; MacNicoll, A.D.; León, V.; Song, K.J.; Jäkel, T.; Oldenburg, J.; Müller, C.R. Novel mutations in the VKORC1 gene of wild rats and mice—A response to 50 years of selection pressure by warfarin? *BMC Genet.* **2009**, *10*, 4. [CrossRef] [PubMed]
74. Watzka, M.; Geisen, C.; Bevans, C.G.; Sittinger, K.; Spohn, G.; Rost, S.; Seifried, E.; Müller, C.R.; Oldenburg, J. Thirteen novel VKORC1 mutations associated with oral anticoagulant resistance: Insights into improved patient diagnosis and treatment. *J. Thromb. Haemost. JTH* **2011**, *9*, 109–118. [CrossRef] [PubMed]
75. Fregin, A.; Czogalla, K.J.; Gansler, J.; Rost, S.; Taverna, M.; Watzka, M.; Bevans, C.G.; Müller, C.R.; Oldenburg, J. A new cell culture-based assay quantifies vitamin K 2,3-epoxide reductase complex subunit 1 function and reveals warfarin resistance phenotypes not shown by the dithiothreitol-driven VKOR assay. *J. Thromb. Haemost. JTH* **2013**, *11*, 872–880. [CrossRef] [PubMed]
76. Czogalla, K.J.; Biswas, A.; Wendeln, A.C.; Westhofen, P.; Müller, C.R.; Watzka, M.; Oldenburg, J. Human VKORC1 mutations cause variable degrees of 4-hydroxycoumarin resistance and affect putative warfarin binding interfaces. *Blood* **2013**, *122*, 2743–2750. [CrossRef] [PubMed]
77. Tie, J.K.; Jin, D.Y.; Tie, K.; Stafford, D.W. Evaluation of warfarin resistance using transcription activator-like effector nucleases-mediated vitamin K epoxide reductase knockout HEK293 cells. *J. Thromb. Haemost. JTH* **2013**, *11*, 1556–1564. [CrossRef] [PubMed]
78. Haque, J.; McDonald, M.; Kulman, J.; Rettie, A.E. A cellular system for quantitation of vitamin K cycle activity: Structure-activity effects on vitamin K antagonism by warfarin metabolites. *Blood* **2013**, *123*, 582–589. [CrossRef] [PubMed]
79. Itoh, S.; Onishi, S. Developmental changes of vitamin K epoxidase and reductase activities involved in the vitamin K cycle in human liver. *Early Hum. Dev.* **2000**, *57*, 15–23. [CrossRef]
80. Ko, M.S.; Threat, T.A.; Wang, X.; Horton, J.H.; Cui, Y.; Wang, X.; Pryor, E.; Paris, J.; Wells-Smith, J.; Kitchen, J.R.; *et al.* Genome-wide mapping of unselected transcripts from extraembryonic tissue of 7.5-day mouse embryos reveals enrichment in the *t*-complex and under-representation on the X chromosome. *Hum. Mol. Genet.* **1998**, *7*, 1967–1978. [CrossRef] [PubMed]
81. Diez-Roux, G.; Banfi, S.; Sultan, M.; Geffers, L.; Anand, S.; Rozado, D.; Magen, A.; Canidio, E.; Pagani, M.; Peluso, I.; *et al.* A high-resolution anatomical atlas of the transcriptome in the mouse embryo. *PLoS Biol.* **2011**, *9*, e1000582. [CrossRef] [PubMed]
82. Caspers, M.; Czogalla, K.J.; Liphardt, K.; Müller, J.; Westhofen, P.; Watzka, M.; Oldenburg, J. Two enzymes catalyze vitamin K 2,3-epoxide reductase activity in mouse: VKORC1 is highly expressed in exocrine tissues while VKORC1L1 is highly expressed in brain. *Thromb. Res.* **2015**, *135*, 977–983. [CrossRef] [PubMed]
83. Fernández, I.; Vijayakumar, P.; Marques, C.; Cancela, M.L.; Gavaia, P.J.; Laizé, V. Zebrafish vitamin K epoxide reductases: Expression *in vivo*, along extracellular matrix mineralization and under phylloquinone and warfarin *in vitro* exposure. *Fish Physiol. Biochem.* **2015**, *41*, 745–759. [CrossRef] [PubMed]
84. Vijayakumar, P.; Laizé, V.; Cardeira, J.; Trindade, M.; Cancela, M.L. Development of an *in vitro* cell system from zebrafish suitable to study bone cell differentiation and extracellular matrix mineralization. *Zebrafish* **2013**, *10*, 500–509. [CrossRef] [PubMed]
85. Zou, D.; Ma, L.; Yu, J.; Zhang, Z. Biological Databases for Human Research. *Genomics Proteomics Bioinform.* **2015**, *13*, 55–63. [CrossRef] [PubMed]
86. Su, A.I.; Wiltshire, T.; Batalov, S.; Lapp, H.; Ching, K.A.; Block, D.; Zhang, J.; Soden, R.; Hayakawa, M.; Kreiman, G.; *et al.* A gene atlas of the mouse and human protein-encoding transcriptomes. *Proc. Natl. Acad. Sci. USA* **2004**, *101*, 6062–6067. [CrossRef] [PubMed]

87. Blaveri, E.; Kelly, F.; Mallei, A.; Harris, K.; Taylor, A.; Reid, J.; Razzoli, M.; Carboni, L.; Piubelli, C.; Musazzi, L.; *et al.* Expression profiling of a genetic animal model of depression reveals novel molecular pathways underlying depressive-like behaviours. *PLoS ONE* **2010**, *5*, e12596. [CrossRef] [PubMed]
88. Freeman, T.C.; Ivens, A.; Baillie, J.K.; Beraldi, D.; Barnett, M.W.; Dorward, D.; Downing, A.; Fairbairn, L.; Kapetanovic, R.; Raza, S.; *et al.* A gene expression atlas of the domestic pig. *BMC Biol.* **2012**, *10*, 90. [CrossRef] [PubMed]
89. Lui, J.C.K.; Andrade, A.C.; Forcinito, P.; Hegde, A.; Chen, W.; Baron, J.; Nilsson, O. Spatial and temporal regulation of gene expression in the mammalian growth plate. *Bone* **2010**, *46*, 1380–1390. [CrossRef] [PubMed]
90. Forcinito, P.; Andrade, A.C.; Finkielstain, G.P.; Baron, J.; Nilsson, O.; Lui, J.C. Growth-inhibiting conditions slow growth plate senescence. *J. Endocrinol.* **2011**, *208*, 59–67. [CrossRef] [PubMed]
91. Wu, C.; Orozco, C.; Boyer, J.; Leglise, M.; Goodale, J.; Batalov, S.; Hodge, C.L.; Haase, J.; Janes, J.; Huss, J.W.; *et al.* BioGPS: An extensible and customizable portal for querying and organizing gene annotation resources. *Genome Biol.* **2009**, *10*, R130. [CrossRef] [PubMed]
92. The GTEx Consortium; Ardlie, K.G.; Deluca, D.S.; Segre, A.V.; Sullivan, T.J.; Young, T.R.; Gelfand, E.T.; Trowbridge, C.A.; Maller, J.B.; Tukiainen, T.; *et al.* The Genotype-Tissue Expression (GTEx) pilot analysis: Multitissue gene regulation in humans. *Science* **2015**, *348*, 648–660. [CrossRef] [PubMed]
93. Melé, M.; Ferreira, P.G.; Reverter, F.; de Luca, D.S.; Monlong, J.; Sammeth, M.; Young, T.R.; Goldmann, J.M.; Pervouchine, D.D.; Sullivan, T.J.; *et al.* The human transcriptome across tissues and individuals. *Science* **2015**, *348*, 660–665. [CrossRef] [PubMed]
94. Benjamini, Y.; Hochberg, Y. Controlling the False Discovery Rate: A Practical and Powerful Approach to Multiple Testing. *J. R. Stat. Soc. Ser. B Methodol.* **1995**, *57*, 289–300.
95. Thelen, J.J.; Miernyk, J.A. The proteomic future: Where mass spectrometry should be taking us. *Biochem. J.* **2012**, *444*, 169–181. [CrossRef] [PubMed]
96. Kim, M.S.; Pinto, S.M.; Getnet, D.; Nirujogi, R.S.; Manda, S.S.; Chaerkady, R.; Madugundu, A.K.; Kelkar, D.S.; Isserlin, R.; Jain, S.; *et al.* A draft map of the human proteome. *Nature* **2014**, *509*, 575–581. [CrossRef] [PubMed]
97. Wilhelm, M.; Schlegl, J.; Hahne, H.; Moghaddas Gholami, A.; Lieberenz, M.; Savitski, M.M.; Ziegler, E.; Butzmann, L.; Gessulat, S.; Marx, H.; *et al.* Mass-spectrometry-based draft of the human proteome. *Nature* **2014**, *509*, 582–587. [CrossRef] [PubMed]
98. Ravasi, T.; Suzuki, H.; Cannistraci, C.V.; Katayama, S.; Bajic, V.B.; Tan, K.; Akalin, A.; Schmeier, S.; Kanamori-Katayama, M.; Bertin, N.; *et al.* An atlas of combinatorial transcriptional regulation in mouse and man. *Cell* **2010**, *140*, 744–752. [CrossRef] [PubMed]
99. FANTOM Consortium; Suzuki, H.; Forrest, A.R.R.; van Nimwegen, E.; Daub, C.O.; Balwierz, P.J.; Irvine, K.M.; Lassmann, T.; Ravasi, T.; Hasegawa, Y.; *et al.* The transcriptional network that controls growth arrest and differentiation in a human myeloid leukemia cell line. *Nat. Genet.* **2009**, *41*, 553–562.
100. Arnold, P.; Erb, I.; Pachkov, M.; Molina, N.; van Nimwegen, E. MotEvo: Integrated Bayesian probabilistic methods for inferring regulatory sites and motifs on multiple alignments of DNA sequences. *Bioinform. Oxf. Engl.* **2012**, *28*, 487–494. [CrossRef] [PubMed]
101. Note 4: Data for *VKORC1* and *VKORC1L1* from EdgeExpress DB; http://fantom.gsc.riken.jp/4/edgeexpress/view/#5540409 and #5561011, accessed on 1 May 2015.
102. Pelz, H.J.; Rost, S.; Hünerberg, M.; Fregin, A.; Heiberg, A.C.; Baert, K.; MacNicoll, A.D.; Prescott, C.V.; Walker, A.S.; Oldenburg, J.; *et al.* The genetic basis of resistance to anticoagulants in rodents. *Genetics* **2005**, *170*, 1839–1847. [CrossRef] [PubMed]
103. Oldenburg, J.; Müller, C.R.; Rost, S.; Watzka, M.; Bevans, C.G. Comparative genetics of warfarin resistance. *Hämostaseologie* **2014**, *34*, 143–159. [CrossRef] [PubMed]
104. Note 5: Data for *VKORC1* and *VKORC1L1* can be viewed at http://fantom.gsc.riken.jp/4/gev/gbrowse/hg18/; accessed on 1 May 2010.
105. Ohno, S. *Evolution by Gene Duplication*; Allen & Unwin: London, UK; Springer-Verlag: New York, NY, USA, 1970.
106. Lynch, M.; Force, A. The probability of duplicate gene preservation by subfunctionalization. *Genetics* **2000**, *154*, 459–473. [PubMed]
107. Holland, N.D.; Holland, L.Z.; Holland, P.W.H. Scenarios for the making of vertebrates. *Nature* **2015**, *520*, 450–455. [CrossRef] [PubMed]

108. Diogo, R.; Kelly, R.G.; Christiaen, L.; Levine, M.; Ziermann, J.M.; Molnar, J.L.; Noden, D.M.; Tzahor, E. A new heart for a new head in vertebrate cardiopharyngeal evolution. *Nature* **2015**, *520*, 466–473. [CrossRef] [PubMed]
109. Doolittle, R.F. Coagulation in vertebrates with a focus on evolution and inflammation. *J. Innate Immun.* **2011**, *3*, 9–16. [CrossRef] [PubMed]

9

Long-Chain Metabolites of Vitamin E: Metabolic Activation as a General Concept for Lipid-Soluble Vitamins?

Martin Schubert [1,2,†], Stefan Kluge [1,2,†], Lisa Schmölz [1,2], Maria Wallert [1,3], Francesco Galli [4], Marc Birringer [5] and Stefan Lorkowski [1,2,*]

1 Department of Biochemistry and Physiology of Nutrition, Friedrich-Schiller-University Jena, 07743 Jena, Germany; m.schubert@uni-jena.de (M.S.); s.kluge@uni-jena.de (S.K.); lisa.schmoelz@uni-jena.de (L.S.); maria.wallert@uni-jena.de (M.W.)
2 Competence Center for Nutrition and Cardiovascular Health (nutriCARD), Halle-Jena-Leipzig, 07743 Jena, Germany
3 Baker IDI Heart and Diabetes Institute, Melbourne VIC 3004, Australia
4 Department of Pharmaceutical Sciences, Laboratory of Nutrition and Clinical Biochemistry, University of Perugia, 06123 Perugia, Italy; francesco.galli@unipg.it
5 Department of Nutrition, Food and Consumer Sciences, University of Applied Sciences Fulda, 36037 Fulda, Germany; marc.birringer@oe.hs-fulda.de
* Correspondence: stefan.lorkowski@uni-jena.de
† These authors contributed equally.

Abstract: Vitamins E, A, D and K comprise the class of lipid-soluble vitamins. For vitamins A and D, a metabolic conversion of precursors to active metabolites has already been described. During the metabolism of vitamin E, the long-chain metabolites (LCMs) 13′-hydroxychromanol (13′-OH) and 13′-carboxychromanol (13′-COOH) are formed by oxidative modification of the side-chain. The occurrence of these metabolites in human serum indicates a physiological relevance. Indeed, effects of the LCMs on lipid metabolism, apoptosis, proliferation and inflammatory actions as well as tocopherol and xenobiotic metabolism have been shown. Interestingly, there are several parallels between the actions of the LCMs of vitamin E and the active metabolites of vitamin A and D. The recent findings that the LCMs exert effects different from that of their precursors support their putative role as regulatory metabolites. Hence, it could be proposed that the mode of action of the LCMs might be mediated by a mechanism similar to vitamin A and D metabolites. If the physiological relevance and this concept of action of the LCMs can be confirmed, a general concept of activation of lipid-soluble vitamins via their metabolites might be deduced.

Keywords: vitamin E; long-chain metabolites of vitamin E; 13′-hydroxychromanol (13′-OH); 13′-carboxychromanol (13′-COOH); vitamin E metabolism; biological activity

---

1. The Biological Significance of Vitamin E

The term vitamin E comprises eight lipophilic molecules, which can be classified as tocopherols (TOHs) and tocotrienols (T3). Both classes share two common features: (i) the phytyl-like side chain, which is bound to (ii) the chroman ring system. A saturated side chain characterizes the TOHs, while the T3s carry three double bonds in this substructure. Further, the methylation pattern of the chroman ring determines the classification as α-, β-, γ- or δ-TOH or T3, respectively. Vitamin E is found in oils, nuts, germs, seeds and a variety of other plant products. The naturally found vitamin E forms exist either in *RRR*-configuration (TOHs) or in *R*-configuration (T3s), whereas only synthetically produced forms contain a mixture of the different possible stereoisomers [1].

Vitamin E was discovered in 1922 as vital factor for the fertility of rats, indicating its essentiality for animal and human health, and was therefore classified as a vitamin [2]. Nevertheless, the benefits of vitamin E for human health are still a contentious issue. However, several disease conditions, such as anemia, erythrocyte rupture and neuronal degeneration, as well as muscle degeneration, are linked to vitamin E deficiency or malabsorption (extensively reviewed in [3]). Further, vitamin E was shown in human intervention trials to slow down the progression of age-related neurodegenerative pathologies such as Alzheimer's disease, maybe due to its antioxidative properties [4,5]. Vitamin E is also an essential factor for the development of the central nervous system and cognitive functions of the embryo [6,7]. Next, vitamin E may play a supportive role in the prevention of neural tube defects in humans along with folic acid [8,9]. Initially, the effects of vitamin E were only attributed to its antioxidant properties, however more recent work unveiled non-antioxidant regulatory effects. There is growing evidence that vitamin E modulates gene expression and enzyme activities and interferes with signaling cascades independent of its capacity as an antioxidant [10]. Over time, several functions of vitamin E, such as suppression of inflammatory mediators, reactive oxygen species, and adhesion molecules, the induction of scavenger receptors, and the activation of nuclear factor kappa-light-chain-enhancer of activated B cells (NF_kB) (reviewed in [11]) were revealed. Based on these observations, it was concluded that vitamin E likely plays a role in several inflammatory but also other diseases. However, further research is required, as the results obtained from clinical trials with TOHs are inconsistent with respect to beneficial effects on the development of chronic diseases such as cancer and cardiovascular diseases [12].

2. Absorption and Distribution of Vitamin E

Like for all macro- and micronutrients, intestinal absorption is the limiting factor for the bioavailability of vitamin E in humans. As a fat-soluble vitamin, intestinal absorption, hepatic metabolism and cellular uptake of vitamin E follows that of other lipophilic molecules [13]. The absorption rate of vitamin E varies between 20% and 80% [13,14], and is thus generally lower than for vitamins A and D [15,16]. Differences in the rates of absorption of vitamin E and the other fat-soluble vitamins may result also from the parallel intake of additional food ingredients. For example, retinoic acid [17], plant sterols [18], eicosapentaenoic acid [14], alcohol (chronic consumption) [14], and dietary fiber [19] are natural food components that may compete with the absorption of vitamin E. In addition, it has been shown that the supplied form of vitamin E, either as a free molecule or coupled to other compounds like acetate, is also crucial for its bioavailability [20].

For optimal absorption, fat must be consumed along with the ingested vitamin E. This is a general requirement for all types of fat-soluble vitamins and is therefore also applicable for vitamins A, D and K [16,21]. The absorption of triacylglycerides and esterified fat-soluble molecules starts with enzymatic processing in the stomach by the action of gastric lipases [15]. The following digestion of dietary lipids appears in the intestinal lumen by the action of various enzymes, including pancreatic lipase, carboxyl esterase and phospholipase A_2 [22]. Since most of the vitamin E in the human diet is not esterified, lipolytic degradation is scarce [14]. In contrast, the human diet contains significantly more esterified vitamin A and D, mostly in the form of retinyl-esters and vitamin D_3 oleate, which can be hydrolyzed by the above mentioned enzymes [16,21]. A key step of the intestinal absorption of fat-soluble vitamins is the emulsification, i.e., the incorporation into micelles formed with phospholipids and bile acids. Under normal conditions, bile salts facilitate the absorption of all three vitamins, but especially the vitamin D forms differ in their dependency for bile salt availability, i.e., vitamin D_3 absorption is more dependent on the presence of bile salts than 25-hydroxyvitamin D (OHD) [23]. After emulsification, vitamin E is taken up into the intestinal enterocytes by passive diffusion or receptor-mediated transport via scavenger receptor class B type 1 (SRB1) [24], or Niemann–Pick C1-like protein 1 [25], which is also involved in the uptake of the vitamins A, D and K as well as cholesterol [16,26,27]. Since no specific plasma transport protein for α-TOH is known, the subsequent transport of vitamin E in blood follows largely that of cholesterol [25], meaning that under normal physiological conditions, α-TOH is transported via chylomicrons. This transport is independent of the type of stereoisomer [28,29]. In addition, retinol, unconverted pro-retinoid carotenoids (β-carotene), non-pro-retinoid carotenoids (lycopene), vitamin D_3 and phylloquinone (representing the main dietary form of vitamin K) are also incorporated into chylomicrons [16,21,30]. After entering the circulation, chylomicrons undergo a process of remodeling that involves primarily the hydrolysis of triglycerides by lipoprotein lipase, resulting in the formation of chylomicron remnants [25]. Vitamins E, A, D and K are not affected by hydrolysis and remain in the lipoprotein particle for further transport to the liver [31]. The different forms of vitamin E are discriminated in the liver by the α-tocopherol transfer protein (α-TTP), which promotes the incorporation of 2*R*- or *RRR*-α-TOH into very low-density lipoproteins (VLDL) [32,33], whereas other forms and stereoisomers are either metabolized or secreted into bile [34]. Besides α-TTP, the TOH-associated protein and the TOH-binding protein are known mediators of the intracellular transport of vitamin E. Interestingly, α-TOH secretion from the liver is apparently not necessarily dependent on VLDL assembly and secretion, thus oxysterol-binding proteins [35] and ATP-binding cassette transporter A1 (ABCA1) [36] have been suggested to contribute to the release from the liver. Furthermore, ABCA1 mediates the efflux of vitamin E in the intestine, macrophages, and fibroblasts [36], and multidrug resistance P-glycoprotein has been identified as a transporter for the excretion of α-TOH via bile [37]. After the release of vitamin E-carrying VLDL into blood circulation and action of lipoprotein lipase as well as hepatic lipase, receptors such as SRB1, low-density lipoprotein (LDL) receptor as well as LDL receptor-related protein mediate the uptake of vitamin E into peripheral tissues and the liver [31,38].

3. Metabolism of Vitamin E

The metabolism of vitamin E is primarily localized in the liver (Figure 1) (reviewed in [39]), whereas extrahepatic pathways have been also suggested [40,41]. The degradation processes of hepatic metabolism remain poorly understood, but the initial mechanisms are generally accepted, i.e., all vitamers are degraded to vitamer-specific physiological metabolites with an intact chromanol ring and a shortened side-chain. Interestingly, accumulation of vitamin E to toxic levels is prevented by increased metabolism in response to higher vitamin E levels. Due to the preferential binding to α-TTP, α-TOH is the prevalent form of vitamin E in humans. It is speculated that α-TTP protects the α-form from degradation, thus leading to the accumulation of α-TOH. With the lower affinities of the other vitamin E forms to α-TTP taken into consideration, γ- and δ-forms are likely catabolized faster [42]. Despite of the different catabolic rates, all forms of vitamin E follow the same metabolic route, as confirmed by the detection of the respective end products of hepatic metabolism, α-, β-, γ-, and δ-carboxyethylhydroxychromanol (CEHC) [43,44]. However, the rate of catabolism is different for the vitamin E forms, possibly due to distinct affinities to key enzymes [42,45]. The chroman ring is not modified during catabolism (the catabolic end products are still classified as α-, β-, γ- and δ-forms); it is rather the aliphatic side chain where modifications are introduced. Metabolism of T3 follows the same principle, albeit further enzymes such as 2,4 dienoyl-coenzyme A (CoA) reductase and 3,2-enoyl-CoA isomerase (necessary for the metabolism of unsaturated fatty acids) are likely required for the degradation of the unsaturated side chain [46].

The catabolism of the vitamin E molecule takes place in different cell compartments: endoplasmic reticulum, peroxisomes, and mitochondria. However, the mechanism of metabolite transfer between the compartments is not well understood and requires further investigation. The initial step at the endoplasmic reticulum leads to the formation of 13′-hydroxychromanol (13′-OH) metabolites via ω-hydroxylation by cytochrome P450 (CYP) 4F2 or CYP3A4, respectively [45,47]. The following ω-oxidation, which is probably mediated by alcohol and aldehyde dehydrogenases (an aldehyde intermediate is formed), results in 13′-carboxychromanol (COOH) metabolites. In general, the resulting metabolites with carboxy function are degraded like branched-chain fatty acids. Hence, the side chain is shortened by β-oxidation, and the formed propionyl-CoA or acetyl-CoA is eliminated. The intermediate-chain metabolites 11′-COOH and 9′-COOH are formed in peroxisomes during the first two cycles of β-oxidation. Three additional cycles of β-oxidation are carried out in the mitochondria, resulting in the short-chain metabolites (SCMs) 7′-COOH and 5′-COOH as well as the end-product CEHC or 3′-COOH. Moreover, conjugation of the metabolites takes place during metabolism, resulting predominantly in sulfated and glucuronidated metabolites. However, glycine-, glycine–glucuronide-, and taurine-modified metabolites of vitamin E have also been identified [48].

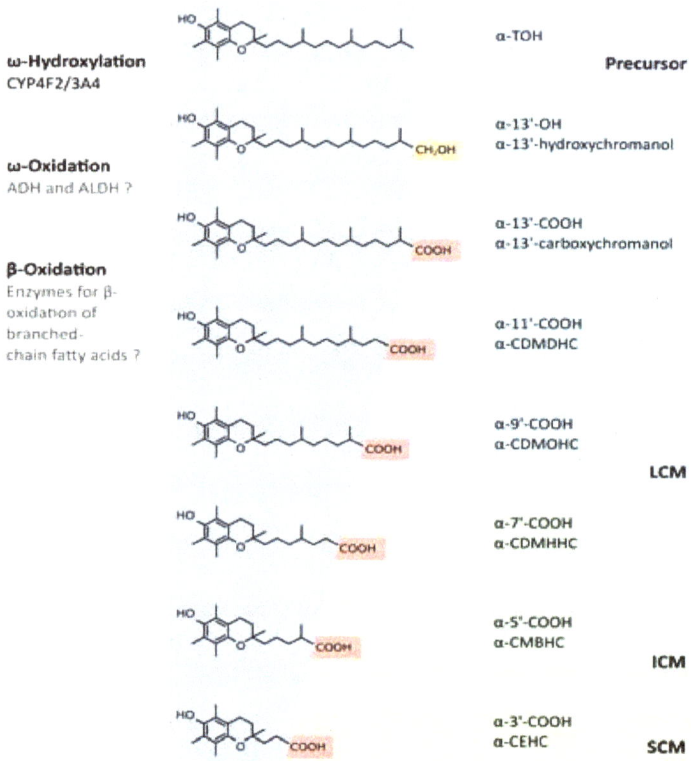

Figure 1. Metabolism of vitamin E. The metabolism of vitamin E is initiated by a terminal ω-hydroxylation of the side-chain via CYP4F2 and CYP3A4. The resulting hydroxychromanol is further modified by ω-oxidation, resulting in the formation of carboxychromanol, possibly by alcohol and aldehyde dehydrogenases. As a consequence, the metabolite can be subjected to β-oxidation. Five cycles of β-oxidation lead to the formation of the short-chain metabolite CEHC. However, this review focuses on the LCMs 13′-OH and 13′-COOH as these molecules have been synthesized in sufficient amounts for in vitro and in vivo investigations. The following abbreviations are used: ADH, alcohol dehydrogenase; ALDH, aldehyde dehydrogenase; CDMDHC, carboxydimethyldecylhydroxychromanol; CDMOHC, carboxymethyloctylhydroxychromanol; CDMHHC, carboxymethylhexylhydroxychromanol; CMBHC, carboxymethylbutylhydroxychromanol; CEHC, carboxyethylhydroxychromanol.

The conjugated SCMs are more hydrophilic and thus mainly found in glucuronidated form in human urine [44]. In contrast, the long-chain metabolites (LCMs) and their metabolic precursors are secreted via bile into the intestine and the metabolites in fecal samples are not conjugated. The fecal route is considered as the major pathway of vitamin E excretion [12,49].

Like vitamin E, other fat-soluble vitamins, such as the vitamins A (i), D (ii) and K (iii) are also metabolized in the human body:

(i). Under physiological conditions, retinyl esters (in the intestinal lumen) and carotenoids (in enterocytes) are converted into retinol before or during their intestinal absorption, respectively. Inside the enterocytes, retinol is re-esterified by lecithin-retinol acyl transferase or acyl-CoA:retinol-acyltransferase and packed into chylomicrons for transport. The retinyl esters are transferred to the liver and stored in hepatic parenchymal and non-parenchymal cells.

Vitamin A is mobilized from liver stores by the retinol-binding protein, a specific transporter allowing the transport of retinol in blood circulation [50]. These results suggest that vitamin A has an active (retinol) and a storage form (retinyl ester). In addition, the oxidation of retinol leads to the formation of retinal, another active form of vitamin A, which is primarily bound to opsins in the photoreceptors of the retina [51]. More current research indicates that all-*trans* retinoic acid (ATRA), 9-*cis*-RA, and all-*trans*-4-oxo-RA are the vitamin A metabolites with the highest biological activity. These active vitamin A metabolites serve as ligands for nuclear receptors, called retinoic acid receptors (RARs) [52] and retinoid receptors (RXRs) [53], which act as ligand-activated transcription factors controlling the expression of their respective target genes. Therefore, hepatic retinol is transferred to extrahepatic tissues and metabolized to retinoic acid by different enzymatic systems. LAMPEN and co-workers found that ATRA is also formed in the small intestine via direct oxidation of vitamin A. Based on this result, they hypothesized that biologically active retinoids are formed in the gastrointestinal tract and act as retinoid-receptor ligands controlling various processes in the intestinal mucosa via RAR [53].

(ii). The human metabolism of vitamin D is primarily located in liver and kidney. Metabolism of vitamin D_2 and D_3 starts with the formation of 25-OHD, the major circulating vitamin D metabolite, by vitamin D-25 hydroxylase. Afterwards, 25-OHD is transferred to the kidney and further catabolized by 25-OHD-1α-hydroxylase to 1,25-dihydroxyvitamin $D_{2/3}$. These molecules serve as ligands for the vitamin D receptor (VDR), a transcription factor expressed in various tissues. Vitamin D receptor binds to specific regions in the promoter regions of genes, the so-called vitamin D responsive elements, thus controlling the expression of respective target genes. Therefore, 1,25-dihydroxyvitamin D is the active metabolic form of vitamin D [54,55].

(iii). Phylloquinone (vitamin K_1) and menaquinone (vitamin K_2) are summarized by the term vitamin K. Phylloquinone is synthesized in plants, while menaquinone is derived from animal and bacterial origins [30,56]. Both compounds share a 2-methyl-1,4-naphthoquinone structure, called menadione, and a side chain at the 3′-position. The side chain of phylloquinone is composed of three isopentyl units and one isopentenyl unit, while the side chain of menaquinone contains a variable number of only isopentenyl units (2–13) [30]. The metabolism of vitamin K is localized in the liver and has not been studied in detail so far [57]. Nevertheless, the metabolic pathway of phylloquinone and menaquinone degradation likely follows that of vitamin E. Hence, the degradation starts with an initial ω-oxidation, which is mediated by CYP. While the ω-oxidation of vitamin E is catalyzed primarily by CYP4F2, CYP3A4 has been described as the possible mediator for the ω-oxidation of vitamin K. Next, the following degradation of the side chain of vitamin K occurs via β-oxidation [30,56,58]. A 5-carbon carboxylic acid metabolite termed K acid 2 has been identified as the end-product of either phylloquinone or menaquinone metabolism and is excreted via urine and bile [30,58]. In addition to their metabolic degradation, it has been suggested that phylloquinones could also be converted to menaquinones [59,60]. For this, phylloquinone is likely transformed to the intermediate menadione by removing its side chain, which is subsequently replaced by a newly synthesized isopentenyl side chain to form menaquinone [30]. While menaquinone is considered as the physiologically active form of vitamin K in humans [56], almost nothing is known about a possible biological activity of the vitamin K metabolites. Further studies are needed to unravel whether vitamin K must be included into the general concept of a metabolic pre-activation of lipid-soluble vitamins.

Although the metabolisms of vitamin A and D differ in location and the involved enzymatic systems, the formation of active metabolites seems to be a key element of both metabolic pathways, i.e., both vitamins mediate their gene regulatory effects by metabolic pre-activation. Therefore, the discovery of vitamin E metabolism in animals and humans and the emerging evidence for important biological functions of vitamin E metabolites could indicate a general metabolic activation mechanism of fat-soluble vitamins in the human body.

In Vivo Verification of Systemic LCM Availability

Since the discovery of vitamin E by EVANS and BISHOP in 1922 [2], α-TOH has been accounted as an antioxidant capable to scavenge reactive oxygen species, and decreased α-TOH levels have been associated with several diseases including different types of cancer, cardiovascular diseases and diabetes [61]. It took 80 years since AZZI and co-workers set up the hypothesis for an additional gene regulatory role of α-TOH in the human body [62]. In addition, the discovery of vitamin E metabolism in animals and humans and the emerging evidence for important biological functions of the vitamin E metabolites [63,64], suggested that the TOHs may gain biological activity after metabolism (as confirmed for vitamin A and D). This prompted studies that investigated also the putative functions of the LCMs of TOH. In 2014, Wallert and co-workers showed the occurrence of α-13′-COOH in human serum, which has been confirmed later by others [65,66]. For these studies, serum obtained from a healthy, middle-aged (39 years), non-smoking male, who received a balanced diet with no additional vitamin E supplementation was used for the detection of α-13′-COOH via liquid chromatography coupled mass spectrometry [63]. The analyses revealed for the first time that α-TOH metabolites are transferred into blood circulation following metabolism of α-TOH in the liver. Furthermore, cell experiments showed that α-13′-OH and α-13′-COOH are more potent regulators of gene expression than their metabolic precursor α-TOH [63]. Taken together, the results of Wallert et al. provided the first evidence that the LCMs are an active form of their metabolic precursor [63], promoting regulatory effects in peripheral tissues of the human body. However, while the role of vitamin E as a lipophilic antioxidant in vitro is widely accepted, the relevance in vivo is still a matter of debate [67–69].

4. Biological Activity

Not much is known about the biological activity of the LCMs. However, the publications on this topic published during the last ten years can be categorized by the biological effects of the LCMs as follows: (i) anti-inflammatory actions [64,70–75]; (ii) anti-carcinogenic effects [72,76,77]; (iii) regulation of cellular lipid homeostasis [63,64]; (iv) interaction with pharmaceuticals [78]; and (v) regulation of their own metabolism [79] (Figure 2).

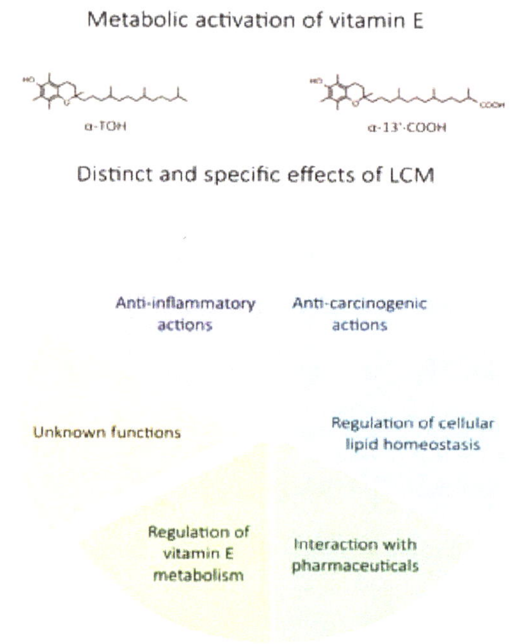

Figure 2. Reported biological functions of the LCMs of vitamin E.

4.1. Anti-Inflammatory Actions

Investigations on anti-inflammatory actions often focus on the regulation of pro-inflammatory enzymes, such as inducible cyclooxygenase 2 (COX2) [70–72,74], inducible nitric oxide synthase (iNOS or nitric oxide synthase, NOS2) [64,71,74,75], or 5-lipoxygenase (5-LO) [72,73], as well as mediators such as chemokines or cytokines. For this purpose, cells were treated with the LCMs and challenged with a pro-inflammatory stimulus or alternatively, isolated enzymes were used. Several LCMs (α-, γ-, δ-13′-COOH; δ-9′-COOH; α-13′-OH) have been tested and reduced the stimulus-induced expression (mRNA or protein) or enzyme activity. In general, 13′-COOH are more potent than the shorter LCMs and the conjugation of LCMs with sulfate abrogates their anti-inflammatory effects [64,70].

Jiang et al. gained first hints on the anti-inflammatory actions of LCMs [70]. A549 cells, which are capable of metabolizing vitamin E, were incubated with TOHs and an inhibition of the arachidonic acid-stimulated COX activity was reported. When the metabolism of vitamin E was suppressed by sesamin, the effects were less pronounced, indicating the involvement of the LCMs as regulatory molecules. For further experiments, the LCMs were extracted from the cell culture medium and their inhibitory capacity on COX activity was tested (half maximal inhibitory concentration (IC_{50}): δ-13′-COOH: 4 μM; δ-9′-COOH: 6 μM). The impact of conjugation was tested, and the sulfate LCM conjugates were unable to exert anti-inflammatory effects. In 2016, a comparison of the different types of LCMs was performed, and the LCMs showed similar effects regardless of their origin (isolated from cell culture medium or semisynthetic isolation from *Garcinia kola*) [72]. In RAW264.7 macrophages, the anti-inflammatory action on lipopolysaccharide (LPS)-stimulated COX2 mRNA and protein expression, as well as prostaglandin (PG) release was reported for α-13′-OH [71] and α-13′-COOH [74].

The regulation of iNos by the LCMs was studied in RAW264.7 macrophages [64,71,74,75]. The LPS-stimulated iNos mRNA and protein expression as well as release of nitric oxide were reduced by the LCMs tested (α- and δ-13′-OH, α- and δ-13′-COOH) [64]. The inhibitory effect of the LCMs was highly dependent on the structure of the LCMs. The 13′-COOH were more effective than the 13′-OH, while the substitution of the chromanol ring system (α- vs. δ-LCMs) had no influence.

The inhibition of ionophore-induced leukotriene release (leukotriene B_4) in HL-60 cells and neutrophils was reported with IC_{50} values of 4–7 μM [73]. Furthermore, the activity of isolated 5-LO was inhibited by δ-13′-COOH with IC_{50} values of 0.5–1 μM, which is more effective than the synthetic 5-LO inhibitor zileuton (IC_{50}: 3–5 μM) [73]. The inhibition of 5-LO activity by δ-13′-COOH was also confirmed by Jang et al. [72]. An overview of the known anti-inflammatory actions of the different LCMs of vitamin E studied so far is provided in Table 1.

Table 1. Overview of anti-inflammatory actions of the LCMs of vitamin E.

Targets	Cells	Effects	Substances	Refs.
COX2	A549 cells	Reduced activity in arachidonic acid-pre-induced cells	γ-13′-COOH δ-13′-COOH δ-9′-COOH	[70] [70,72] [70]
	Isolated enzyme	Inhibition of activity	δ-13′-COOH δ-9′-COOH	[70]
	RAW264.7	Inhibition of LPS-stimulated mRNA and protein expression, as well as reduced PG release	α-13′-OH α-13′-COOH	[71] [74]
iNos	RAW264.7	Inhibition of LPS-stimulated mRNA and protein expression, as well as reduced release of nitric oxide	α-13′-OH α-13′-COOH δ-13′-OH δ-13′-COOH	[64,71,74,75]
5-LO	Isolated enzyme HL-60 neutrophils	Inhibition of activity Reduced activity and LT release in pre-induced cells	δ-13′-COOH δ-13′-COOH	[72,73] [73]

PG, prostaglandin; LT, leukotriene.

The metabolites of vitamin K have also been shown to exert anti-inflammatory functions. First experiments were carried out with a synthetic 7-carbon carboxylic acid vitamin K metabolite (2-methyl, 3-(2′methyl)-hexanoic acid-1,4-naphthoquinone; K acid 1), which was a more effective inhibitor of LPS-induced IL-6 release from fibroblast than the precursors phylloquinone and menaquinon-4 [80]. In LPS-challenged MG63 osteoblasts the 7-carbon carboxylic acid metabolite as well as the 5-carbon carboxylic acid metabolite (K acid 2) attenuated the expression of IL-6 [81]. Later, the long-chain metabolites of vitamin K (10 to 20-carbon carboxylic acid metabolites) were also synthesized and examined for their anti-inflammatory activity. In LPS-challenged mouse macrophages, these compounds reduced the induction of gene-expression of the inflammatory markers IL-1β, IL-6 and TNFα [82]. However, K acid 1 and K acid 2 were also effective in this study; and it is not possible to estimate, which vitamin K metabolite (either long-chain or short-chain) is the most effective [82]. Interestingly, the minor 7-carbon carboxylic acid metabolite was more effective in MG63 osteoblasts than the 5-carbon carboxylic acid metabolite, and a replacement of the carboxy function by a methyl group made the two metabolites less effective [81]. This is in line with findings for the LCMs of vitamin E. Here, the carboxy metabolite is more effective than the respective TOH precursor with respect to the anti-inflammatory actions (vide supra). However, the in vivo relevance of the regulatory activities of the vitamin K metabolites is a matter of debate, as they increase with vitamin K intake in urine [83], but have not yet been found in human blood or other tissues to the best of our knowledge.

4.2. Cancerogenesis and Chemoprevention

The metabolites of vitamin E were investigated with respect to putative anti-cancerogenic, i.e., anti-proliferative and pro-apoptotic, properties in several studies. First experiments revealed that the SCMs inhibit cell proliferation in different cell lines [84,85]. Interestingly, the metabolites as well as the precursor molecules showed different efficiencies, depending on the methylation pattern of the chroman ring and also on the cell type tested [84,85]. Based on the anti-proliferative effects of the SCMs, the interest in the effects of the LCMs aroused. Hence, Birringer et al. investigated the effects of the LCMs α-13′-COOH and δ-13′-COOH as well as α-13′-OH and δ-13′-OH on the proliferation of the human hepatocyte carcinoma cell line HepG2 [77]. Interestingly, both 13′-COOH metabolites effectively caused cell growth arrest, but the hydroxy metabolites did not exhibit anti-proliferative effects. Thus, the introduction of the carboxy group during TOH metabolism renders the molecule active with respect to cell growth arrest. This is supported by the finding that the metabolic precursors, i.e., TOHs, did not affect proliferation of HepG2 cells [77]. As mentioned above, the methylation of the chroman ring alters the efficiency of the molecules. With an effective concentration of 6.5 μM in HepG2 cells regarding the effects on cell growth, the δ-metabolite is more effective than its α-counterpart with 13.5 μM [77]. At first glance, contradictory results were reported for human prostate cancer cells. Here, not only δ-13′-COOH inhibited cell proliferation, but also the hydroxy metabolite α-13′-OH. The LCMs as well as the tested SCMs α-CEHC and γ-CEHC inhibited the proliferation by about 60% in a concentration of 10 μM [76]. Hence, the efficiency of the hydroxy metabolite is likely dependent on the cell type. It is possible that the differences in TOH metabolism in different cell types lead to divergent effects. Interestingly, even differences between different cancer and non-cancer cell lines have been described. The proliferation of the colon cancer cell lines HCT-116 and HT-29 was inhibited by δ-13′-COOH, with IC_{50} values of 8.9 μM and 8.6 μM, respectively [72]. While 10 μM of the LCMs reduce the viability of the cancer cells by around 60%, normal colon epithelial cells showed a reduction of 10–20% at this concentration. Comparable effects were found for the δ-T3 LCM δ-T3-13′-COOH (δ-garcinoic acid), which reduced the viability of the colon cancer cells by about 75%, but the viability of normal colon cells merely by 10–20% [72].

The actions of the vitamin E metabolites are comparable to that of the metabolites of vitamin D and vitamin A. The active vitamin D metabolite $1,25(OH)_2D_3$ has been shown to modulate differentiation and proliferation of colon cancer cells and prostate cancer cells [86]. However, $1,25(OH)_2D_3$ led to an arrest of most cells that express a functional vitamin D receptor in G0/G1 phase [87]. The actions are mediated by interference with several regulatory proteins, such as epidermal growth factor receptor (EGFR), insulin-like growth factors (IGFs), p21, p27 as well as cyclins and cyclin-dependent kinases (CDKs) [87]. The retinoids are also known for their modulation of the cell cycle. In several cancer cell lines, retinoic acid (RA) led to a cell cycle arrest in the G0/G1 phase via direct or indirect modulation of cyclins, CDKs and cell-cycle inhibitors [88]. Interestingly, TOHs and TOH SCMs have also been linked to cyclins and CDKs. In the human prostate cancer cell line PC3, γ-TOH as well as γ-CEHC led to a strong decrease in cyclin D1 protein expression. In line with this observation, CDK4 and p27 expression are reduced, albeit less pronounced [85]. Moreover, α-TOH and α-CEHC are ineffective with respect to anti-proliferative actions as well as suppression of cyclin D1 and CDK4 [85]. However, to date, no data is available on the action of the vitamin E LCMs on cell cycle regulators, although strong anti-proliferative effects have been shown for this class of metabolites.

More detailed investigations were carried out on the pro-apoptotic effects of the vitamin E LCMs. Birringer et al. found a significant induction of apoptosis in HepG2 cells treated with 20 μM of α-13′-COOH, δ-13′-COOH or δ-13′-OH [77]. The LCMs induced the cleavage of caspases 3, 7 and 9, and in line with this, the cleavage of the downstream mediator poly-ADP ribose polymerase-1 (PARP-1). Again, the 13′-COOH were more effective in caspase-cleavage and apoptosis induction than the hydroxy metabolite [77]. Moreover, induction of mitochondrial apoptosis by the LCMs was identified as the process leading to apoptosis. This process is accompanied by the formation of reactive oxygen species (ROS). Birringer et al. observed a significant increase in ROS production in cells treated with α- and δ-13′-COOH but not with the hydroxy metabolites and the TOHs [77]. The augmented ROS production was not only measured intracellularly but also intramitochondrial, hence providing evidence for mitochondrial-derived apoptosis. Alterations in the mitochondrial membrane potential supported this finding. Treatment with 20 μM of the LCMs led to a significant reduction of the mitochondrial membrane potential. Interestingly, in this particular case, the α-metabolite was more potent than the δ-metabolites with 60% reduction vs. 20% reduction [77]. The pro-apoptotic actions of the δ-LCMs of vitamin E were confirmed in colon cancer cells [72]. Early and late apoptosis were induced by δ-13′-COOH and δ-T3-13′-COOH. The activation of caspase-9 and cleavage of PARP found by Birringer et al. [77] were confirmed in colon cancer cells [72]. Moreover, an induction of the autophagy marker microtubule-associated protein 1A/1B-light chain 3 (LC3)-II was found. Jang et al. assumed that alterations in sphingolipid metabolism caused by the carboxy-LCMs are the reason for the induction of apoptosis. Indeed, both δ-13′-COOH and δ-T3-13′-COOH increased total ceramides, dihydroceramides and dihydrosphingosines, while all measured sphingomyelins were decreased. Inhibition of sphingosine biosynthesis revealed that LC3-II expression but not PARP-cleavage is modulated by the LCMs via alterations in sphingolipid metabolism [72].

Taken together, there are several similarities between the metabolites of vitamins A, D and E with respect to anti-cancerogenic properties. Data on anti-cancerogenic effects of vitamin K metabolites, however, are sparse. Merely synthetic carboxylic derivatives of menaquinone with different side-chain lengths have been studied [89]. The biologically most abundant 5-carbon carboxylic acid metabolite (K acid 2) was not included in this study and the 7-carbon carboxylic acid metabolite (K acid 1) was the structure with the shortest side-chain. Interestingly, the growth-suppressing effect on hepatocellular carcinoma cells increased with the length of the side chain of the carboxy derivatives, except for the full-length metabolite, which was as effective as the 7-carbon carboxylic acid metabolite. Conversely, menaquinone itself was completely ineffective, showing nicely that the introduction of a carboxy function activates the compound. Blocking of the effects with chemical antagonists suggested that the derivatives act through caspase/transglutaminase-related signaling [89]. The above mentioned disruption of mitochondrial function by the LCMs of vitamin E has also been described for the metabolites of vitamin A [90], and induction of apoptosis by $1,25(OH)_2D_3$ via mitochondrial pathways (e.g., via B-cell lymphoma (BCL)-2 and BCL-xL) in breast, colon and prostate cancer cells are also known [87]. Based on their anti-proliferative and pro-differentiation actions but also due to the induction of cell death, retinoids are used for treating certain types of cancer [91]. Vitamin A metabolites were successfully used in the treatment of acute promyelocytic leukemia (ATRA and 13-*cis*-RA, 13*c*RA), squamous cell skin cancer and neuroblastoma (13*c*RA), lung cancer (ATRA) and Kaposi's sarcoma (9-*cis*-RA, 9*c*RA). Beneficial effects of retinoids in cancer prevention have also been observed.

These properties can be explained by the targeting of regulators of cell cycle progression by retinoids. The expression of the CDK inhibitors p21 and p27 is regulated by ATRA via RARβ2 upregulation, and retinoic acid has been shown to stimulate the degradation of cyclin D1, leading to a suppression of CDK activity [91]. Interestingly, TOHs as well as SCMs of vitamin E modulate cyclins, CDKs and CDK inhibitors [85]. Albeit the LCMs of vitamin E efficiently suppress proliferation, the identification of effects on regulators of cell cycle progression is pending. However, given that 'decreased proliferation is one of the best biomarkers of a cancer preventive effect' [91], vitamin E and its metabolites are promising compounds for cancer prevention.

4.3. Cellular Lipid Homeostasis

To date, the effects of the LCMs of vitamin E on cellular lipid homeostasis have not been investigated extensively. However, the regulation of key metabolic pathways in foam cell development of macrophages by the LCMs were of particular interest in a study by Wallert et al. [63]. Here, the regulation of the expression of the cluster of differentiation 36 (CD36), the uptake of oxidized low density lipoprotein (oxLDL), phagocytosis and the intracellular storage of lipids were investigated [63]. For this, the monocytic THP-1 cell line, which can be differentiated to macrophage-like cells, was used. In differentiated macrophages, the LCMs α-13′-OH and α-13′-COOH induced the expression of CD36 mRNA and consequently CD36 protein levels. In contrast, the precursor α-TOH exerted opposite effects on CD36 mRNA and protein. Whereas α-TOH reduced the expression of CD36 at a concentration of 100 μM, the α-LCMs induced the expression of CD36 in concentrations of 5 and 10 μM, respectively [63]. Thus, the α-LCMs not only act in a different way than their precursors, but appeared to be also significantly more potent. Interestingly, similar effects were described for the lipid soluble vitamin A. Langmann et al. found that the precursor β-carotene is less effective in inducing expression of CD36 than its metabolites ATRA and 9*c*RA in human monocytes and macrophages [92]. The authors stated that the metabolites 9*c*RA and ATRA displayed high biological activity [92], while the precursors retinol and β-carotene were only marginally metabolized, an observation that parallels the characteristics of the LCMs of vitamin E with respect to their reported serum concentrations [63,93]. The effects of vitamin A metabolites are better characterized than that of the LCMs of vitamin E. It was repeatedly shown that the metabolites of vitamin A regulate CD36 expression in macrophage cell models. The metabolite 9*c*RA induced CD36 mRNA [94,95] and protein expression [95] in human THP-1 macrophages. ATRA increases expression of CD36 mRNA in THP-1 cells [96] and CD36 protein in THP-1 and HL60 macrophages [96,97]. The induction of CD36 expression by ATRA and 9*c*RA has been confirmed in primary human monocytes and macrophages [92,96] to show the physiological relevance in non-cancer cells. With the same intention, it was also shown that the LCMs of vitamin E induced CD36 expression in peripheral blood mononuclear cell (PBMC)-derived primary human macrophages [63].

The scavenger receptor CD36 mediates the uptake of the modified lipoprotein oxLDL [98], a process that in turn stimulates CD36 expression [99]. Given the induction of the expression of CD36 by the LCMs of vitamin E under basal conditions (vide supra), a further stimulation by oxLDL treatment could be expected. As the uptake of oxLDL is a hallmark of macrophage foam cell formation, Wallert et al. examined whether preincubation of THP-1 macrophages with the LCMs of vitamin E affects the oxLDL-induced expression of CD36 [63]. As expected, CD36 expression was induced by oxLDL treatment. Pre-treatment with α-TOH suppressed the induction by oxLDL. In contrast, the pre-incubation with the LCMs augmented the induction of CD36 expression by oxLDL. These findings resemble the reaction of the cells in the absence of oxLDL to α-TOH and its LCMs. Given the higher CD36 expression in the presence of the LCMs, the uptake of oxLDL should in turn be induced in LCM-treated macrophages. However, pre-incubation of the macrophages with the LCMs for 24 h led to decreased oxLDL uptake. Incubation with both, α-13′-OH or α-13′-COOH, decreased the uptake by about 20%. This effect was again confirmed in PBMC-derived macrophages. Here, oxLDL uptake was decreased by α-13′-OH pre-treatment by 24% and by α-13′-COOH pre-treatment by 20%, respectively [63]. The LCMs of vitamin E thus exerted unexpected effects on oxLDL uptake. As mentioned before, vitamin A metabolites also caused increased CD36 expression, but the metabolite 9*c*RA induced the binding and uptake of oxLDL in THP-1 macrophages as expected [94]. Generally, an activation of RXR leads to an augmented association of oxLDL to THP-1 macrophages [100]. However, 9*c*RA also promoted the degradation of oxLDL and the cholesterol efflux via ATP binding cassette transporters, thus leading to a net depletion of cholesterol esters. Triglyceride levels were apparently not affected, neither by oxLDL treatment nor combination with 9*c*RA [94]. In contrast, in the study of Wallert et al. on the LCMs of vitamin E, oxLDL treatment of the macrophages led to an increase of neutral lipids in the cells. Preincubation with the LCMs diminished the oxLDL-induced neutral lipid accumulation [63]. However, the contradictory results on the effects of the LCMs on CD36 expression and oxLDL uptake required an alternative explanation how the LCMs decrease oxLDL uptake. Thus, Wallert et al. focused on phagocytosis as an alternative uptake mechanism for oxLDL [101]. Indeed, treatment of the macrophages with α-13′-OH led to an inhibition of phagocytotic activity of 16% and with α-13′-COOH of 41%, respectively [63]. Hence, the inhibition of phagocytosis by the LCMs might explain the discrepancy between their effects on CD36 expression and oxLDL uptake in this study.

Taken together, the metabolites of vitamin E and vitamin A induce the expression of CD36 in macrophages. However, their effects on oxLDL uptake are different. While the vitamin A metabolite 9*c*RA induces oxLDL uptake, the LCMs of vitamin E reduce it. In contrast to vitamin A and vitamin E metabolites, the metabolite of vitamin D, $1{,}25(OH)_2D_3$ has been shown to reduce the expression of CD36 mRNA and protein in oxLDL-treated macrophages obtained from diabetic subjects. Concomitantly, oxLDL and cholesterol uptake are decreased [102,103]. Hence, the vitamin D metabolite as well as the vitamin E LCMs suppress macrophage foam cell formation and may thus exert positive effects in the context of atherosclerosis prevention.

4.4. Interaction with Pharmaceuticals

The interaction of the vitamin E LCMs with pharmaceuticals was tested by analyzing the regulation of P-glycoprotein (P-gp). P-gp regulates, inter alia, the intracellular concentration of pharmaceuticals and its expression is regulated by various transcription factors, including heat shock transcription factor 1, nuclear factor Y and the pregnane X receptor (PXR) [104,105].

Several vitamin E forms and their metabolites (α-TOH, α-T3, α-13′-COOH, α-CEHC, γ-TOH, γ-T3, γ-CEHC and plastochromanol-8) were used and the regulation of P-gp expression was analyzed in human epithelial-like colon LS180 cells [78]. Only α-13′-COOH and γ-T3 induced P-gp expression and α-T3, α-13′-COOH as well as γ-T3 induced the activity of PXR in a reporter gene assay. In case of vitamin E supplementation, an interaction with the metabolic handling of pharmaceuticals might be possible.

4.5. Regulation of LCM Formation

The regulatory processes, which modulate the metabolism of vitamin E, are largely unknown. In this context, two key issues are important: (i) Apart from CYP4F2 and CYP3A4, the full set of enzymes involved in the first steps of the catabolism of vitamin E remains to be identified, and (ii) the mechanisms by which vitamin E metabolism is regulated have not yet been sufficiently unraveled. However, the upregulation of CYP4F2 protein expression by α-13′-OH in human HepG2 liver cells was reported recently [79], pointing to a positive regulatory feedback loop. If this concept holds true, the enhancement of metabolism by products would be a new facet for the fat-soluble vitamins, as the metabolism of vitamin A and D is mainly regulated negatively by their metabolic products [54,106].

The aldehyde- and alcohol-dehydrogenases have been suggested to be responsible for the ω-oxidation steps and the enzymes for branched-chain fatty acids might catalyze the subsequent β-oxidation [107]. Following the identification of the specific set of enzymes required for vitamin E metabolism, a major aim will be the characterization of the regulatory factors, which modulate the metabolism of vitamin E.

5. Structure-Specific Effects

To get deeper insights into the specificity of the regulatory effects of the LCMs of vitamin E, a structure-activity study was conducted [64]. For this purpose, substances were used that represent specific substructures of the LCMs or their precursors. The chromanol ring system was mirrored by the SCM α-CEHC and the modified side-chain was represented by the branched-chain fatty acid pristanic acid. Furthermore, the α- and δ-forms of 13′-OH and 13′-COOH were used to study the influence of the side-chain modification. Overall, the application of α- and δ-forms of LCMs and their precursors (α-TOH, α-13′-OH, α-13′-COOH, δ-TOH, δ-13′-OH, δ-13′-COOH) should clarify the importance of the substitution of the ring-system. The regulation of CD36 and iNos by the test compounds was similar for all of the LCMs, but neither the precursors nor their substructures were able to cause the same effects on the expression of the target genes as the LCMs. The substitution of the chromanol ring system had no influence (α- and δ-forms), while the modification of the side-chain (oxidation of TOH to 13′-OH and 13′-COOH) was highly relevant for the effects. Overall, the 13′-COOH was most potent in this study. Based on these specific regulations the existence of specific regulatory molecular pathways for the LCMs has been suggested.

6. Receptors of Vitamin Metabolites

As indicated above, the lipid-soluble vitamins A and D need a conversion to their active metabolites to exert their effects. These metabolites are either bound intracellularly and transferred to the receptor or directly bind the receptor. The receptors for the vitamin A metabolites, RARs and RXRs, were identified in the late 1980s [108–111]. Evidence for binding proteins for the active vitamin D metabolite 1,25$(OH)_2D_3$ was already provided in the 1970's [112,113]; however, cloning of the human vitamin D receptor also succeeded in the late 1980's [114]. In contrast, no specific receptor for vitamin E and/or its metabolites has been identified yet. Interestingly, the metabolites of vitamin A and D act through nuclear receptors. This class of transcription factors can roughly be divided into more specific and rather unspecific members. The vitamin D receptor can be categorized as a more specific receptor, as it is activated by its endogenous ligand 1,25$(OH)_2D_3$ already at sub-nanomolar concentrations [115,116]. This feature is also shared by steroid hormone receptors (estrogen receptor, androgen receptor, ergosterone receptor, cortisol receptor), the thyroid hormone receptor and RARs. The RARs specifically bind ATRA, and also 9*c*RA with lower affinity [117]. The specificity of the nuclear receptors is mainly determined by the structure of the ligand binding pocket. Specific receptors have a relatively small ligand binding pocket, which allows only a limited number of molecules to interact. In contrast, the so-called adopted orphan receptors have a larger ligand binding pocket, allowing the activation of the receptor by a larger number of ligands [115]. Members of this group are the liver X receptors (LXRs), farnesoid X receptor (FXR), peroxisome proliferator-activated receptors (PPARs) and RXRs. The latter have been shown to bind the vitamin A metabolite 9*c*RA [118]. However, it is not entirely accepted that 9*c*RA represents the endogenous ligand for RXR [119]. Nonetheless, the example of 9*c*RA opens the possibility that vitamin metabolites act through highly specific receptors but also through rather unspecific ones.

Following the concept that the LCMs of vitamin E represent biologically active metabolites similar to 1,25$(OH)_2D_3$, ATRA and 9*c*RA, these molecules might also exert their effects through nuclear receptors. Indeed, Podszun et al. reported an activation of PXR by α-13′-COOH in the human colon adenocarcinoma cell line LS180 [78] (for detailed information, the reader is referred to the section 'Interaction with pharmaceuticals'). Interestingly, α-T3 and γ-T3 were also able to activate PXR, while α-TOH and γ-TOH as well as the SCMs α-CEHC and γ-CEHC failed to activate PXR [78]. These findings confirm earlier findings in HepG2 cells only in part. In HepG2 cells transfected with PXR and a CAT (chloramphenicol acetyltransferase) reporter gene, α-T3 and γ-T3 efficiently activated PXR-mediated gene transcription, but α-TOH, γ-TOH and δ-TOH were also able to induce the expression of the reporter gene via PXR [120]. In contrast, the SCMs α-CEHC and α-CMBHC were not able to activate PXR in this study and the LCMs were not tested [120]. Taken together, the T3s reliably activate PXR but the effects of the TOHs need further investigation. Possibly, LS180 and HepG2 metabolize TOH with different efficiency, in turn determining the amounts of LCMs formed as PXR-activating metabolites. Hence, the observed effects of TOHs in HepG2 might be explained by the intracellular formation of the LCMs. However, further investigations on the cell-type specific metabolism of TOH are needed to confirm this hypothesis. Further, with PXR a rather unspecific nuclear receptor is identified for TOHs and their LCMs. As a general sensor for toxic compounds and xenobiotics, PXR has a large ligand binding cavity, which allows the binding of a wide range of ligands [121]. Thus, it is not surprising that PXR has been described as a receptor of vitamin K [122,123], and it has been reported that several menaquinone derivatives activate PXR [124]. Unfortunately, the biologically occurring carboxy derivatives were not included in this study. Hence, merely speculations about the activity based on structure-function-relationships are possible. A reporter gene assay revealed that a terminal phenyl group enhances the activity of the derivatives, while a terminal hydroxy group diminished it compared to the unmodified menaquinone [124]. In conclusion, a more hydrophobic side chain leads to an increased activity on PXR. Hence, the natural metabolic products in humans bearing a terminal carboxy group are likely less potent with respect to the activation of PXR. However, this concept is in contrast to the findings for vitamin E. The TOH precursors are unable to activate PXR, while the LCM α-13′-COOH activates it [78]. Hence, further studies are needed to clarify whether vitamin K metabolites are physiological ligands for the rather unspecific nuclear receptor PXR, like their metabolic precursor menaquinone and the LCMs of vitamin E.

Given that RXR as a receptor for the vitamin A metabolite 9*c*RA is also rather unspecific, it might be possible that the LCMs of vitamin E also act through PXR. However, it is questionable whether all of the reported biological effects of the LCMs, i.e., anti-inflammatory actions, anti-cancerogenic features, and effects on cellular lipid homeostasis (please refer to the respective sections here) can be ascribed to PXR activation. Hence, further investigations aiming at the identification and characterization of receptors for the LCMs of vitamin E LCMs are highly required. Strategies for the identification of further receptors or a receptor specific for the LCMs of vitamin E might be the use of target fishing approaches, gene expression arrays, knockdown/knockout studies, as well as reporter gene assays and ligand binding studies.

7. Conclusions

With the detection of the LCMs of vitamin E in human serum, an important hint for the possible action of these metabolites as signaling molecules was provided. Several studies reinforced this hypothesis by the characterization of the biological effects of the LCMs, as summarized in Figure 2. Interestingly, the LCMs act more potent and in part even contrary to their metabolic precursors. Some of the controversial effects reported for vitamin E might be therefore explained by the action of the LCMs. The evidence of circulating α-LCM in human blood (nanomolar concentrations) provides a new perspective in vitamin E research [63]. Therefore, the LCMs must be seriously considered to correctly interpret the effects of vitamin E in humans, beside the better studied TOHs and T3s. So far, only a few studies have focused on this class of compounds. However, based on our current knowledge and our studies in progress, we speculate that the LCMs comprise a new class of regulatory molecules. These molecules can exert effects that are different from their metabolic precursors, complicating the interpretation of studies on the effects of vitamin E in vivo. Nevertheless, the LCMs share properties with their precursors but also exert unique or even adverse effects. It is evident that the LCMs and their precursors act in the same manner with respect to the modulation of COX2 and 5-LOX activity, but it is of note that the LCMs are significantly more potent than their precursors. Furthermore, the LCM can act in areas where the TOHs are virtually not effective. A prime example is the regulation of COX2 expression. Hence, the LCMs may indeed play a role in mediating some of the effects of vitamin E in the human body although blood concentrations are significantly lower than those of TOH. So far, blood concentrations are the only valid value for the systemic distribution of the LCMs of vitamin E in the human body. However, based on preliminary data of unpublished in vitro and in vivo studies of our group, we can hypothesize that the LCMs of vitamin E may also accumulate in different parts of the human body, where they reach concentrations higher than in blood. Further studies are required to study this issue in more detail and to differentiate between physiologic (at low concentrations) and pharmacologic (at high concentrations) actions of the LCMs.

To sum up, the LCMs could be regarded as the metabolically activated forms of vitamin E. This is in line with the metabolic activation of the other lipid-soluble vitamins A and D. Consequently, the concept of metabolic activation established for vitamin A and D could now be extended to vitamin E. Thus, a general concept for the biological activity and modes of action of the lipid-soluble vitamins could be defined.

Acknowledgments: The work of Stefan Lorkowski is supported by grants from the Federal Ministry of Education and Research (01EA1411A), the Deutsche Forschungsgemeinschaft (DFG; RTG 1715) and the German Ministry of Economics and Technology (AiF 16642 BR) via AiF (the German Federation of Industrial Research Associations) and FEI (the Research Association of the German Food Industry), and by the Free State of Thuringia and the European Social Fund (2016 FGR 0045). The work of Lisa Schmölz is supported by the Free State of Thuringia and the European Social Fund (2016 FGR 0045). The work of Maria Wallert is funded by the DFG (Wa 3836/1-1).

Author Contributions: Martin Schubert, Stefan Kluge, Lisa Schmölz, Maria Wallert, Francesco Galli, Marc Birringer and Stefan Lorkowski wrote the paper.

References

1. Horn, M.; Gunn, P.; van Emon, M.; Lemenager, R.; Burgess, J.; Pyatt, N.A.; Lake, S.L. Effects of natural (*RRR* alpha-tocopherol acetate) or synthetic (all-*rac*-alpha-tocopherol acetate) vitamin E supplementation on reproductive efficiency in beef cows. *J. Anim. Sci.* **2010**, *88*, 3121–3127. [CrossRef] [PubMed]
2. Evans, H.M.; Bishop, K.S. On the existence of a hitherto unrecognized dietary factor essential for reproduction. *Science* **1922**, *56*, 650–651. [CrossRef] [PubMed]
3. Kluge, S.; Schubert, M.; Schmölz, L.; Birringer, M.; Wallert, M.; Lorkowski, S. Garcinoic Acid: A Promising Bioactive Natural Product for Better Understanding the Physiological Functions of Tocopherol Metabolites. *Stud. Nat. Prod. Chem.* **2016**, *51*, 435–481. [CrossRef]
4. Sano, M.; Ernesto, C.; Thomas, R.G.; Klauber, M.R.; Schafer, K.; Grundman, M.; Woodbury, P.; Growdon, J.; Cotman, C.W.; Pfeiffer, E.; et al. A controlled trial of selegiline, alpha-tocopherol, or both as treatment for Alzheimer's disease. The Alzheimer's Disease Cooperative Study. *N. Engl. J. Med.* **1997**, *336*, 1216–1222. [CrossRef] [PubMed]
5. Dysken, M.W.; Guarino, P.D.; Vertrees, J.E.; Asthana, S.; Sano, M.; Llorente, M.; Pallaki, M.; Love, S.; Schellenberg, G.D.; McCarten, J.R.; et al. Vitamin E and memantine in Alzheimer's disease: Clinical trial methods and baseline data. *Alzheimer Dement. J. Alzheimer Assoc.* **2014**, *10*, 36–44. [CrossRef] [PubMed]
6. Jishage, K.; Arita, M.; Igarashi, K.; Iwata, T.; Watanabe, M.; Ogawa, M.; Ueda, O.; Kamada, N.; Inoue, K.; Arai, H.; et al. Alpha-tocopherol transfer protein is important for the normal development of placental labyrinthine trophoblasts in mice. *J. Biol. Chem.* **2001**, *276*, 1669–1672. [CrossRef] [PubMed]
7. Shichiri, M.; Yoshida, Y.; Ishida, N.; Hagihara, Y.; Iwahashi, H.; Tamai, H.; Niki, E. α-Tocopherol suppresses lipid peroxidation and behavioral and cognitive impairments in the Ts65Dn mouse model of Down syndrome. *Free Radic. Biol. Med.* **2011**, *50*, 1801–1811. [CrossRef] [PubMed]
8. Czeizel, A.E.; Dudás, I. Prevention of the first occurrence of neural-tube defects by periconceptional vitamin supplementation. *N. Engl. J. Med.* **1992**, *327*, 1832–1835. [CrossRef] [PubMed]
9. Chandler, A.L.; Hobbs, C.A.; Mosley, B.S.; Berry, R.J.; Canfield, M.A.; Qi, Y.P.; Siega-Riz, A.M.; Shaw, G.M. Neural tube defects and maternal intake of micronutrients related to one-carbon metabolism or antioxidant activity. *Birth Defects Res. Part A Clin. Mol. Teratol.* **2012**, *94*, 864–874. [CrossRef] [PubMed]
10. Brigelius-Flohé, R. Vitamin E: The shrew waiting to be tamed. *Free Radic. Biol. Med.* **2009**, *46*, 543–554. [CrossRef] [PubMed]

11. Wallert, M.; Schmölz, L.; Galli, F.; Birringer, M.; Lorkowski, S. Regulatory metabolites of vitamin E and their putative relevance for atherogenesis. *Redox Biol.* **2014**, *2*, 495–503. [CrossRef] [PubMed]
12. Jiang, Q. Natural forms of vitamin E: Metabolism, antioxidant, and anti-inflammatory activities and their role in disease prevention and therapy. *Free Radic. Biol. Med.* **2014**, *72*, 76–90. [CrossRef] [PubMed]
13. Rigotti, A. Absorption, transport, and tissue delivery of vitamin E. *Mol. Asp. Med.* **2007**, *28*, 423–436. [CrossRef] [PubMed]
14. Bjørneboe, A.; Bjørneboe, G.E.; Drevon, C.A. Absorption, transport and distribution of vitamin E. *J. Nutr.* **1990**, *120*, 233–242. [CrossRef] [PubMed]
15. Borel, P.; Pasquier, B.; Armand, M.; Tyssandier, V.; Grolier, P.; Alexandre-Gouabau, M.C.; Andre, M.; Senft, M.; Peyrot, J.; Jaussan, V.; et al. Processing of vitamin A and E in the human gastrointestinal tract. *Am. J. Physiol.-Gastrointest. Liver Physiol.* **2001**, *280*, G95–G103. [CrossRef] [PubMed]
16. Reboul, E. Intestinal absorption of vitamin D: From the meal to the enterocyte. *Food Funct.* **2015**, *6*, 356–362. [CrossRef] [PubMed]
17. Bieri, J.G.; Wu, A.L.; Tolliver, T.J. Reduced intestinal absorption of vitamin E by low dietary levels of retinoic acid in rats. *J. Nutr.* **1981**, *111*, 458–467. [PubMed]
18. Richelle, M.; Enslen, M.; Hager, C.; Groux, M.; Tavazzi, I.; Godin, J.-P.; Berger, A.; Métairon, S.; Quaile, S.; Piguet-Welsch, C.; et al. Both free and esterified plant sterols reduce cholesterol absorption and the bioavailability of beta-carotene and alpha-tocopherol in normocholesterolemic humans. *Am. J. Clin. Nutr.* **2004**, *80*, 171–177. [PubMed]
19. Doi, K.; Matsuura, M.; Kawara, A.; Tanaka, T.; Baba, S. Influence of dietary fiber (konjac mannan) on absorption of vitamin B12 and vitamin E. *Tohoku J. Exp. Med.* **1983**, *141*, 677–681. [CrossRef] [PubMed]
20. Burton, G.W.; Ingold, K.U.; Foster, D.O.; Cheng, S.C.; Webb, A.; Hughes, L.; Lusztyk, E. Comparison of free alpha-tocopherol and alpha-tocopheryl acetate as sources of vitamin E in rats and humans. *Lipids* **1988**, *23*, 834–840. [CrossRef] [PubMed]
21. D'Ambrosio, D.N.; Clugston, R.D.; Blaner, W.S. Vitamin A metabolism: An update. *Nutrients* **2011**, *3*, 63–103. [CrossRef] [PubMed]
22. Weng, W.; Li, L.; van Bennekum, A.M.; Potter, S.H.; Harrison, E.H.; Blaner, W.S.; Breslow, J.L.; Fisher, E.A. Intestinal absorption of dietary cholesteryl ester is decreased but retinyl ester absorption is normal in carboxyl ester lipase knockout mice. *Biochemistry* **1999**, *38*, 4143–4149. [CrossRef] [PubMed]
23. Maislos, M.; Shany, S. Bile salt deficiency and the absorption of vitamin D metabolites. In vivo study in the rat. *Isr. J. Med. Sci.* **1987**, *23*, 1114–1117. [PubMed]
24. Reboul, E.; Klein, A.; Bietrix, F.; Gleize, B.; Malezet-Desmoulins, C.; Schneider, M.; Margotat, A.; Lagrost, L.; Collet, X.; Borel, P. Scavenger receptor class B type I (SR-BI) is involved in vitamin E transport across the enterocyte. *J. Biol. Chem.* **2006**, *281*, 4739–4745. [CrossRef] [PubMed]
25. Hacquebard, M.; Carpentier, Y.A. Vitamin E: Absorption, plasma transport and cell uptake. *Curr. Opin. Clin. Nutr. Metab. Care* **2005**, *8*, 133–138. [CrossRef] [PubMed]
26. Yamanashi, Y.; Takada, T.; Kurauchi, R.; Tanaka, Y.; Komine, T.; Suzuki, H. Transporters for the Intestinal Absorption of Cholesterol, Vitamin E, and Vitamin K. *J. Atheroscler. Thromb.* **2017**, *24*, 347–359. [CrossRef] [PubMed]
27. Reboul, E. Absorption of vitamin A and carotenoids by the enterocyte: Focus on transport proteins. *Nutrients* **2013**, *5*, 3563–3581. [CrossRef] [PubMed]
28. Traber, M.G.; Burton, G.W.; Ingold, K.U.; Kayden, H.J. RRR- and SRR-alpha-tocopherols are secreted without discrimination in human chylomicrons, but RRR-alpha-tocopherol is preferentially secreted in very low density lipoproteins. *J. Lipid Res.* **1990**, *31*, 675–685. [PubMed]
29. Traber, M.G.; Burton, G.W.; Hughes, L.; Ingold, K.U.; Hidaka, H.; Malloy, M.; Kane, J.; Hyams, J.; Kayden, H.J. Discrimination between forms of vitamin E by humans with and without genetic abnormalities of lipoprotein metabolism. *J. Lipid Res.* **1992**, *33*, 1171–1182. [PubMed]
30. Shearer, M.J.; Newman, P. Metabolism and cell biology of vitamin K. *Thromb. Haemost.* **2008**. [CrossRef]
31. Cooper, A.D. Hepatic uptake of chylomicron remnants. *J. Lipid Res.* **1997**, *38*, 2173–2192. [PubMed]
32. Kiyose, C.; Muramatsu, R.; Kameyama, Y.; Ueda, T.; Igarashi, O. Biodiscrimination of alpha-tocopherol stereoisomers in humans after oral administration. *Am. J. Clin. Nutr.* **1997**, *65*, 785–789. [CrossRef] [PubMed]

33. Weiser, H.; Riss, G.; Kormann, A.W. Selective biodiscrimination of alpha-tocopherol stereoisomers. Similar enrichment of all 2R forms in rat tissues after oral all-rac-alpha-tocopheryl acetate. *Ann. N. Y. Acad. Sci.* **1992**, *669*, 393–395. [CrossRef] [PubMed]
34. Traber, M.G.; Kayden, H.J. Alpha-tocopherol as compared with gamma-tocopherol is preferentially secreted in human lipoproteins. *Ann. N. Y. Acad. Sci.* **1989**, *570*, 95–108. [CrossRef] [PubMed]
35. Arita, M.; Nomura, K.; Arai, H.; Inoue, K. alpha-tocopherol transfer protein stimulates the secretion of alpha-tocopherol from a cultured liver cell line through a brefeldin A-insensitive pathway. *Proc. Natl. Acad. Sci. USA* **1997**, *94*, 12437–12441. [CrossRef] [PubMed]
36. Oram, J.F.; Vaughan, A.M.; Stocker, R. ATP-binding cassette transporter A1 mediates cellular secretion of alpha-tocopherol. *J. Biol. Chem.* **2001**, *276*, 39898–39902. [CrossRef] [PubMed]
37. Mustacich, D.J.; Shields, J.; Horton, R.A.; Brown, M.K.; Reed, D.J. Biliary secretion of alpha-tocopherol and the role of the mdr2 P-glycoprotein in rats and mice. *Arch. Biochem. Biophys.* **1998**, *350*, 183–192. [CrossRef] [PubMed]
38. Lemaire-Ewing, S.; Desrumaux, C.; Néel, D.; Lagrost, L. Vitamin E transport, membrane incorporation and cell metabolism: Is alpha-tocopherol in lipid rafts an oar in the lifeboat? *Mol. Nutr. Food Res.* **2010**, *54*, 631–640. [CrossRef] [PubMed]
39. Schmölz, L.; Birringer, M.; Lorkowski, S.; Wallert, M. Complexity of vitamin E metabolism. *World J. Biol. Chem.* **2016**, *7*, 14–43. [CrossRef] [PubMed]
40. Abe, C.; Uchida, T.; Ohta, M.; Ichikawa, T.; Yamashita, K.; Ikeda, S. Cytochrome P450-dependent metabolism of vitamin E isoforms is a critical determinant of their tissue concentrations in rats. *Lipids* **2007**, *42*, 637–645. [CrossRef] [PubMed]
41. Bardowell, S.A.; Ding, X.; Parker, R.S. Disruption of P450-mediated vitamin E hydroxylase activities alters vitamin E status in tocopherol supplemented mice and reveals extra-hepatic vitamin E metabolism. *J. Lipid Res.* **2012**, *53*, 2667–2676. [CrossRef] [PubMed]
42. Grebenstein, N.; Schumacher, M.; Graeve, L.; Frank, J. α-Tocopherol transfer protein is not required for the discrimination against γ-tocopherol in vivo but protects it from side-chain degradation in vitro. *Mol. Nutr. Food Res.* **2014**, *58*, 1052–1060. [CrossRef] [PubMed]
43. Chiku, S.; Hamamura, K.; Nakamura, T. Novel urinary metabolite of d-delta-tocopherol in rats. *J. Lipid Res.* **1984**, *25*, 40–48. [PubMed]
44. Swanson, J.E.; Ben, R.N.; Burton, G.W.; Parker, R.S. Urinary excretion of 2,7,8-trimethyl-2-(beta-carboxyethyl)-6-hydroxychroman is a major route of elimination of gamma-tocopherol in humans. *J. Lipid Res.* **1999**, *40*, 665–671. [PubMed]
45. Sontag, T.J.; Parker, R.S. Cytochrome P450 omega-hydroxylase pathway of tocopherol catabolism. Novel mechanism of regulation of vitamin E status. *J. Biol. Chem.* **2002**, *277*, 25290–25296. [CrossRef] [PubMed]
46. Birringer, M.; Pfluger, P.; Kluth, D.; Landes, N.; Brigelius-Flohé, R. Identities and differences in the metabolism of tocotrienols and tocopherols in HepG2 cells. *J. Nutr.* **2002**, *132*, 3113–3118. [PubMed]
47. Parker, R.S.; Sontag, T.J.; Swanson, J.E. Cytochrome P4503A-dependent metabolism of tocopherols and inhibition by sesamin. *Biochem. Biophys. Res. Commun.* **2000**, *277*, 531–534. [CrossRef] [PubMed]
48. Johnson, C.H.; Slanař, O.; Krausz, K.W.; Kang, D.W.; Patterson, A.D.; Kim, J.-H.; Luecke, H.; Gonzalez, F.J.; Idle, J.R. Novel metabolites and roles for α-tocopherol in humans and mice discovered by mass spectrometry-based metabolomics. *Am. J. Clin. Nutr.* **2012**, *96*, 818–830. [CrossRef] [PubMed]
49. Zhao, Y.; Lee, M.-J.; Cheung, C.; Ju, J.-H.; Chen, Y.-K.; Liu, B.; Hu, L.-Q.; Yang, C.S. Analysis of multiple metabolites of tocopherols and tocotrienols in mice and humans. *J. Agric. Food Chem.* **2010**, *58*, 4844–4852. [CrossRef] [PubMed]
50. Goodman, D.S. Overview of current knowledge of metabolism of vitamin A and carotenoids. *J. Natl. Cancer Inst.* **1984**, *73*, 1375–1379. [PubMed]
51. Zhong, M.; Kawaguchi, R.; Kassai, M.; Sun, H. Retina, retinol, retinal and the natural history of vitamin A as a light sensor. *Nutrients* **2012**, *4*, 2069–2096. [CrossRef] [PubMed]
52. Petkovich, M.; Brand, N.J.; Krust, A.; Chambon, P. A human retinoic acid receptor which belongs to the family of nuclear receptors. *Nature* **1987**, *330*, 444–450. [CrossRef] [PubMed]
53. Lampen, A.; Meyer, S.; Arnhold, T.; Nau, H. Metabolism of vitamin A and its active metabolite all-trans-retinoic acid in small intestinal enterocytes. *J. Pharmacol. Exp. Ther.* **2000**, *295*, 979–985. [PubMed]

54. Bikle, D.D. Vitamin D metabolism, mechanism of action, and clinical applications. *Chem. Biol.* **2014**, *21*, 319–329. [CrossRef] [PubMed]
55. Urrutia-Pereira, M.; Solé, D. Vitamin D deficiency in pregnancy and its impact on the fetus, the newborn and in childhood. *Rev. Paul. Pediatr.* **2015**, *33*, 104–113. [CrossRef]
56. Landes, N.; Birringer, M.; Brigelius-Flohé, R. Homologous metabolic and gene activating routes for vitamins E and K. *Mol. Asp. Med.* **2003**, *24*, 337–344. [CrossRef]
57. Hodges, S.J.; Pitsillides, A.A.; Ytrebø, L.M.; Soper, R. Anti-inflammatory actions of vitamin K. In *Vitamin K2—Vital for Health and Wellbeing*; Gordeladze, J.O., Ed.; InTech: Rijeka, Croatia, 2017.
58. Traber, M.G. Vitamin E and K interactions—A 50-year-old problem. *Nutr. Rev.* **2008**, *66*, 624–629. [CrossRef] [PubMed]
59. Yamamoto, R.; Komai, M.; Kojima, K.; Furukawa, Y.; Kimura, S. Menaquinone-4 accumulation in various tissues after an oral administration of phylloquinone in Wistar rats. *J. Nutr. Sci. Vitaminol.* **1997**, *43*, 133–143. [CrossRef] [PubMed]
60. Okano, T.; Shimomura, Y.; Yamane, M.; Suhara, Y.; Kamao, M.; Sugiura, M.; Nakagawa, K. Conversion of phylloquinone (Vitamin K1) into menaquinone-4 (Vitamin K2) in mice: Two possible routes for menaquinone-4 accumulation in cerebra of mice. *J. Biol. Chem.* **2008**, *283*, 11270–11279. [CrossRef] [PubMed]
61. Brigelius-Flohé, R.; Kelly, F.J.; Salonen, J.T.; Neuzil, J.; Zingg, J.-M.; Azzi, A. The European perspective on vitamin E: Current knowledge and future research. *Am. J. Clin. Nutr.* **2002**, *76*, 703–716. [PubMed]
62. Azzi, A.; Ricciarelli, R.; Zingg, J.-M. Non-antioxidant molecular functions of α-tocopherol (vitamin E). *FEBS Lett.* **2002**, *519*, 8–10. [CrossRef]
63. Wallert, M.; Mosig, S.; Rennert, K.; Funke, H.; Ristow, M.; Pellegrino, R.M.; Cruciani, G.; Galli, F.; Lorkowski, S.; Birringer, M. Long-chain metabolites of α-tocopherol occur in human serum and inhibit macrophage foam cell formation in vitro. *Free Radic. Biol. Med.* **2014**, *68*, 43–51. [CrossRef] [PubMed]
64. Schmölz, L.; Wallert, M.; Rozzino, N.; Cignarella, A.; Galli, F.; Glei, M.; Werz, O.; Koeberle, A.; Birringer, M.; Lorkowski, S. Structure-Function Relationship Studies in vitro Reveal Distinct and Specific Effects of Long-Chain Metabolites of Vitamin E. *Mol. Nutr. Food Res.* **2017**. [CrossRef] [PubMed]
65. Torquato, P.; Ripa, O.; Giusepponi, D.; Galarini, R.; Bartolini, D.; Wallert, M.; Pellegrino, R.; Cruciani, G.; Lorkowski, S.; Birringer, M.; et al. Analytical strategies to assess the functional metabolome of vitamin E. *J. Pharm. Biomed. Anal.* **2016**, *124*, 399–412. [CrossRef] [PubMed]
66. Giusepponi, D.; Torquato, P.; Bartolini, D.; Piroddi, M.; Birringer, M.; Lorkowski, S.; Libetta, C.; Cruciani, G.; Moretti, S.; Saluti, G.; et al. Determination of tocopherols and their metabolites by liquid-chromatography coupled with tandem mass spectrometry in human plasma and serum. *Talanta* **2017**, *170*, 552–561. [CrossRef] [PubMed]
67. Munteanu, A.; Zingg, J.-M.; Azzi, A. Anti-atherosclerotic effects of vitamin E—Myth or reality? *J. Cell. Mol. Med.* **2004**, *8*, 59–76. [CrossRef] [PubMed]
68. Traber, M.G.; Atkinson, J. Vitamin E, antioxidant and nothing more. *Free Radic. Biol. Med.* **2007**, *43*, 4–15. [CrossRef] [PubMed]
69. Brigelius-Flohé, R.; Davies, K.J.A. Is vitamin E an antioxidant, a regulator of signal transduction and gene expression, or a 'junk' food? Comments on the two accompanying papers: "Molecular mechanism of alpha-tocopherol action" by A. Azzi and "Vitamin E, antioxidant and nothing more" by M. Traber and J. Atkinson. *Free Radic. Biol. Med.* **2007**, *43*, 2–3. [CrossRef] [PubMed]
70. Jiang, Q.; Yin, X.; Lill, M.A.; Danielson, M.L.; Freiser, H.; Huang, J. Long-chain carboxychromanols, metabolites of vitamin E, are potent inhibitors of cyclooxygenases. *Proc. Natl. Acad. Sci. USA* **2008**, *105*, 20464–20469. [CrossRef] [PubMed]
71. Ciffolilli, S.; Wallert, M.; Bartolini, D.; Krauth, V.; Werz, O.; Piroddi, M.; Sebastiani, B.; Torquato, P.; Lorkowski, S.; Birringer, M.; et al. Human serum determination and in vitro anti-inflammatory activity of the vitamin E metabolite α-(13′-hydroxy)-6-hydroxychroman. *Free Radic. Biol. Med.* **2015**, *89*, 952–962. [CrossRef] [PubMed]
72. Jang, Y.; Park, N.-Y.; Rostgaard-Hansen, A.L.; Huang, J.; Jiang, Q. Vitamin E metabolite 13′-carboxychromanols inhibit pro-inflammatory enzymes, induce apoptosis and autophagy in human cancer cells by modulating sphingolipids and suppress colon tumor development in mice. *Free Radic. Biol. Med.* **2016**, *95*, 190–199. [CrossRef] [PubMed]

73. Jiang, Z.; Yin, X.; Jiang, Q. Natural forms of vitamin E and 13′-carboxychromanol, a long-chain vitamin E metabolite, inhibit leukotriene generation from stimulated neutrophils by blocking calcium influx and suppressing 5-lipoxygenase activity, respectively. *J. Immunol.* **2011**, *186*, 1173–1179. [CrossRef] [PubMed]
74. Wallert, M.; Schmolz, L.; Koeberle, A.; Krauth, V.; Glei, M.; Galli, F.; Werz, O.; Birringer, M.; Lorkowski, S. Alpha-Tocopherol long-chain metabolite alpha-13′-COOH affects the inflammatory response of lipopolysaccharide-activated murine RAW264.7 macrophages. *Mol. Nutr. Food Res.* **2015**, *59*, 1524–1534. [CrossRef] [PubMed]
75. Schmölz, L.; Wallert, M.; Lorkowski, S. Optimized incubation regime for nitric oxide measurements in murine macrophages using the Griess assay. *J. Immunol. Methods* **2017**. [CrossRef] [PubMed]
76. Mazzini, F.; Betti, M.; Netscher, T.; Galli, F.; Salvadori, P. Configuration of the vitamin E analogue garcinoic acid extracted from Garcinia Kola seeds. *Chirality* **2009**, *21*, 519–524. [CrossRef] [PubMed]
77. Birringer, M.; Lington, D.; Vertuani, S.; Manfredini, S.; Scharlau, D.; Glei, M.; Ristow, M. Proapoptotic effects of long-chain vitamin E metabolites in HepG2 cells are mediated by oxidative stress. *Free Radic. Biol. Med.* **2010**, *49*, 1315–1322. [CrossRef] [PubMed]
78. Podszun, M.C.; Jakobi, M.; Birringer, M.; Weiss, J.; Frank, J. The long chain α-tocopherol metabolite α-13′-COOH and γ-tocotrienol induce P-glycoprotein expression and activity by activation of the pregnane X receptor in the intestinal cell line LS 180. *Mol. Nutr. Food Res.* **2017**, *61*. [CrossRef] [PubMed]
79. Torquato, P.; Bartolini, D.; Giusepponi, D.; Saluti, G.; Russo, A.; Barola, C.; Birringer, M.; Galarini, R.; Galli, F. a-13′-OH is the main product of a-tocopherol metabolism and influences CYP4F2 and PPARg: Gene expression in HepG2 human hepatocarcinoma cells. *Free Radic. Biol. Med.* **2016**, *96*, S19–S20. [CrossRef]
80. Reddi, K.; Henderson, B.; Meghji, S.; Wilson, M.; Poole, S.; Hopper, C.; Harris, M.; Hodges, S.J. Interleukin 6 production by lipopolysaccharide-stimulated human fibroblasts is potently inhibited by naphthoquinone (vitamin K) compounds. *Cytokine* **1995**, *7*, 287–290. [CrossRef] [PubMed]
81. Soper, R.J.; Oguz, C.; Emery, R.; Pitsillides, A.A.; Hodges, S.J. Vitamin K catabolite inhibition of ovariectomy-induced bone loss: Structure-activity relationship considerations. *Mol. Nutr. Food Res.* **2014**, *58*, 1658–1666. [CrossRef] [PubMed]
82. Fujii, S.; Shimizu, A.; Takeda, N.; Oguchi, K.; Katsurai, T.; Shirakawa, H.; Komai, M.; Kagechika, H. Systematic synthesis and anti-inflammatory activity of ω-carboxylated menaquinone derivatives—Investigations on identified and putative vitamin K_2 metabolites. *Bioorg. Med. Chem.* **2015**, *23*, 2344–2352. [CrossRef] [PubMed]
83. Harrington, D.J.; Soper, R.; Edwards, C.; Savidge, G.F.; Hodges, S.J.; Shearer, M.J. Determination of the urinary aglycone metabolites of vitamin K by HPLC with redox-mode electrochemical detection. *J. Lipid Res.* **2005**, *46*, 1053–1060. [CrossRef] [PubMed]
84. Conte, C.; Floridi, A.; Aisa, C.; Piroddi, M.; Floridi, A.; Galli, F. Gamma-tocotrienol metabolism and antiproliferative effect in prostate cancer cells. *Ann. N. Y. Acad. Sci.* **2004**, *1031*, 391–394. [CrossRef] [PubMed]
85. Galli, F.; Stabile, A.M.; Betti, M.; Conte, C.; Pistilli, A.; Rende, M.; Floridi, A.; Azzi, A. The effect of alpha- and gamma-tocopherol and their carboxyethyl hydroxychroman metabolites on prostate cancer cell proliferation. *Arch. Biochem. Biophys.* **2004**, *423*, 97–102. [CrossRef] [PubMed]
86. Kennel, K.A.; Drake, M.T. Vitamin D in the cancer patient. *Curr. Opin. Support. Palliat. Care* **2013**, *7*, 272–277. [CrossRef] [PubMed]
87. Vanoirbeek, E.; Krishnan, A.; Eelen, G.; Verlinden, L.; Bouillon, R.; Feldman, D.; Verstuyf, A. The anti-cancer and anti-inflammatory actions of $1,25(OH)_2D_3$. *Best Pract. Res. Clin. Endocrinol. Metab.* **2011**, *25*, 593–604. [CrossRef] [PubMed]
88. Tang, X.-H.; Gudas, L.J. Retinoids, retinoic acid receptors, and cancer. *Ann. Rev. Pathol.* **2011**, *6*, 345–364. [CrossRef] [PubMed]
89. Qin, X.-Y.; Fujii, S.; Shimizu, A.; Kagechika, H.; Kojima, S. Carboxylic Derivatives of Vitamin K2 Inhibit Hepatocellular Carcinoma Cell Growth through Caspase/Transglutaminase-Related Signaling Pathways. *J. Nutr. Sci. Vitaminol.* **2015**, *61*, 285–290. [CrossRef] [PubMed]
90. De Oliveira, M.R. Vitamin A and Retinoids as Mitochondrial Toxicants. *Oxid. Med. Cell. Longev.* **2015**, *2015*, 140267. [CrossRef] [PubMed]
91. Uray, I.P.; Dmitrovsky, E.; Brown, P.H. Retinoids and rexinoids in cancer prevention: From laboratory to clinic. *Semin. Oncol.* **2016**, *43*, 49–64. [CrossRef] [PubMed]

92. Langmann, T.; Liebisch, G.; Moehle, C.; Schifferer, R.; Dayoub, R.; Heiduczek, S.; Grandl, M.; Dada, A.; Schmitz, G. Gene expression profiling identifies retinoids as potent inducers of macrophage lipid efflux. *Biochim. Biophys. Acta* **2005**, *1740*, 155–161. [CrossRef] [PubMed]
93. Galli, F.; Azzi, A.; Birringer, M.; Cook-Mills, J.M.; Eggersdorfer, M.; Frank, J.; Cruciani, G.; Lorkowski, S.; Özer, N.K. Vitamin E: Emerging aspects and new directions. *Free Radic. Biol. Med.* **2017**, *102*, 16–36. [CrossRef] [PubMed]
94. Argmann, C.A.; Sawyez, C.G.; McNeil, C.J.; Hegele, R.A.; Huff, M.W. Activation of peroxisome proliferator-activated receptor gamma and retinoid X receptor results in net depletion of cellular cholesteryl esters in macrophages exposed to oxidized lipoproteins. *Arterioscler. Thromb. Vasc. Biol.* **2003**, *23*, 475–482. [CrossRef] [PubMed]
95. Han, S.; Sidell, N. Peroxisome-proliferator-activated-receptor gamma (PPARgamma) independent induction of CD36 in THP-1 monocytes by retinoic acid. *Immunology* **2002**, *106*, 53–59. [CrossRef] [PubMed]
96. Wuttge, D.M. Induction of CD36 by all-trans retinoic acid: Retinoic acid receptor signaling in the pathogenesis of atherosclerosis. *FASEB J.* **2001**. [CrossRef]
97. Barber, N.; Belov, L.; Christopherson, R.I. All-trans retinoic acid induces different immunophenotypic changes on human HL60 and NB4 myeloid leukaemias. *Leuk. Res.* **2008**, *32*, 315–322. [CrossRef] [PubMed]
98. Endemann, G.; Stanton, L.W.; Madden, K.S.; Bryant, C.M.; White, R.T.; Protter, A.A. CD36 is a receptor for oxidized low density lipoprotein. *J. Biol. Chem.* **1993**, *268*, 11811–11816. [PubMed]
99. Silverstein, R.L.; Li, W.; Park, Y.M.; Rahaman, S.O. Mechanisms of cell signaling by the scavenger receptor CD36: Implications in atherosclerosis and thrombosis. *Trans. Am. Clin. Climatol. Assoc.* **2010**, *121*, 206–220. [PubMed]
100. Tontonoz, P.; Nagy, L.; Alvarez, J.G.; Thomazy, V.A.; Evans, R.M. PPARgamma promotes monocyte/macrophage differentiation and uptake of oxidized LDL. *Cell* **1998**, *93*, 241–252. [CrossRef]
101. Schrijvers, D.M.; De Meyer, G.R.Y.; Herman, A.G.; Martinet, W. Phagocytosis in atherosclerosis: Molecular mechanisms and implications for plaque progression and stability. *Cardiovasc. Res.* **2007**, *73*, 470–480. [CrossRef] [PubMed]
102. Oh, J.; Weng, S.; Felton, S.K.; Bhandare, S.; Riek, A.; Butler, B.; Proctor, B.M.; Petty, M.; Chen, Z.; Schechtman, K.B.; et al. 1,25$(OH)_2$ vitamin D inhibits foam cell formation and suppresses macrophage cholesterol uptake in patients with type 2 diabetes mellitus. *Circulation* **2009**, *120*, 687–698. [CrossRef] [PubMed]
103. Riek, A.E.; Oh, J.; Bernal-Mizrachi, C. Vitamin D regulates macrophage cholesterol metabolism in diabetes. *J. Steroid Biochem. Mol. Biol.* **2010**, *121*, 430–433. [CrossRef] [PubMed]
104. Dewanjee, S.; Dua, T.K.; Bhattacharjee, N.; Das, A.; Gangopadhyay, M.; Khanra, R.; Joardar, S.; Riaz, M.; Feo, V.D.; Zia-Ul-Haq, M. Natural products as alternative choices for P-Glycoprotein (P-gp) inhibition. *Molecules* **2017**, *22*, 871. [CrossRef] [PubMed]
105. Silva, R.; Vilas-Boas, V.; Carmo, H.; Dinis-Oliveira, R.J.; Carvalho, F.; de Lourdes Bastos, M.; Remião, F. Modulation of P-glycoprotein efflux pump: Induction and activation as a therapeutic strategy. *Pharmacol. Ther.* **2015**, *149*, 1–123. [CrossRef] [PubMed]
106. Henry, H.L. Regulation of vitamin D metabolism. *Best Pract. Res. Clin. Endocrinol. Metab.* **2011**, *25*, 531–541. [CrossRef] [PubMed]
107. Mustacich, D.J.; Leonard, S.W.; Patel, N.K.; Traber, M.G. Alpha-tocopherol beta-oxidation localized to rat liver mitochondria. *Free Radic. Biol. Med.* **2010**, *48*, 73–81. [CrossRef] [PubMed]
108. Benbrook, D.; Lernhardt, E.; Pfahl, M. A new retinoic acid receptor identified from a hepatocellular carcinoma. *Nature* **1988**, *333*, 669–672. [CrossRef] [PubMed]
109. Brand, N.; Petkovich, M.; Krust, A.; Chambon, P.; de Thé, H.; Marchio, A.; Tiollais, P.; Dejean, A. Identification of a second human retinoic acid receptor. *Nature* **1988**, *332*, 850–853. [CrossRef] [PubMed]
110. Giguere, V.; Ong, E.S.; Segui, P.; Evans, R.M. Identification of a receptor for the morphogen retinoic acid. *Nature* **1987**, *330*, 624–629. [CrossRef] [PubMed]
111. Zelent, A.; Krust, A.; Petkovich, M.; Kastner, P.; Chambon, P. Cloning of murine alpha and beta retinoic acid receptors and a novel receptor gamma predominantly expressed in skin. *Nature* **1989**, *339*, 714–717. [CrossRef] [PubMed]
112. Brumbaugh, P.F.; Hughes, M.R.; Haussler, M.R. Cytoplasmic and nuclear binding components for 1alpha25-dihydroxyvitamin D3 in chick parathyroid glands. *Proc. Natl. Acad. Sci. USA* **1975**, *72*, 4871–4875. [CrossRef] [PubMed]

113. Tsai, H.C.; Norman, A.W. Studies on calciferol metabolism. 8. Evidence for a cytoplasmic receptor for 1,25-dihydroxy-vitamin D3 in the intestinal mucosa. *J. Biol. Chem.* **1973**, *248*, 5967–5975. [PubMed]
114. Baker, A.R.; McDonnell, D.P.; Hughes, M.; Crisp, T.M.; Mangelsdorf, D.J.; Haussler, M.R.; Pike, J.W.; Shine, J.; O'Malley, B.W. Cloning and expression of full-length cDNA encoding human vitamin D receptor. *Proc. Natl. Acad. Sci. USA* **1988**, *85*, 3294–3298. [CrossRef] [PubMed]
115. Carlberg, C.; Campbell, M.J. Vitamin D receptor signaling mechanisms: Integrated actions of a well-defined transcription factor. *Steroids* **2013**, *78*, 127–136. [CrossRef] [PubMed]
116. Gross, C.; Krishnan, A.V.; Malloy, P.J.; Eccleshall, T.R.; Zhao, X.Y.; Feldman, D. The vitamin D receptor gene start codon polymorphism: A functional analysis of FokI variants. *J. Bone Miner. Res.* **1998**, *13*, 1691–1699. [CrossRef] [PubMed]
117. Allenby, G.; Janocha, R.; Kazmer, S.; Speck, J.; Grippo, J.F.; Levin, A.A. Binding of 9-*cis*-retinoic acid and all-trans-retinoic acid to retinoic acid receptors alpha, beta, and gamma. Retinoic acid receptor gamma binds all-trans-retinoic acid preferentially over 9-cis-retinoic acid. *J. Biol. Chem.* **1994**, *269*, 16689–16695. [PubMed]
118. Heyman, R.A.; Mangelsdorf, D.J.; Dyck, J.A.; Stein, R.B.; Eichele, G.; Evans, R.M.; Thaller, C. 9-*cis*-retinoic acid is a high affinity ligand for the retinoid X receptor. *Cell* **1992**, *68*, 397–406. [CrossRef]
119. Wolf, G. Is 9-*cis*-retinoic acid the endogenous ligand for the retinoic acid-X receptor? *Nutr. Rev.* **2006**, *64*, 532–538. [CrossRef] [PubMed]
120. Landes, N.; Pfluger, P.; Kluth, D.; Birringer, M.; Rühl, R.; Böl, G.-F.; Glatt, H.; Brigelius-Flohé, R. Vitamin E activates gene expression via the pregnane X receptor. *Biochem. Pharmacol.* **2003**, *65*, 269–273. [CrossRef]
121. Kliewer, S.A.; Goodwin, B.; Willson, T.M. The nuclear pregnane X receptor: A key regulator of xenobiotic metabolism. *Endocr. Rev.* **2002**, *23*, 687–702. [CrossRef] [PubMed]
122. Tabb, M.M.; Sun, A.; Zhou, C.; Grün, F.; Errandi, J.; Romero, K.; Pham, H.; Inoue, S.; Mallick, S.; Lin, M.; et al. Vitamin K2 regulation of bone homeostasis is mediated by the steroid and xenobiotic receptor SXR. *J. Biol. Chem.* **2003**, *278*, 43919–43927. [CrossRef] [PubMed]
123. Ichikawa, T.; Horie-Inoue, K.; Ikeda, K.; Blumberg, B.; Inoue, S. Steroid and xenobiotic receptor SXR mediates vitamin K2-activated transcription of extracellular matrix-related genes and collagen accumulation in osteoblastic cells. *J. Biol. Chem.* **2006**, *281*, 16927–16934. [CrossRef] [PubMed]
124. Suhara, Y.; Watanabe, M.; Nakagawa, K.; Wada, A.; Ito, Y.; Takeda, K.; Takahashi, K.; Okano, T. Synthesis of novel vitamin K2 analogues with modification at the ω-terminal position and their biological evaluation as potent steroid and xenobiotic receptor (SXR) agonists. *J. Med. Chem.* **2011**, *54*, 4269–4273. [CrossRef] [PubMed]

10

Structural Modeling Insights into Human VKORC1 Phenotypes

Katrin J. Czogalla [1], Matthias Watzka [1,2] and Johannes Oldenburg [1,2,*]

[1] Institute of Experimental Hematology and Transfusion Medicine, University Clinic Bonn, Bonn 53105, Germany; E-Mails: katrin.czogalla@ukb.uni-bonn.de (K.J.C.); matthias.watzka@ukb.uni-bonn.de (M.W.)

[2] Center for Rare Diseases Bonn (ZSEB), University Clinic Bonn, Bonn 53127, Germany

* Author to whom correspondence should be addressed; E-Mail: johannes.oldenburg@ukb.uni-bonn.de

Abstract: Vitamin K 2,3-epoxide reductase complex subunit 1 (VKORC1) catalyses the reduction of vitamin K and its 2,3-epoxide essential to sustain γ-carboxylation of vitamin K-dependent proteins. Two different phenotypes are associated with mutations in human VKORC1. The majority of mutations cause resistance to 4-hydroxycoumarin- and indandione-based vitamin K antagonists (VKA) used in the prevention and therapy of thromboembolism. Patients with these mutations require greater doses of VKA for stable anticoagulation than patients without mutations. The second phenotype, a very rare autosomal-recessive bleeding disorder caused by combined deficiency of vitamin K dependent clotting factors type 2 (VKCFD2) arises from a homozygous Arg98Trp mutation. The bleeding phenotype can be corrected by vitamin K administration. Here, we summarize published experimental data and *in silico* modeling results in order to rationalize the mechanisms of VKA resistance and VKCFD2.

Keywords: vitamin K epoxide reductase (VKOR); VKORC1; vitamin K; vitamin K 2,3-epoxide; warfarin; VKCFD2; molecular modeling; vitamin K antagonists

---

1. Introduction

Vitamin K 2,3-epoxide reductase complex subunit 1 (VKORC1) is the rate limiting enzyme of the vitamin K cycle [1,2]. VKORC1 is located in the endoplasmic reticulum (ER) membrane and catalyses reduction of vitamin K 2,3-epoxide (K > O) to vitamin K quinone (K) and further to vitamin K hydroquinone (KH_2) [3]. Vitamin K reduction to KH_2 is essential for the enzyme γ-glutamyl carboxylase (GGCX) to modify vitamin K-dependent (VKD) proteins at their Gla domains. During γ-carboxylation, KH_2 is oxidized to K > O. The K > O is reduced to vitamin K quinone and further to KH_2 by VKORC1, completing a recycling mechanism known as the vitamin K cycle [4]. A functional vitamin K cycle including VKORC1 and GGCX is required to enable physiological function of all VKD proteins. VKD proteins are involved in blood coagulation (coagulation factors FII, FVII, FIX, FX, Protein C, S, and Z) as well as in calcium homeostasis (matrix Gla protein, MGP; bone Gla protein, OST) [5,6]. There have been several additional VKD proteins reported to be involved in other pathways including cell-cycle regulation or with unknown functions [7].

Since the *VKORC1* gene was cloned in 2004, genetic analysis has revealed a number of mutations causing one of two different pathological phenotypes [8–10]. To date, 28 human *VKORC1* mutations have been identified that cause resistance to several vitamin K antagonists (VKA) that are used clinically as oral anticoagulants [11,12]. Patients with these mutations require higher VKA doses for stable anticoagulation. Other 4-hydroxycoumarin and indandione derivatives are used as rodenticides. Historically, warfarin has been the most common VKA used in the anticoagulant clinic or as a rodenticide, and it has been common terminology to describe patients and animals with resistance to any VKA as possessing "warfarin resistance" (WR). This convention will be used in this manuscript. Interestingly, there are also several rat and mouse VKORC1 mutations reported to cause WR that affect residues homologous to known warfarin resistance mutations in human VKORC1 (hVKORC1) [13,14].

In contrast, there is only one mutation known to result in the VKCFD2 phenotype. VKORC1:p.Arg98Trp causes diminished vitamin K epoxide reductase (VKOR) activity compared to that of the wild-type enzyme [15]. VKCFD2 patients exhibit severely diminished activities for the VKD coagulation factors and suffer spontaneous or surgery/injury induced bleeding episodes [16,17]. In addition to this haemorrhagic phenotype, abnormalities in epiphyseal growth have been reported in one case [18]. This phenotype is very rare. Worldwide, there are only four unrelated families known to be affected with VKCFD2 [16–18].

This review discusses features of the modeled structure of the human VKORC1 enzyme, putative amino acid sequences involved in warfarin binding, and motifs that influence ER-retention of the enzyme and proposed general mechanisms that can explain the respective phenotypes.

2. The Crystal Structure of *Synechococcus* VKOR—A Homolog to hVKORC1

The first X-ray crystallographic structure of *Synechococcus* sp. VKOR (synVKOR), a bacterial homolog of the hVKORC1 enzyme, was reported by Li *et al.* in 2010 [19]. This enzyme is composed of five transmembrane helices (TMs). The first four TMs form a bundle surrounding a quinone in its interior thereby comprising the catalytic core of synVKOR. The quinone substrate is close to the periplasmic side of the enzyme and in close proximity to the CXXC active site motif located in TM4. There is a long periplasmic loop between TM1 and TM2 that includes a 1⁄2 helix ("1⁄2 segment" in the original article) and a pair of cysteines (Cys50, Cys56) and a serine/threonine residue (Ser62) conserved among all VKOR homologs [20]. The fifth TM of synVKOR is located outside of the four-helix bundle and is connected via a C-terminal linker segment to a thioredoxin (Trx)-like domain. The Trx-like domain is the naturally fused redox partner of synVKOR. Li *et al.* [19] observed a disulfide bridge with strong electron density between Cys50 in the periplasmic loop of the VKOR domain and Cys209 of the Trx-like domain. Thus, the synVKOR structure suggests an electron transfer mechanism that shuttles reducing equivalents from the Trx-like domain, via the conserved cysteines in the loop, to the CXXC active site motif where the bound ubiquinone substrate becomes reduced to the hydroquinone form [21].

3. The Human VKORC1 Homology Model

In the absence of high-resolution X-ray crystallographic or NMR structures of hVKORC1, creation of a homology model based on the synVKOR structure provides an opportunity to gain structure-based insights into hVKORC1 function. Several *in silico* algorithms revealed conflicting topology predictions of either a 3TM, 4TM or 5TM structure for *hVKORC1* [8,9,11,22–24]. There are also conflicting experimental data supporting 3TM or 4TM topologies [25–27]. Nevertheless, all VKOR homologues share conserved functional residues at homologous positions which strongly suggest that all homologs share a common protein fold and topology with respect to the lipid membrane in which they are embedded.

4. Conserved Amino Acid Residues of Human VKORC1

VKORC1 homologues are found in plants, bacteria, archaea and mammals but not in yeast and fungi [20,28,29]. All VKOR homolog enzymes possess a CXXC motif in the active site, essential for reduction of quinone substrates [3,20,30–32]. The cysteines of the CXXC motif form a disulfide bridge that becomes reduced for catalytic activity. There are two additional cysteines (Cys43 and Cys51) that can form a disulfide bond and a conserved serine at amino acid position 57 (or either threonine in some VKORC1 homologues) in the large loop of hVKORC1 [3,19,30,32,33]. These four cysteines and the serine/threonine are absolutely conserved and define proteins of the VKOR family.

The CXXC motif is located in the last TM and is oriented towards the ER lumen in both 3TM and 4TM models for hVKORC1 (Figure 1). All published reports show complete loss of VKOR activity if one of the cysteines in the CXXC motif is mutated (Cys132 and Cys135, Table 1) [3,19,30,31]. These data clearly demonstrate that the CXXC motif is the active center essential for substrate reduction. The functional role of the conserved cysteines in the large loop, Cys43 and Cys51, is not completely clear. Due to their localisation Cys43 and Cys51 are also called "loop cysteines". Of the two topology models, studies proposing the 4TM model claim that the loop cysteines are essential for *in vivo* VKOR activity [27,33], whereas studies supporting the 3TM model argue that they are not necessary [3,26,34]. The main difference between both models is the orientation of the N-terminus, the first TM, and the large loop. In the 3TM model, the loop is located in the cytoplasm, whereas in the 4TM model, the loop is in the ER lumen (Figure 1). In the 4TM model, the loop cysteines are required for electron transfer from redox partners located in the ER lumen to reduce the CXXC motif. This postulated electron transfer pathway is necessary for catalytic VKOR activity and is also present in bacterial VKOR homologues. In synVKOR, the disulfide bridge formed between the loop cysteines is reduced by a periplasmic Trx-like redox partner naturally fused to the VKOR core protein. In vertebrates, this natural fused redox partner is missing. Therefore, Trx-like domain containing proteins are thought to reduce the loop cysteines in vertebrates. Candidate partner oxidoreductases include protein disulfide isomerases (PDIs) that are either separate globular proteins in the ER lumen or type-I ER membrane-anchored proteins with redox-active cysteines facing the ER lumen [27,35]. Thus, electron transfer mediated by the loop cysteines is feasible for the 4TM model only, as most PDIs are resident in the ER lumen. However, for the 3TM model, PDIs would not be able to reduce the loop cysteines if the loop is located in the cytoplasm. Here, the two loop cysteines could not be essential for VKOR activity, and electron transfer would presumably take place through direct reduction of the CXXC motif. Thus, location of the loop cysteines in the ER lumen might not be a strict requirement for hVKORC1 function if the 3TM model were to be correct.

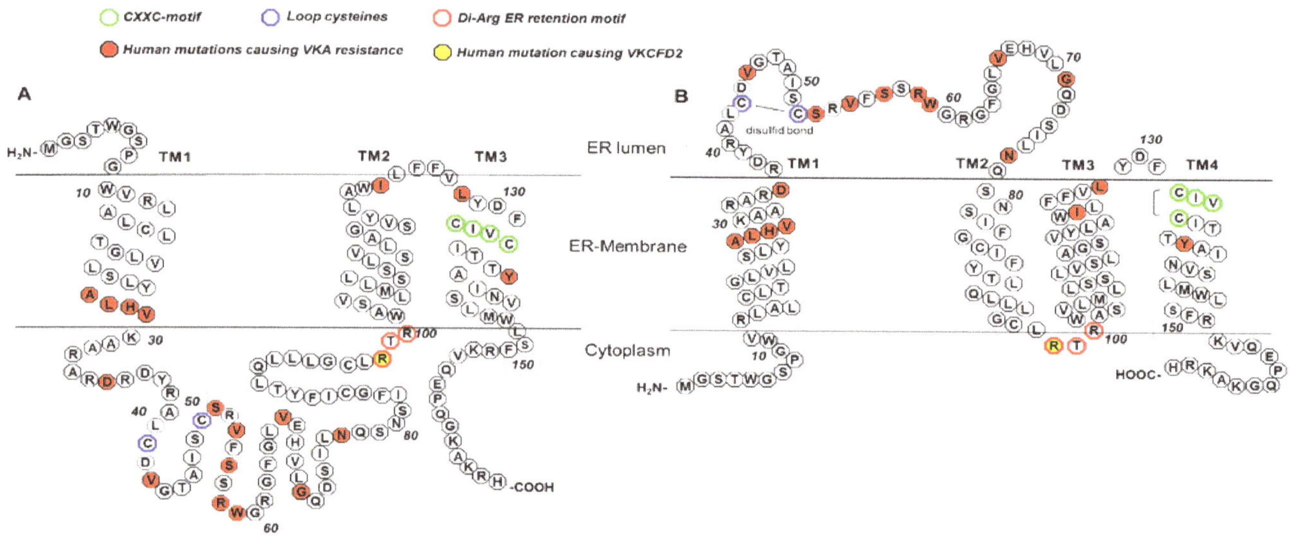

Figure 1. 3TM and 4TM topological models for hVKORC1 (modified from Tie *et al.*, 2012 [26]). In both models, conserved cysteines (Cys132 and Cys135 of the active center (CXXC motif), green; loop cysteines Cys43 and Cys51, blue) and Arg98_Arg100 of the di-arginine endoplasmic reticulum (ER) retention motif (red) are labeled with colored circles. Amino acid positions for which mutations were reported to be associated with either vitamin K antagonist (VKA) resistance or combined deficiency of vitamin K dependent clotting factors type 2 (VKCFD2) are marked by filled circles (mutations causing VKA resistance, red; VKCFD2 mutation, yellow). (**A**) Shows the putative topology for hVKORC1 as a 3 TM membrane-embedded protein with the loop located in the cytoplasm. The N-terminus is located in the ER lumen, whereas the C-terminus is in the cytoplasm. (**B**) Shows the putative 4TM topology for hVKORC1 with the loop containing the conserved cysteines Cys43 and Cys51 in the ER lumen with both termini located in the cytoplasm.

Table 1. Published activities for hVKORC1 conserved cysteines by various functional assays.

Publication	Rost *et al.* [30]	Jin *et al.* [3]	Rishavy *et al.* [33]	Tie *et al.* [26]	Tie *et al.* [34]	Tie *et al.* [36]
Type of VKOR assay	DTT-driven assay	DTT-driven assay	DTT-driven assay	Cell-based assay	DTT-driven assay/cell-based assay	Cell-based assay
Reductant	DTT	DTT	DTT/Trx/TrxR	-	-	-
Cell line	HEK293 cells	Sf9 cells	Sf21 cells	HEK293 cells	HEK293 cells	C1 + L1 DKO HEK cells
Cysteine residue variants:						
Cys43Ala	20%	25%	~85%/0%	<5%	25%/<5%	<5%
Cys43Ser	20%					
Cys51Ala		100%	~50%/0%	95%	100%/100%	105%
Cys51Ser	<5%					
Cys43Ala + Cys51Ala		112%		60%	85%/110%	90%
Cys43_Cys51del		85%			85%/60%	
Cys132Ala/Ser	<5%	0%			0%/0%	
Cys135Ala/Ser	<5%	0%			0%/0%	

This table shows the published vitamin K epoxide reductase (VKOR) activities of human vitamin K 2,3-epoxide reductase complex subunit 1 (hVKORC1) variants in which conserved cysteines were selectively mutated or deleted. In each published study the VKOR activities are presented as a percentage of the activity of the wild-type hVKORC1 reported in the same study. The table also lists the type of VKOR assay, reductant (dithiothreitol (DTT) or thioredoxin/thioredoxin reductase (Trx/TrxR)), and cell line (human embryonic kidney (HEK) cells, *Spodoptera frugiperda* (Sf21) cells, or double knock-out (DKO) HEK cells) used.

It follows from the arguments presented above that VKOR activity measurements of variants affecting the loop cysteines might provide important clues to elucidate the topology and structure of hVKORC1. Reduced activities for amino acid substitutions of loop cysteines would tend to support the 4TM model where loop cysteines would be essential for electron transfer. Alternatively, data revealing unaffected activity for these variants would favour the 3TM topology model where loop cysteines would not be required for CXXC motif reduction. Several research groups have published conflicting activity data regarding the loop cysteines supporting either the 3TM or 4TM topology (Table 1). Rost *et al.* [30] were the first to publish data regarding the loop cysteines of hVKORC1 investigated by the commonly used dithiothreitol (DTT)-driven VKOR assay. They demonstrated a reduction of VKOR activity to 5% for Cys51Ser and to 20% for Cys43Ser with respect to wild-type activity [30]. By contrast, Jin *et al.* published results revealing more than 100% activity for Cys51Ala compared to that of wild-type VKORC1. However, the Cys43Ala variant showed reduced activity to 25% which corresponds well to the data of Rost *et al.* for Cys43Ser. Interestingly, VKOR activity of a variant with both loop cysteines mutated was unaffected (Table 1) [3]. Rishavy *et al.* [33] modified this *in vitro* VKOR assay by replacing the non-physiological DTT with the reductant thioredoxin/thioredoxin reductase (Trx/TrxR). In their study, they demonstrated that VKOR activity assessed by the DTT-driven assay is prone to false positive results. They showed that membrane-permeable DTT directly reduces the active centre of hVKORC1, essentially bypassing the loop cysteines. Thus, the loop cysteine variants showed VKOR activity when DTT was used as reductant. When DTT was replaced by the membrane impermeable Trx/TrxR reductant, VKORC1 loop cysteine mutants did not show VKOR activity (Table 1) [33]. This strongly suggests that loop cysteines are essential for VKOR activity when driven by a biological oxidoreductase enzyme. However, the study was negatively critiqued regarding the relative concentration differences between DTT and Trx/TrxR concentrations used (millimolar for DTT *vs.* micromolar for Trx/TrxR) [22]. Alternatively, loop cysteine variants have been examined in one of the recently reported cell-based assays in which no detergent and extra reductants are used and VKOR activity is indirectly assessed in living cells. Two studies by Tie *et al.* [26,36] revealed very low VKOR activity for Cys43Ala (<5%), whereas Cys51Ala showed activity comparable to that of wild-type VKORC1. Again, they found that mutation of both loop cysteines did not affect VKOR activity (Table 1) [26,36].

Taken together, data from all research groups demonstrated reduction of VKOR activity for all variants affecting Cys43, independent of the type of assay used. However, results regarding activities of Cys51 variants are in disaccord as they range between 0% and 100% relative to wild-type VKOR activity. Moreover, these data do not unequivocally clarify whether or not the loop cysteines are essential for hVKORC1 activity and, thus, do not definitively support either the 3TM or 4TM model.

5. The 3TM VKORC1 Topology Model

The 3TM model is characterized by three transmembrane alpha-helices with a large cytoplasmic loop containing the conserved loop cysteines located between the first and second TMs. The C-terminus is located in the cytoplasm and the N-terminus in the ER lumen (Figure 1A). The 3TM model is supported by several *in silico* topology prediction algorithms and by experimental data from a fluorescence protease protection (FFP) assay of Tie *et al.* [26,37]. In this assay, VKORC1 enzyme was either C- or N-terminal tagged with the green fluorescent protein (GFP). After expression of both GFP tagged variants in HEK293 cells, a GFP digestion was performed using trypsin. The cells were treated before the digestion with digitonin to selectively permeabilize only the plasma membrane so that GFP tags located in the cytoplasm, but not in the ER lumen, become digested by the protease. The FFP assay results revealed a complete digestion of GFP for the C-terminal tagged VKORC1 protein after 90 s, whereas the N-terminal GFP-tagged VKORC1 continued to show a fluorescent signal even after 150 s. These data suggest that N- and C-termini are located on opposite sides of the ER membrane with the C-terminus in the cytoplasm. The N-terminus appears to be located in the ER lumen because it is protected from the proteolysis [26].

6. The 4TM VKORC1 Topology Model

The putative 4TM topology for hVKORC1 is composed of 4TM domains and includes the large ER lumenal loop between TM1 and TM2 with the two conserved loop cysteines. Both termini are located in the cytoplasm (Figure 1B). The CXXC motif is located in 4TM close to the ER lumen, equivalent to its placement in the third and final TM for the 3TM model. The crystal structure of the bacterial synVKOR enzyme strongly suggests a 4TM topology for hVKORC1. The membrane embedded four-helix bundle of synVKOR is homologous to hVKORC1 which shares ~24% primary sequence identity [19].

Wajih *et al.* [35] performed a knock-down of PDI expression by using siRNA silencing. This revealed reduced VKOR activity to 25% in HEK293 cells. In addition, they demonstrated by sodium dodecyl sulfate polyacrylamide gel electrophoresis (SDS-PAGE) that PDIs form a complex with VKORC1 [35]. This was the first convincing evidence that PDIs may be physiological redox partners for hVKORC1. Further immunoprecipitation data by Li *et al.* [27] confirmed which PDI family member interacts with hVKORC1 [27]. The interaction was only present if Cys51 of hVKORC1 and the second active site cysteine of the Trx-like domain of PDI were both mutated to alanine. These amino acid substitutions were necessary because the native cysteine pairs of VKORC1 and PDI are self-reducing during redox cycling and do not form stable disulfide bonds. As a result of the mutagenesis, the "donor" cysteine of PDI and the "acceptor" cysteine (Cys43) of hVKORC1 form a stable disulfide bond that remains oxidized during immunoprecipitation and detection. These results indicate that at least three PDIs identified can transfer electrons to the loop cysteines of hVKORC1. *In silico* modeling of hVKORC1 on the X-ray crystallographic structure of synVKOR also suggests a 4TM topology [19,23]. Additionally, *in silico* docking of warfarin on this model disclosed three putative binding interfaces. All human, as well as rodent, VKORC1 mutations associated with warfarin resistance are located in or close to these putative binding interfaces, supporting the plausibility of our *in silico* analysis (see detailed information in the next section) [23].

Taken together, data from the PDI knock-down, immunoprecipitation interaction studies, and *in silico* modeling of hVKORC1 with the identification of putative warfarin binding interfaces are largely consistent with a 4TM topology for hVKORC1 (Table 2).

Table 2. Overview of published experimental data supporting 3TM or 4TM topological models for hVKORC1.

Arguments for 3TM hVKORC1 Structure	Arguments for 4TM hVKORC1 Structure
Location of the C-Terminus of VKORC1 in the cytoplasm and of the N-Terminus in the ER-lumen; FFP assay [26]	siRNA knock-down of PDI located in the ER lumen results in reduced VKOR activity [35]
Cys51Ala exhibits VKOR activity = Cys51 is not required for VKOR activity, DTT and cell-based assays [3,26,36]	Cys43Ala/Ser and Cys51Ala/Ser exhibit no VKOR activity = Cys43 and Cys51 are required for VKOR activity, DTT and Trx/TrxR assays [30,33]
hVKOR model, prediction program TOPCONS [37]	Cys43 forms a disulfide bond with four PDIs, immunoprecipitation [27] 3.6 Å crystal structure of the bacterial homologue of VKOR from *Synechococcus* sp. in conjunction with multiple sequence alignments [19] hVKORC1 model based on crystal structure of synVKOR and putative warfarin binding interfaces that correspond to the reported WR mutations [23]

The left- and right-hand columns present brief summaries of the experimental data obtained from structural studies and assays of VKOR activity (together with literature citations) that support either the 3TM or 4TM topology for hVKORC1 respectively.

7. Warfarin Binding and Mutations Causing Warfarin Resistance

VKA such as warfarin, are direct inhibitors of VKORC1 and are used in the prevention and therapy of thromboembolic disorders [4,29]. It is widely believed that warfarin binds to VKORC1 irreversibly [38]. To date, genetic analysis of *VKORC1* has implicated a total of 28 mutations to be associated with WR in humans (Table 3) [8,11,12]. Affected patients require greater doses of VKA drugs for stable oral anticoagulation compared to wild-type VKORC1 probands. Some WR patients even exhibit an apparent complete resistance leading to ineffective control or to the abandonment of anticoagulation therapy with VKA [11,12].

Table 3. Comparison of warfarin inhibition for hVKORC1 variants determined by *in vitro* assays of vitamin K 2,3-epoxide reductase (VKOR) in cell fractions or in cultured cells.

hVKORC1 Variant	Mean Patient Dosage in HDT Multiples [Drug] for n = Number of Reported Patients [11]	Warfarin IC_{50} by DTT-Driven VKOR Assay [8,12]	Warfarin IC_{50} by Cell Based Assay [23]	Warfarin Phenotypes by Cell Based Assay [36]
Wild-type	1.0 [W, P] (n = 77)			
Ala26Pro	>3.0 [W] (n = 1)	11.2-fold increased K_i [12]	49.6-fold increased IC_{50}	n.d.
Ala26Thr	>2.0 [P] (n = 1)	sensitive as wt [12]	3.0-fold increased IC_{50}	n.d.
Leu27Val	>3.0 [F], 1.0 [W] (n = 1) *	sensitive as wt [12]	2.5-fold increased IC_{50}	n.d.
His28Gln	3.5 [P] (n = 1)	more sensitive than wt [12]	2.9-fold increased IC_{50}	n.d.
Val29Leu	2.0 [W] (n = 1)	absence of expression [12]/low VKOR activity and more sensitive than wt [8]	5.5-fold increased IC_{50}	n.d.
Ala34Pro	3.8 [W] (n = 1)	n.d.	n.d.	n.d.
Asp36Gly	3.0 [W] (n = 1)	more sensitive than wt [12]	3.2-fold increased IC_{50}	n.d.
Asp36Tyr	1.5–3.5 [W] (n = 10)	sensitive as wt [12]	3.8-fold increased IC_{50}	n.d.
Val45Ala	>2.0 [W] (n = 1)	low VKOR activity [8], more sensitive than wt [8,12]	6.2-fold increased IC_{50}	n.d.
Ser52Leu	>3.0 [P] (n = 1)	low VKOR activity, K_i determination not possible [12]	7.4-fold increased IC_{50}	moderate resistance
Ser52Trp	3.5 [P] (n = 1)	low VKOR activity, K_i determination not possible [12]	5.7-fold increased IC_{50}	sensitive as wt
Val54Leu	1.5–5.5 [W] (n = 2)	4.6-fold increased K_i [12]	4.5-fold increased IC_{50}	n.d.
Ser56Phe	>5.0 [P] (n = 1)	more sensitive than wt [12]	6.8-fold increased IC_{50}	n.d.
Arg58Gly	5.0 [W] (n = 1)	low VKOR activity [8], more sensitive than wt [8,12]	3.4-fold increased IC_{50}	n.d.
Trp59Arg	7.0 [P] (n = 1)	low VKOR activity, K_i determination not possible [12]	17.5-fold increased IC_{50}	high resistance
Trp59Cys	>3.5 [P] (n = 1)	more sensitive than wt [12]	7.6-fold increased IC_{50}	n.d.

Table 3. *Cont.*

hVKORC1 Variant	Mean Patient Dosage in HDT Multiples [Drug] for n = Number of Reported Patients [11]	Warfarin IC_{50} by DTT-Driven VKOR Assay [8,12]	Warfarin IC_{50} by Cell Based Assay [23]	Warfarin Phenotypes by Cell Based Assay [36]
Trp59Leu	>5.0 [P] (n = 1)	low VKOR activity, K_i determination not possible [12]	75.2-fold increased IC_{50}	high VKOR activity, high resistance
Val66Gly	2.5 [P] (n = 1)	low VKOR activity, K_i determination not possible [12]	2.8-fold increased IC_{50}	sensitive as wt
Val66Met	3.0–6.0 [W] (n = 7)	low VKOR activity, K_i determination not possible [12]	5.4-fold increased IC_{50}	sensitive as wt
Gly71Ala	>2.0 [P] (n = 1)	low VKOR activity, K_i determination not possible [12]	5.1-fold increased IC_{50}	sensitive as wt
Asn77Ser	>3.0 [P] (n = 1)	low VKOR activity, K_i determination not possible [12]	5.3-fold increased IC_{50}	moderate resistance
Asn77Tyr	3.5 [W] (n = 1)	low VKOR activity, K_i determination not possible [12]	3.9-fold increased IC_{50}	sensitive as wt
Ile123Asn	>7.0 [P] (n = 1)	2.4-fold increased K_i [12]	8.5-fold increased IC_{50}	n.d.
Leu128Arg	>4.0–7.0 [W] (n = 5)	low VKOR activity [8,12], K_i determination not possible [12]/more sensitive than wt [8]	49.7-fold increased IC_{50}	high VKOR activity, high resistance
Tyr139His	>3.0 [W] (n = 1)	3.6-fold increased K_i [12]	4.6-fold increased IC_{50}	n.d.

This table shows patient data as well as *in vitro* results from the DTT-driven and cell culture-based VKOR assays for VKORC1 variants reported to cause resistance to VKA. Patient data from Watzka *et al.* [11] and Hodroge *et al.* [12], with [P] = phenprocoumon, [W] = warfarin; HDT = High Dosage Threshold which is equivalent to the mean patient population dosage divided by that for the control group (homozygous wild-type *VKORC1* alleles with *VKORC1*:c.-1639GG haplotype). The patient marked with an asterisk (*) and Leu27Val mutation had additionally the CYP2C9*2*3 haplotype which results in a reduced warfarin dosage requirement to achieve a stable, therapeutic INR compared to patients with wild-type CYP2C9*1*1 haplotype. Variants investigated by the DTT-driven assay by Hodroge *et al.* [12] and Rost *et al.* [8] were summarized in one column, followed by data from Czogalla *et al.* [23] and Tie *et al.* [36]. n.d. = not determined.

Investigation by *in vitro* assays of these mutations is challenging and the results often do not correlate with patient phenotypes [39]. Rost *et al.* (2004) first investigated warfarin inhibition of six WR variants heterologously expressed in HEK293 cells using the DTT-driven VKOR assay but none of these mutations showed an *in vitro* resistance phenotype [8]. Similarly, Hodroge *et al.* (2012) expressed human WR variants in *Pichia pastoris* and found that only four of 25 mutations investigated revealed resistance phenotypes by the DTT-driven VKOR assay [12]. Nineteen variants were either non-functional or did not show a resistance phenotype [12]. Ten of the mutations that had essentially no *in vitro* VKOR activity in the study of Hodroge *et al.* (2012) [12] were re-examined by Tie *et al.* (2013) [36] using a cell-based assay. This assay indirectly reports activity of hVKORC1 using carboxylation of a coexpressed chimeric VKD protein in a HEK293 cell line constitutively knocked-out for both endogenous *VKORC1* and its paralog enzyme *VKORC1L1* [36]. For all the variants investigated, Tie *et al.* [36] detected VKOR activity as great as or greater than that of wild-type VKORC1. Five mutations exhibited a warfarin resistance phenotype by their cell culture-based assay, consistent with reported patient WR phenotypes [35]. However, five other WR mutations were not resistant to warfarin in their assay [36]. Hodroge *et al.* (2012) [12] and Tie *et al.* (2013) [36] both speculated that therapeutic doses of warfarin in these patients possibly have impact alternative enzyme targets other than the hVKORC1 mutated variants. In contrast, our group showed that all known hVKORC1 mutations associated with WR revealed *in vitro* WR phenotypes by a similar cell culture-based assay [23,39]. In all cases, we measured *in vitro* WR phenotypes ranging from mild to total resistance, in agreement with elevated patient dosages previously reported (Table 3) [11]. Discrepancies detected for WR phenotypes by the cell culture-based assays of Tie *et al.* [36] and of Czogalla *et al.* [23,39] might be explained by differences in the experimental setting. The genomic background of the HEK293T cell strains used was a wild-type in the study of Czogalla *et al.* [23] and a *VKORC1/VKORC1L1* double knock-out in the study of Tie *et al.* [36]. Additionally, our group [23,39] used wild-type FIX as a coexpressed VKD reporter protein to measure VKORC1 function, whereas Tie and co-workers [36] used a chimeric construct comprising protein C with its Gla domain replaced by that of FIX. Similar differences in the ability of DTT-based and cell culture-based assays to report *in vitro* WR phenotypes for mouse and rat VKORC1 have been reported [13,14,40].

To gain further insight into the binding and inhibitory action of warfarin, we performed *in silico* docking of warfarin on our model of hVKORC1. Molecular docking analysis revealed three putative warfarin binding interfaces on hVKORC1 comprising linear sequences of the ER-lumenal loop (Ser52-Phe55), and the first (Leu22-Lys30) and fourth (Phe131-Thr137) transmembrane helices of hVKORC1 [23]. Twenty-four human and nine rodent VKORC1 mutations confirmed to be WR are located at or near to the predicted binding interfaces. In addition, all amino acid substitutions causing WR, except for Tyr139His, were found to have their side chains on the ER lumenal side of the enzyme, thereby potentially influencing warfarin binding. Furthermore, our data suggest that warfarin might inhibit hVKORC1 in three possible ways. Firstly, binding of warfarin may interfere with the redox cycling of the disulfide bridge between the loop cysteines (Cys43 and Cys51). Secondly, warfarin binding might hinder the close approach of the reduced loop cysteines to the active centre of VKORC1 (CXXC motif). Thirdly, binding of warfarin might also hinder access of the K > O substrate to its binding pocket in the hVKORC1 active site. In summary, the insight gained through comparative modeling of hVKORC1 based on the synVKOR X-ray crystallographic structure has led to further investigation of the molecular mechanisms of warfarin inhibition of hVKORC1 and warfarin resistance.

8. VKCFD2

To date, there have been only three unrelated families reported with probands suffering from VKCFD2 who harbour homozygous VKORC1:p.Arg98Trp alleles [16,17]. Instead of WR, this mutation causes spontaneous bleedings due to reduced VKOR activity of 20%–60% compared to that for homozygous wild-type hVKORC1 individuals [8,16–18]. A previous study confirmed diminished, warfarin-sensitive VKOR activity of ~10%, relative to that of wild-type enzyme by the DTT-driven VKOR assay [30]. However, the haemorrhagic phenotype of these patients can be corrected by vitamin K administration which results in restoration of activities for the vitamin K-dependent clotting factors to normal ranges. Until recently, the pathophysiological mechanism underlying the single mutation causing VKCFD2 was unknown.

In a recent study, we modeled hVKORC1 and performed *in silico* analysis of the region of interest. We found that the Arg98Trp mutation might be part of a putative di-arginine ER retention motif [15]. To confirm these *in silico* results experimentally, different variants affecting Arg98 and/or Arg100 of the putative ER retention motif were expressed in HEK293T cells and analysed by fluorescence confocal microscopy. As expected, wild-type hVKORC1 was exclusively located in the ER, whereas all variants affecting the di-arginine ER retention motif revealed reduced ER localization to only 9% compared to that of wild-type hVKORC1. The naturally occurring variant Arg98Trp resulted in 20% ER-localization compared to that of the wild-type. We further observed that the protein variants affecting the di-arginine ER retention motif were directed to the cytoplasm. If the residual amount of hVKORC1:Arg98Trp in the ER is not functionally impaired with respect to VKOR activity, this would explain phenotype correction by vitamin K administration for VKCFD2 patients [41].

Interestingly, our identified di-arginine ER retention motif (Arg98_Arg100) is consistent with both the 3TM and 4TM topology models for hVKORC1. Di-arginine based ER retention motifs are generally present in cytosolic domains of proteins at approximately 16–46 A° from the lipid bilayer and allows for interaction with ER retention proteins [42,43]. This is observed for both hVKORC1 models, in which the guanidyl groups of Arg98 and Arg100 are exposed to the cytoplasm. In the 4TM model, these arginines are located in the small cytoplasm-exposed loop connecting TM2 with TM3 (Figure 1B) [42,43]. However, our results would also support the alternative 3TM model for hVKORC1 where the di-arginine ER retention motif would be located at the end of the large putative cytoplasmic loop just before the TM2 helix (Figure 1A).

9. Conclusions

The identification of the human *VKORC1* gene in 2004 was a major step towards understanding the molecular and genetic mechanisms of the vitamin K cycle. Since then, 28 mutations causing WR and a single mutation responsible for VKCFD2 have been identified and functionally confirmed by *in vitro* studies. *In silico* analysis has provided insight into structural requirements for warfarin binding and the pathophysiological mechanism of VKCFD2.

Acknowledgments: This work was supported, in part, by funding from BONFOR grant 2014-1-3 (KJC), Baxter Germany GmbH (JO, MW) and from the Deutsche Forschungsgemeinschaft (DFG) grant Ol100 5-1 (JO, MW).

Author Contributions: Katrin J. Czogalla, Matthias Watzka and Johannes Oldenburg conceived and wrote the article. Katrin J. Czogalla provided the figure and tables.

References

1. Wajih, N.; Sane, D.C.; Hutson, S.M.; Wallin, R. Engineering of a recombinant vitamin K-dependent gamma-carboxylation system with enhanced gamma-carboxyglutamic acid forming capacity: Evidence for a functional CXXC redox center in the system. *J. Biol. Chem.* **2005**, *280*, 10540–10547. [CrossRef] [PubMed]
2. Oldenburg, J.; Bevans, C.G.; Müller, C.R.; Watzka, M. Vitamin K epoxide reductase complex subunit 1 (VKORC1): The key protein of the vitamin K cycle. *Antioxid. Redox Signal.* **2006**, *8*, 347–353. [CrossRef] [PubMed]
3. Jin, D.-Y.; Tie, J.-K.; Stafford, D.W. The conversion of vitamin K epoxide to vitamin K quinone and vitamin K quinone to vitamin K hydroquinone uses the same active site cysteines. *Biochemistry* **2007**, *46*, 7279–7283. [CrossRef] [PubMed]
4. Oldenburg, J.; Marinova, M.; Müller-Reible, C.; Watzka, M. The vitamin K cycle. *Vitam. Horm.* **2008**, *78*, 35–62. [PubMed]
5. Gundberg, C.M.; Lian, J.B.; Booth, S.L. Vitamin K-dependent carboxylation of osteocalcin: Friend or foe? *Adv. Nutr.* **2012**, *3*, 149–157. [CrossRef] [PubMed]
6. Cancela, M.L.; Laizé, V.; Conceição, N. Matrix Gla protein and osteocalcin: From gene duplication to neofunctionalization. *Arch. Biochem. Biophys.* **2014**, *561*, 56–63. [CrossRef] [PubMed]
7. Ferland, G. Vitamin K and the nervous system: An overview of its actions. *Adv. Nutr.* **2012**, *3*, 204–212. [CrossRef] [PubMed]
8. Rost, S.; Fregin, A.; Ivaskevicius, V.; Conzelmann, E.; Hörtnagel, K.; Pelz, H.J.; Lappegard, K.; Seifried, E.; Scharrer, I.; Tuddenham, E.G.; *et al.* Mutations in VKORC1 cause warfarin resistance and multiple coagulation factor deficiency type 2. *Nature* **2004**, *427*, 537–541. [CrossRef] [PubMed]
9. Li, T.; Chang, C.Y.; Jin, D.Y.; Lin, P.J.; Khvorova, A.; Stafford, D.W. Identification of the gene for vitamin K epoxide reductase. *Nature* **2004**, *427*, 541–544. [CrossRef] [PubMed]
10. Fregin, A.; Rost, S.; Wolz, W.; Krebsova, A.; Muller, C.R.; Oldenburg, J. Homozygosity mapping of a second gene locus for hereditary combined deficiency of vitamin K-dependent clotting factors to the centromeric region of chromosome 16. *Blood* **2002**, *100*, 3229–3232. [CrossRef] [PubMed]
11. Watzka, M.; Geisen, C.; Bevans, C.G.; Sittinger, K.; Spohn, G.; Rost, S.; Seifried, E.; Müller, C.R.; Oldenburg, J. Thirteen novel VKORC1 mutations associated with oral anticoagulant resistance: Insights into improved patient diagnosis and treatment. *J. Thromb. Haemost.* **2011**, *9*, 109–118. [CrossRef] [PubMed]
12. Hodroge, A.; Matagrin, B.; Moreau, C.; Fourel, I.; Hammed, A.; Benoit, E.; Lattard, V. VKORC1 mutations detected in patients resistant to vitamin K antagonists are not all associated with a resistant VKOR activity. *J. Thromb. Haemost.* **2012**, *10*, 2535–2543. [CrossRef] [PubMed]
13. Pelz, H.-J.; Rost, S.; Hünerberg, M.; Fregin, A.; Heiberg, A.C.; Baert, K.; MacNicoll, A.D.; Prescott, C.V.; Walker, A.S.; Oldenburg, J.; *et al.* The genetic basis of resistance to anticoagulants in rodents. *Genetics* **2005**, *170*, 1839–1847. [CrossRef] [PubMed]

14. Rost, S.; Pelz, H.-J.; Menzel, S.; MacNicoll, A.D.; León, V.; Song, K.J.; Jäkel, T.; Oldenburg, J.; Müller, C.R. Novel mutations in the VKORC1 gene of wild rats and mice—A response to 50 years of selection pressure by warfarin? *BMC Genet.* **2009**, *10*, 4. [CrossRef] [PubMed]
15. Czogalla, K.J.; Biswas, A.; Rost, S.; Watzka, M.; Oldenburg, J. The Arg98Trp mutation in human VKORC1 causing VKCFD2 disrupts a di-Arginine-based ER retention motif. *Blood* **2014**, *124*, 1354–1362. [CrossRef] [PubMed]
16. Oldenburg, J.; von Brederlow, B.; Fregin, A.; Rost, S.; Wolz, W.; Eberl, W.; Eber, S.; Lenz, E.; Schwaab, R.; Brackmann, H.H.; *et al.* Congenital deficiency of vitamin K dependent coagulation factors in two families presents as a genetic defect of the vitamin K-epoxide-reductase-complex. *Thromb. Haemost.* **2000**, *84*, 937–941. [PubMed]
17. Marchetti, G.; Caruso, P.; Lunghi, B.; Pinotti, M.; Lapecorella, M.; Napolitano, M.; Canella, A.; Mariani, G.; Bernardi, F. Vitamin K-induced modification of coagulation phenotype in VKORC1 homozygous deficiency. *J. Thromb. Haemost.* **2008**, *6*, 797–803. [CrossRef] [PubMed]
18. Pauli, R.M.; Lian, J.B.; Mosher, D.F.; Suttie, J.W. Association of congenital deficiency of multiple vitamin K-dependent coagulation factors and the phenotype of the warfarin embryopathy: Clues to the mechanism of teratogenicity of coumarin derivatives. *Am. J. Hum. Genet.* **1987**, *41*, 566–583. [PubMed]
19. Li, W.; Schulman, S.; Dutton, R.J.; Boyd, D.; Beckwith, J.; Rapoport, T.A. Structure of a bacterial homologue of vitamin K epoxide reductase. *Nature* **2010**, *463*, 507–512. [CrossRef] [PubMed]
20. Goodstadt, L.; Ponting, C.P. Vitamin K epoxide reductase: Homology, active site and catalytic mechanism. *Trends Biochem. Sci.* **2004**, *29*, 289–292. [CrossRef] [PubMed]
21. Liu, S.; Cheng, W.; Fowle Grider, R.; Shen, G.; Li, W. Structures of an intramembrane vitamin K epoxide reductase homolog reveal control mechanisms for electron transfer. *Nat. Commun.* **2014**, *5*, 3110. [CrossRef] [PubMed]
22. Van Horn, W.D. Structural and functional insights into human vitamin K epoxide reductase and vitamin K epoxide reductase-like1. *Crit. Rev. Biochem. Mol. Biol.* **2013**, *48*, 357–372. [CrossRef] [PubMed]
23. Czogalla, K.J.; Biswas, A.; Wendeln, A.C.; Westhofen, P.; Müller, C.R.; Watzka, M.; Oldenburg, J. Human VKORC1 mutations cause variable degrees of 4-hydroxycoumarin resistance and affect putative warfarin binding interfaces. *Blood* **2013**, *122*, 2743–2750. [CrossRef] [PubMed]
24. Wu, S.; Liu, S.; Davis, C.H.; Stafford, D.W.; Kulman, J.D.; Pedersen, L.G. A hetero-dimer model for concerted action of vitamin K carboxylase and vitamin K reductase in vitamin K cycle. *J. Theor. Biol.* **2011**, *279*, 143–149. [CrossRef] [PubMed]
25. Tie, J.K.; Nicchitta, C.; von Heijne, G.; Stafford, D.W. Membrane topology mapping of vitamin K epoxide reductase by *in vitro* translation/cotranslocation. *J. Biol. Chem.* **2005**, *280*, 16410–16416. [CrossRef] [PubMed]
26. Tie, J.K.; Jin, D.Y.; Stafford, D.W. Human vitamin K epoxide reductase and its bacterial homologue have different membrane topologies and reaction mechanisms. *J. Biol. Chem.* **2012**, *287*, 33945–33955. [CrossRef] [PubMed]
27. Schulman, S.; Wang, B.; Li, W.; Rapoport, T.A. Vitamin K epoxide reductase prefers ER membrane-anchored thioredoxin-like redox partners. *Proc. Natl. Acad. Sci. USA* **2010**, *107*, 15027–15032. [CrossRef] [PubMed]
28. Robertson, H.M. Genes encoding vitamin-K epoxide reductase are present in Drosophila and trypanosomatid protists. *Genetics* **2004**, *168*, 1077–1080. [CrossRef] [PubMed]
29. Oldenburg, J.; Müller, C.R.; Rost, S.; Watzka, M.; Bevans, C.G. Comparative genetics of warfarin resistance. *Hamostaseologie* **2014**, *34*, 143–159. [CrossRef] [PubMed]
30. Rost, S.; Fregin, A.; Hünerberg, M.; Bevans, C.G.; Müller, C.R.; Oldenburg, J. Site-directed mutagenesis of coumarin-type anticoagulant-sensitive VKORC1: Evidence that highly conserved amino acids define structural requirements for enzymatic activity and inhibition by warfarin. *Thromb. Haemost.* **2005**, *94*, 780–786. [PubMed]
31. Du, J.J.; Zhan, C.Y.; Lu, Y.; Cui, H.R.; Wang, X.Y. The conservative cysteines in transmembrane domain of AtVKOR/LTO1 are critical for photosynthetic growth and photosystem II activity in Arabidopsis. *Front. Plant Sci.* **2015**, *6*, 238. [CrossRef] [PubMed]
32. Yang, X.J.; Cui, H.R.; Yu, Z.B.; Du, J.J.; Xu, J.N.; Wang, X.Y. Key amino acids of arabidopsis VKOR in the activity of phylloquinone reduction and disulfide bond formation. *Pro. Pept. Lett.* **2015**, *22*, 81–86. [CrossRef]

33. Rishavy, M.A.; Usubalieva, A.; Hallgren, K.W.; Berkner, K.L. Novel insight into the mechanism of the vitamin K oxidoreductase (VKOR): Electron relay through Cys43 and Cys51 reduces VKOR to allow vitamin K reduction and facilitation of vitamin K-dependent protein carboxylation. *J. Biol. Chem.* **2011**, *286*, 7267–7278. [CrossRef] [PubMed]
34. Tie, J.K.; Jin, D.Y.; Stafford, D.W. Mycobacterium tuberculosis vitamin K epoxide reductase homologue supports vitamin K-dependent carboxylation in mammalian cells. *Antioxid. Redox. Signal.* **2012**, *16*, 329–338. [CrossRef] [PubMed]
35. Wajih, N.; Hutson, S.M.; Wallin, R. Disulfide-dependent protein folding is linked to operation of the vitamin K cycle in the endoplasmic reticulum. A protein disulfide isomerase-VKORC1 redox enzyme complex appears to be responsible for vitamin K1 2,3-epoxide reduction. *J. Biol. Chem.* **2007**, *282*, 2626–2635. [CrossRef] [PubMed]
36. Tie, J.K.; Jin, D.Y.; Tie, K.; Stafford, D.W. Evaluation of warfarin resistance using transcription activator-like effector nucleases-mediated vitamin K epoxide reductase knockout HEK293 cells. *J. Thromb. Haemost.* **2013**, *11*, 1556–1564. [CrossRef] [PubMed]
37. Wu, S.; Tie, J.K.; Stafford, D.W.; Pedersen, L.G. Membrane topology for human vitamin K epoxide reductase. *J. Thromb. Haemost.* **2014**, *12*, 112–114. [CrossRef] [PubMed]
38. Fasco, M.J.; Principe, L.M.; Walsh, W.A.; Friedman, P.A. Warfarin inhibition of vitamin K 2,3-epoxide reductase in rat liver microsomes. *Biochemistry* **1983**, *22*, 5655–5660. [CrossRef] [PubMed]
39. Fregin, A.; Czogalla, K.J.; Gansler, J.; Rost, S.; Taverna, M.; Watzka, M.; Bevans, C.G.; Müller, C.R.; Oldenburg, J. A new cell culture-based assay quantifies vitamin K 2,3-epoxide reductase complex subunit 1 function and reveals warfarin resistance phenotypes not shown by the dithiothreitol-driven VKOR assay. *J. Thromb. Haemost.* **2013**, *11*, 872–880. [CrossRef] [PubMed]
40. Müller, E.; Keller, A.; Fregin, A.; Müller, C.R.; Rost, S. Confirmation of warfarin resistance of naturally occurring VKORC1 variants by coexpression with coagulation factor IX and in silico protein modelling. *BMC Genet.* **2014**, *15*, 17. [CrossRef] [PubMed]
41. Van Horn, W.D. VKORC1 ER mislocalization causes rare disease. *Blood* **2014**, *124*, 1215–1216. [CrossRef] [PubMed]
42. Michelsen, K.; Yuan, H.; Schwappach, B. Hide and run. Arginine-based endoplasmic-reticulum-sorting motifs in the assembly of heteromultimeric membrane proteins. *EMBO Rep.* **2005**, *6*, 717–722. [CrossRef] [PubMed]
43. Shikano, S.; Li, M. Membrane receptor trafficking: Evidence of proximal and distal zones conferred by two independent endoplasmic reticulum localization signals. *Proc. Natl. Acad. Sci. USA* **2003**, *100*, 5783–5788. [CrossRef] [PubMed]

11

Vitamin E as an Antioxidant in Female Reproductive Health

Siti Syairah Mohd Mutalip [1,*], Sharaniza Ab-Rahim [2] and Mohd Hamim Rajikin [2]

1 Faculty of Pharmacy, Universiti Teknologi MARA (UiTM) Puncak Alam Campus, Selangor 42300, Malaysia
2 Faculty of Medicine, Universiti Teknologi MARA (UiTM) Sg. Buloh Campus, Selangor 42300, Malaysia; sharaniza_abrahim@salam.uitm.edu.my (S.A.-R.); hamim400@salam.uitm.edu.my (M.H.R.)
* Correspondence: syairah@puncakalam.uitm.edu.my

Abstract: Vitamin E was first discovered in 1922 as a substance necessary for reproduction. Following this discovery, vitamin E was extensively studied, and it has become widely known as a powerful lipid-soluble antioxidant. There has been increasing interest in the role of vitamin E as an antioxidant, as it has been discovered to lower body cholesterol levels and act as an anticancer agent. Numerous studies have reported that vitamin E exhibits anti-proliferative, anti-survival, pro-apoptotic, and anti-angiogenic effects in cancer, as well as anti-inflammatory activities. There are various reports on the benefits of vitamin E on health in general. However, despite it being initially discovered as a vitamin necessary for reproduction, to date, studies relating to its effects in this area are lacking. Hence, this paper was written with the intention of providing a review of the known roles of vitamin E as an antioxidant in female reproductive health.

Keywords: vitamin E; reproduction; antioxidant; tocopherol; tocotrienol

---

1. Vitamin E

Vitamin E was first discovered by Evans and Bishop in 1922, and it was initially denoted as an "anti-sterility factor X" that was necessary for reproduction [1]. Since then, vitamin E has been well characterized as a powerful lipid-soluble antioxidant through extensive research. The antioxidant activities of vitamin E were reported following findings on its ability to scavenge reactive oxygen species (ROS) in cellular membranes [2–4].

1.1. Sources of Vitamin E

Vitamin E, which consists of a mixture of tocopherols (TOCs) and tocotrienols (TCTs), is available in a number of foods and plants, ranging from edible oils to nuts. Some vitamin E-containing foods include wheat, rice bran, barley, oat, coconut, palm and annatto [5,6]. Other sources include rye, amaranth, walnut, hazelnut, poppy, safflower, maize and the seeds of grape and pumpkins. Vitamin E derivatives have also been detected in human milk [7] and palm dates (*Phoenix canariensis*) [8]. Among the many sources of vitamin E, rice bran, palm oil and annatto oil have been described as the richest sources of TCTs [9].

1.2. Structure of Vitamin E

Vitamin E consists of a mixture of tocopherols (TOCs) and tocotrienols (TCTs) that are synthesized by plants from homogenestic acid [10]. These substances are present in eight different homologues; namely, α-tocopherol, β-tocopherol, γ-tocopherol, δ-tocopherol, α-tocotrienol, β-tocotrienol, γ-tocotrienol and δ-tocotrienol [11]. The four TOC homologues (α-, β-, γ-, δ-TOC) have a fully saturated 16-carbon isoprenoid sidechain, while TCT homologues have a similar isoprenoid chain, containing three double bonds (an unsaturated side chain). The TOC homologues are named with respect to the position and number of the methyl groups on the phenol ring. The α-, β-, γ- and δ-homologues contain three, two, two and one methyl groups, respectively (Figure 1). These structural differences and the isomerism determine the biological activity, with α-homologues being the most biologically active [12]. However, it has been reported that light, temperature, and oxygen availability could promote rancidity in vegetable oils [13]. According to a study [13], soybean oil that was stored in the dark for 56 days had increased peroxide value. In addition, its exposure to light in a 12 h light/darkness cycle over for 56 days resulted in an increase in peroxide values of around 1473%.

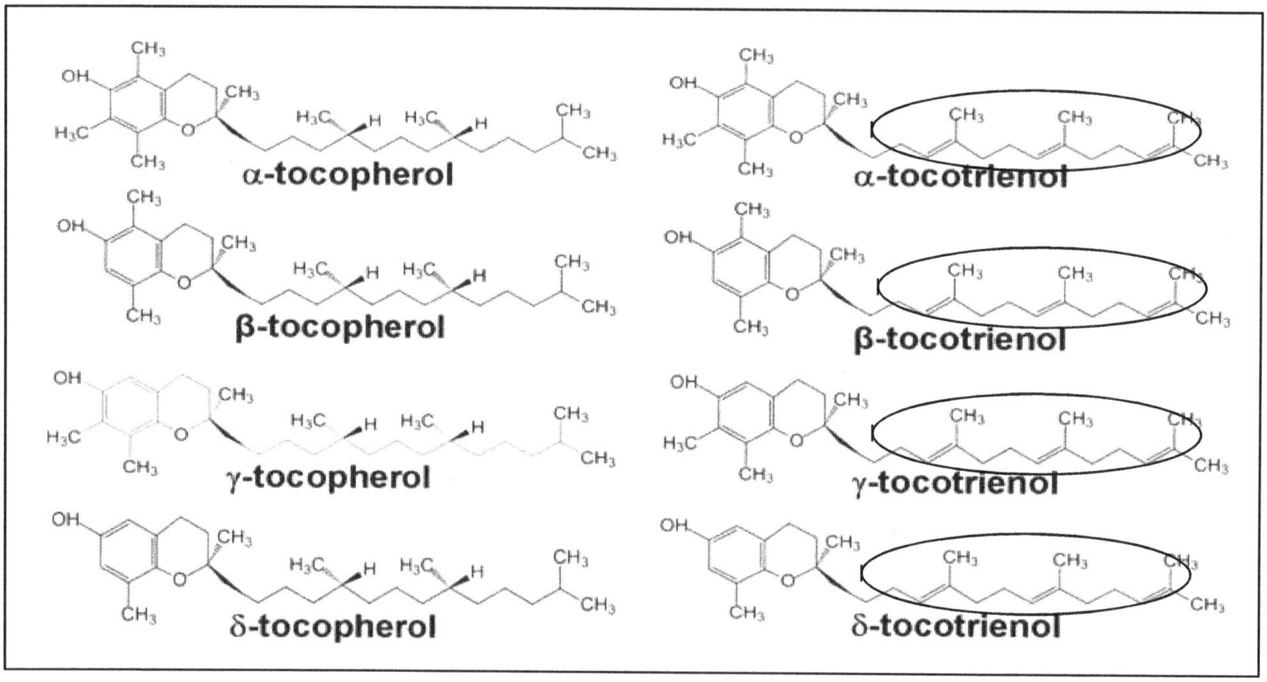

Figure 1. Structure differences between tocopherols (TOCs) and tocotrienols (TCTs). TOCs have saturated side chains, while TCTs have unsaturated side chains. The latter are shown by the presence of three double bonds in TCTs (circled) [14].

2. Reproductive Disorders: The Risk Factors

A number of risk factors contributing to reproductive- and pregnancy-related disorders have been previously reported [15–17]. These factors are generally categorized into two major groups: environmental and lifestyle factors. Examples of major environmental pollutants include hazardous man-made chemicals, industrial discharge, agricultural run-off, human and animal waste, municipal and domestic effluents, and spillage of vessels and oil spills [17]. Exposure to these pollutants during the time of periconceptional period (periconceptional period refers to the time of preconception, conception, implantation, placentation and embryogenesis (or organogenesis) stages of pregnancy) were reported to have adverse effects on the development of conceptus and the neonatal health [15]. These include the risks of embryonic mortality and fetal loss, intrauterine growth restriction (IUGR), birth defects, childhood diseases, premature sexual maturation and a few types of adult cancers [15]. Additionally, Rider et al. [16] also reported that exposure of conceptus to multiple environmental pollutants *in utero* during pregnancy could affect embryonic implantation and the developmental course in a cumulative dose-additive manner.

Exposure to multicomponent mixtures of endocrine-disturbing chemicals may act as hormone mimics or antagonists, leading to the disruption of estrogen, androgen and other hormonal pathways [18]. Furthermore, exposure to multiple environmental pollutants may also result in reactive oxygen species (ROS)-induced oxidative stress (OS) [19–21]. The presence of high levels of OS may be a risk factor for a number of pregnancy-related disorders, such as embryonic mortality, early spontaneous abortion, IUGR, fetal death, premature delivery and low birth weight [22,23].

Lifestyle factors represent another category of major risk factors for reproductive and pregnancy-related disorders. Unhealthy lifestyle behaviors, including cigarette smoking, alcohol consumption, and/or drug abuse, have negative impacts, particularly on female fertility [24,25]. The underlying mechanism of the developmental defects following these unhealthy lifestyle behaviors is mainly a result of an increase in ROS production and associated OS-induced cellular damage [26]. There are also extensive epidemiological studies which have reported on a number of factors such as exposure to tobacco and alcohol, diet, stress, and gestational diabetes as the factors influencing fetal development including miscarriages [27–29].

Much evidence-based epidemiological, clinical, and experimental data on the adverse effects of cigarette smoking on female reproductive health has been reported [30]. The effects of smoking on steroidogenesis, folliculogenesis embryo transport, endometrial receptivity, endometrial angiogenesis, uterine blood flow, and uterine myometrium, all of which are related to delayed or failed implantation and pregnancy loss, have been reported. This is in line with an animal study on the effects of alcohol on reproductive health and pregnancy that indicated that prenatal exposure to ethanol in rats induced hypothalamic OS and neuroendocrine alterations in offspring [31]. Furthermore, excess ethanol administration to pregnant mice [32] and rats [33] caused disturbances in embryogenesis and increased the rate of malformations and fetal death by inducing high levels of OS. Medication use or drug abuse during pregnancy has also been associated with OS [34,35]. Phenytoin [36], thalidomide [37], valproic acid [38], almokalant, dofetilide, cisapride and astemizole [39] are the examples of identified medical drugs known to induce OS and affect the embryonic development leading to birth defects.

To explain further, maternal smoking during pregnancy has been widely recognized as one of the most common factors of reproductive- and pregnancy-related disorders. Cigarette smoke contains a complex mixture of numerous toxic constituents including nicotine, polycyclic aromatic hydrocarbons, and cadmium [30,40]. The different constituents of the mixture cause an increased level of OS and adversely affect the cell proliferation and differentiation during embryonic development in pregnant female smokers [41]. This is supported by studies on the effects of maternal smoking during pregnancy, showing that cigarette smoking is associated with spontaneous abortion [42], placenta previa and placental abruption [43–45], low birth weight and preterm birth [46–48], stillbirth [49,50] and sudden infant death syndrome (SIDS) [51].

One of the most important cigarette smoke constituents, nicotine, has been reported to reduce fertility during adulthood in women [52]. In addition, cotinine (a metabolite of nicotine), cadmium, and benzo[a]pyrene have also been detected in the follicular fluid of smoking women [53–55], suggesting that the chemicals present in cigarette smoke can accumulate in the ovary. The results of these studies suggested that smoking women might develop impaired fertility, resulting from the combination of deteriorated oocyte function and viability [53,56,57].

In addition, laboratories studies have indicated that maternal exposure to cigarette smoke or cigarette smoke condensate (CSC) for 4 weeks results in the increased oocyte fragmentation or delayed fertilization, thus reducing the embryonic development to blastocysts in vitro [58]. Additionally, fragmented oocytes also showed increased production of ROS. Another study on the effects of nicotine on early embryogenesis in murine embryos reported that embryos treated with 3–6 μM of nicotine were smaller than control embryos [59]. Meanwhile, embryos treated with 6 μM of nicotine showed severe defects in the posterior trunk, resembling caudal dysplasia [59]. In addition, excessive apoptosis was also observed in the deformed structures and this was associated with the increased levels of ROS [59]. Nicotine exposure during fetal and neonatal development was also reported to cause reduction in fertility, dysregulation in ovarian steroidogenesis, and alterations in follicle dynamics in female offspring [60]. This has been further supported by another study which reported that treatment with 5 mg/mL nicotine beginning from day 1 of pregnancy throughout gestation decreased the pregnancy rates by 33.3% in Sprague-Dawley rats [61]. Another study by Rajikin et al. [62] reported that the ultrastructure of oocytes from nicotine-exposed mice showed a non-spherical shape with rough surface and torn *zona pellucida*. In addition, treatment with 5 mg/kg nicotine for 30 days increased the apoptosis rate in oocytes [63]. Meanwhile, productions of hatched blastocysts were decreased following injection with 1 mg/kg and 3 mg/kg of nicotine, and embryonic development ceased at the morula stage following exposure to 5 mg/kg of nicotine [64]. This was in line with the work of Phoebe et al. [65], which showed that after 12 weeks of cigarette smoking (directly to the lungs) in mice, the retrieved oocytes had a significantly thicker *zona pellucida*, and also shorter and wider meiotic spindles.

Oxidative Stress (OS) as One of the Risk Factors in Reproductive Disorders

Oxidative stress (OS) is widely recognized as the key element in the pathogenesis of most of the diseases [66], and occurs when there is an imbalance in the presence of antioxidants and pro-oxidants [20,22,67]. Excess pro-oxidants induce OS by either generating reactive oxygen species (ROS) or by inhibiting antioxidant systems [68]. ROS are highly reactive and unstable. They acquire electrons from nucleic acids, lipids, proteins, carbohydrates, or any other nearby molecule causing a string of chain reactions to become stable. These chain reactions result in cellular damage and diseases [69].

In the female reproductive system, ROS can impair cellular functions and subsequently interrupt intracellular homeostasis and furthermore lead to cell damages. The presence of excess ROS can influence early embryonic development through modification of the key transcription factors that modify gene expressions [70]. High concentrations of ROS in the female reproductive tract could also negatively affect the fertilization of oocytes and cause inhibition of embryonic implantation [71,72]. Additionally, earlier studies reported that OS is involved in defective and retarded embryonic development due to OS-induced cell-membrane damage, DNA damage, and apoptosis [73,74]. Apoptosis results in the formation of fragmented embryos which have limited chances of implantation and growth [75].

Previous studies on the effect of OS during the periconceptional period have shown that the placenta could be the key source of OS because of the high metabolic rate and increase in the mitochondrial activities [76,77]. During the first trimester, placental tissues contain low concentrations and activities of principle antioxidant enzymes including catalase, glutathione peroxidase, and superoxide dismutase. This condition may expose the embryonic trophoblast cells to oxygen-mediated damage [78]. An earlier study reported that due to the increase in the oxygen tension during the onset of maternal arterial flow during the beginning of second trimester, a burst of OS was observed in the placenta [79]. The study suggested that this oxidative injury could adversely impair placental remodeling and functions that would subsequently affect the course of gestation [79]. This was further supported by Jauniaux et al. [80], who found that high production of ROS and reduced antioxidant defense capability might cause the developing fetus to be exposed to increased OS.

According to other reports, macromolecule damage mediated by OS has been suggested as a mechanism of thalidomide-induced embryopathy and other embryopathies [81,82]. This suggestion was supported by an experimental finding on untreated pregnant mutant mice with a hereditary glucose-6-phosphate dehydrogenase (G6PD) deficiency that resulted in decreased litter size at birth and increased pre- and post-natal (pre-weaning) death. G6PD is a cytoprotective enzyme for OS. This result indicated that a physiological level of endogenous OS due to a dysfunctional G6PD enzyme during development can cause embryopathy that might lead to both infertility and death [83].

Oxidative stress in the female reproductive system is generally reported in most reproductive- and pregnancy-related disorders. For instance, OS has been associated with endometriosis. Although there is no established information on the involvement of OS in endometriosis, a number of studies have reported on the increased level of OS markers in patients with endometriosis [84–90]. Additionally, OS also has been reported to be involved in cases of spontaneous abortion and idiopathic recurrent pregnancy loss [66,78,80,91], unexplained infertility [92–94], preeclampsia [95–97], intrauterine growth restriction (IUGR) [98,99] and preterm labor [100–103].

3. Antioxidants and Their Roles in Reproductive Disorders

Antioxidants regulate the overproduction of ROS. They are present in two types, enzymatic and non-enzymatic forms. Enzymatic antioxidants, including superoxide dismutase (SOD), catalase, glutathione (GSH) peroxidase and glutathione (GSH) reductase are also known as natural antioxidants or endogenous antioxidants [66,104]. The non-enzymatic antioxidants, also known as exogenous antioxidants, are obtained from dietary fruits and vegetables. These include taurine, hypotaurine, β-carotene, selenium, zinc, vitamin C and vitamin E [66].

The roles of antioxidants during the periconceptional period have been previously reported [105,106]. Endogenous antioxidants play important roles within the placenta as well as in the protection of trophoblast cells from OS [106]. It has been reported that SOD has a primary role in cellular protection, metabolizing two molecules of superoxide (O_2^-) to produce hydrogen peroxide (H_2O_2) and molecular oxygen (O_2). Meanwhile, catalase (predominantly located in the peroxisomes) catalyzes the conversion of H_2O_2 to O_2 and water (H_2O). GSH peroxidase and GSH reductase are involved in oxidizing glutathione peroxides by removing H_2O_2 and lipid hydroperoxides [106].

Another antioxidant system that is highly available in the placental cells is the thioredoxin system [105]. This system consists of three antioxidant enzymes; namely, thioredoxin peroxidase, thioredoxin, and thioredoxin reductase. Thioredoxin peroxidase catalyzes the conversion of H_2O_2 and alkyl hydroperoxides to H_2O and corresponding alcohols. This reaction results in the oxidation of thioredoxin peroxidases to an inactive state requiring reduction by thioredoxin [105]. Thioredoxins have been reported to be involved in a number of cellular functions, including cell growth [107], reduction of thioredoxin peroxidase [105], inhibition of apoptosis through the binding of apoptosis signal-regulating kinase-1 (ASK-1) [108], and the supply of electrons for the synthesis of deoxyribonucleotides by ribonucleotide reductase [109].

Exogenous antioxidants, in line with their endogenous counterparts, also play a prime role in cellular defense against OS. The effects of maternal taurine deficiency, including growth retardation of the offspring, impaired perinatal development of the central nervous and pancreatic endocrine systems, impaired glucose tolerance, and vascular dysfunction, were reported by Aerts and Van [110]. Another exogenous antioxidant, zinc (Zn) is used in assisting the fetal brain development and also as an aid to the mothers in labor [111]. According to one study, an early and progressive decline in serum Zn occurs during pregnancy, and therefore the capacity for metabolic adaptation of pregnant mothers may be limited if the maternal Zn status is poor [112]. This is supported by a meta-analysis study on zinc-supplementation in women, which resulted in 14% of reduction in premature delivery [113].

Vitamin C acts as a reducing agent to protect cells against the adverse effects of OS [114]. Zhang et al. [115] reported that pregnant women who consumed vitamin C at levels lower than the recommended daily allowance (85 mg) had a 2-fold higher risk of developing preeclampsia, suggesting the importance of vitamin C supplementation in pregnant women. One randomized controlled clinical trial on patients with luteal phase defects reported that pregnancy rates were higher in the group supplemented with vitamin C (750 mg/day) than in the control group (no treatment) [116]. Another double-blinded, placebo-controlled pilot study on the effect of supplementation containing vitamin E, iron, zinc, selenium and L-arginine resulted in an increase in ovulation and pregnancy rates [117].

Maternal (preeclampsia, abortion, and hypertension) and neonatal outcomes following antioxidant supplementation for 8 to 12 weeks in pregnancy for women with low antioxidant status were reported by Rumiris et al. [118]. This study was a randomized, double-blind, placebo-controlled trial of daily antioxidant supplementation. The supplementation included vitamins A (1000 international unit (IU)), B6 (2.2 mg), B12 (2.2 μg), C (200 mg), and E (400 IU), folic acid (400 μg), N-acetylcysteine (200 mg), Cu (2 mg), Zn (15 mg), Mn (0.5 mg), Fe (30 mg), Ca (800 mg), and selenium

(100 μg). Meanwhile, the control subjects were given ferum (30 mg) and folic acid (400 μg). Results from this study indicated that antioxidant supplementation was associated with better maternal and perinatal outcomes in pregnant women with low antioxidant status as compared to control supplementation with iron and folate alone [118].

In addition, vitamin E functioning as a chain-breaking antioxidant was reported to protect cellular membranes against ROS, for example through defending polyunsaturated fatty acids (PUFAs) from auto-oxidation [119]. Antioxidants such as vitamin C and vitamin E have been reported to be efficient, and their uses in reproductive- and pregnancy-related disorders have been the subject of significant clinical trials [120]. For instance, a randomized clinical trial was conducted from January 2007 to February 2008 at the Women's Hospital of Tabriz University of Medical Sciences, Iran. This study was conducted in response to the inadequate available evidence about the role of supplementary vitamin E in normal pregnancy, and assessed the potential benefit of vitamin E supplementation on health in pregnancy [121]. This trial involved 104 pregnant women who were treated with vitamin E supplementation, and 168 women (control) who were not treated with the supplementation. Treated women were administered 400 IU vitamin E from week 14 to the end of the pregnancy. The study result indicated a non-significant relationship between supplementation and maternal and perinatal outcomes and birth weight, in which preeclampsia was reported to occur in 1% of treated women as compared to 1.78% of women in the control group. From these results, the authors concluded that the administration of supplementary vitamin E starting from the second trimester of pregnancy did not show any risks with respect to pregnancy outcomes and the occurrence of preeclampsia [121].

This is also supported by earlier studies on the possible beneficial effects of supplementary vitamin E during pregnancy, which investigated the changes in vitamin E levels in normal versus problematic pregnancies. Oxidative stability of vitamin E levels was shown to increase in maternal blood during normal pregnancies [122]. Moreover, it has also been shown that vitamin E requirements may increase in some circumstances, such as in smoking during pregnancy [123]. In a comparative study between abnormal and normal pregnancies, the mean levels of vitamin E were reported to increase from 12.9 μg/mL in early pregnancy to 22.5 μg/mL at term in normal pregnancies. However, vitamin E levels were lower than in normal pregnancies at the corresponding gestational age in abnormal pregnancies [124]. Another study by Tamura et al. [125] on 289 pregnant women in Birmingham, United Kingdom reported that there were no significant associations between vitamin E serum concentrations and pregnancy outcomes. All of these reports suggest that vitamin E is essential for normal and healthy pregnancy, and supplementation of vitamin E does not cause any detrimental effects on pregnancy outcomes.

Another recent study was conducted on the effects of vitamin E on the treatment outcomes of women with unexplained infertility who were undergoing controlled ovarian stimulation and intrauterine insemination (IUI) [126]. The study was conducted between June 2011 and December 2011 in Zekai Tahir Burak Women's Training and Research Hospital, Reproductive Endocrinology and Infertility Department, Ankara, Turkey. The study groups were divided into Group A (n = 53) and Group B (n = 50). Group A underwent controlled ovarian stimulation with clomiphene citrate with vitamin E administration at 400 IU/day, while Group B (control) underwent ovulation induction without the vitamin E administration. The results of the study showed that the difference in the endometrial thickness on the day of human chorionic gonadotropin (hCG) administration was significant between the two groups; however, there was no significant association observed between vitamin E administration and implantation and pregnancy rates. Based on these results, it was concluded that vitamin E administration could improve endometrial response in women with unexplained infertility through the antioxidant and anticoagulant effects. Vitamin E may also modulate the anti-estrogenic effect of clomiphene citrate. Moreover, the issue of thin endometrium in patients may also be improved by vitamin E [126].

As discussed above, vitamin E has been proven to be beneficial in pregnancy and neonatal health. This is in line with previous studies that reported, for instance, plasma α-tocopherol concentrations that is below than 12 mmol/L are associated with increased infection, anemia, growth retardation and poor pregnancy outcomes in both mothers and infants (reviewed in [127]). These problems occur mainly because when low dietary amounts of α-tocopherol are consumed, the requirements for tissue α-tocopherol will exceed the available amounts, resulting in increased damages of the tissues [127].

Vitamin E as an Antioxidant in Female Reproduction: The Reported Studies

Following the first publication by Evans and Bishop [1], a later report discussed the role of vitamin E in reproduction after observations in which a vitamin-E deficient diet resulted in uterine discolorations in rats [128]. Decades later, research on the role of vitamin E in reproductive physiology was re-initiated, and it was reported to have beneficial effects against stress-induced oxidative stress (OS) [129–133].

In another study, a population of women suffering habitual abortion was observed to have high levels of lipid peroxidation and decreased levels of plasma vitamin E [129]. Another study conducted in Egypt also reported that vitamin E to be a key missing micronutrient in children with stunted growth [130]. The study showed that 78.2% of children with stunted growth had vitamin E deficiency, where plasma α-TOC concentrations were recorded at 7.7 μmol/L as compared to 14.1 μmol/L in control (normal) children. In addition, a recent report by [131] also indicated that vitamin A, E, and D deficiencies were very common in very-low-birthweight Tunisian neonates and were associated with preeclampsia.

In more detailed experiments using in vivo laboratory animal models supplemented with palm-tocotrienol rich fractions (TRF), Mokhtar et al. [61] reported that co-administration with 5 mg/kg body weight (bw) of nicotine and 60 mg/kg of tocotrienol-rich fraction (TRF) increased the rates of pregnancy to 83.3% in rats, compared to those treated with nicotine alone, who had pregnancy rates of 33.3%. About 25.7% of the embryos developed into 2- and 4-cell stage in rats treated with both nicotine and TRF [61]. In addition, there was also a report stating that supplementation with γ-TCT in nicotine-induced mice reduced the detrimental effects of nicotine on the ultrastructure of the oocytes [62]. Another study conducted using concurrent treatment with corticosterone (CORT) and TCT reported that the numbers of abnormal embryos were reduced following supplementation with 90 mg/kg and 120 mg/kg of TCT [134]. Meanwhile, co-administration with γ-TCT improved the embryonic development in nicotine-induced mice [64]. Moreover, as reported in more recent findings, using co-incubation in media supplemented with γ-TCT and hydrogen peroxide (H_2O_2), γ-TCT improved the development of porcine embryos through modulation of the apoptotic BCL-XL and BAX genes [135]. The beneficial effects of TCTs were also supported by the reports on the concomitant supplementation of TRF with the anti-cancer prodrug, cyclophosphamide (CPA) on ovarian cells, which was reported to provide protection against OS-induced apoptosis in the ovaries [132,133].

An earlier study using supplementation with annatto-TCTs in pregnant Wistar rats reported that no adverse effects, no increase in embryo lethality and no reduction in fetal body weight were observed [136]. These findings were in line with our recent findings, together with our observations on the anti-survival effects of annatto-delta tocotrienol and soy alpha-tocopherol on the preimplantation embryos of nicotine-treated female mice [137–140]. Furthermore, a recent study also reported that annatto-TCTs suppressed cell growth in human prostate cancer cells through inhibition of the *Src* and *Stat3* genes [141].

In addition to the studies in human and laboratory animals, the benefits of vitamin E have also been studied in domestic animals. An earlier study using the culture of bovine embryos (embryos were derived from the in vitro matured-and-fertilized oocytes) with vitamin E, vitamin C, and ethylenediaminetetraacetic acid (EDTA) showed that more zygotes were developed to the expanded blastocyst stage in culture medium containing 100 μM of vitamin E compared to the control medium. The development to the early, expanded, and hatched blastocyst stages were also lower in the culture medium supplemented with both vitamin E and C, compared to the medium supplemented with vitamin E alone [142]. Moreover, the in vitro-produced embryos were cultured for 5.5 days in medium with or without 100 μM of vitamin E and were non-surgically transferred to recipient cows. After 7 days of transfer, the embryos were non-surgically collected, and the results indicated that embryos cultured with vitamin E were approximately 63% larger in surface area than in the control embryos [142]. Another study by [143] also reported on the effects of antioxidants such as beta-mercaptoethanol (beta-ME) and vitamin E where both suppressed oxidative damage and improved the developmental ability in the porcine embryos.

The beneficial effects of vitamin E were also studied in buffalos. A study was conducted to find whether the supplementation of vitamin E in the culture medium could ameliorate the developmental competence of preimplantation buffalo embryos. The study results indicated that under the culture condition of 20% of O_2 level, the frequency of blastocyst formation and the total cell count were enhanced, and the formation of comet tail (DNA fragmentation) was significantly reduced following supplementation with 100 μM of vitamin E [144]. Another similar study was also conducted in sheep with the aim of determining the effects of α-TOC supplementation of the oocyte maturation media and embryo culture media on the yield of the embryos. Findings from the study showed that supplementation with 200 μM of α-TOC in the embryo culture medium at 20% of O_2 level significantly increased the rates of cleavage, formation of morula and blastocysts, and the total cell number of blastocysts, as compared to the control groups [145].

4. Conclusions

Vitamin E has received much attention in recent years due to its ability to improve reproductive health. As discussed in the present paper, vitamin E has been reported to exert beneficial effects as an antioxidant against the reproductive disorders. Hence, it is highly recommended for women to consume vitamin E regularly, especially those who are in their reproductive age. However, available study reports on the effects of vitamin E on reproduction, pregnancy, and preimplantation embryonic development are still lacking. Many future studies are necessary in order to gain a greater understanding of the antioxidative role of vitamin E, especially with respect to female reproductive health.

Acknowledgments: We are deeply grateful to the **Ministry of Higher Education (MOHE)** Malaysia for providing the financial support through the Fundamental Research Grant Scheme (FRGS) (600-IRMI/FRGS 5/3 (037/2017). Thanks are given to all staff and members of the Faculty of Pharmacy, UiTM Selangor, Puncak Alam Campus, and the Faculty of Medicine, UiTM Selangor, Sg. Buloh Campus, Malaysia for all the assistance and support given in the completion of this paper.

Author Contributions: All authors contributed equally to the completion of this paper. Siti Syairah Mohd Mutalip conceived the idea, collected sources of information, and initiated and contributed to manuscript writing. Mohd Hamim Rajikin and Sharaniza Ab-Rahim contributed to manuscript analysis and review; as well as contributed to the manuscript writing.

References

1. Evans, H.M.; Bishop, K.S. On the existence of a hitherto unrecognized dietary factor essential for reproduction. *Science* **1922**, *56*, 650–651. [CrossRef] [PubMed]
2. Tappel, A.L. Vitamin E as the biological lipid antioxidant. *Vitam. Horm.* **1962**, *20*, 493–510.
3. Burton, G.W.; Ingold, K.U. Vitamin E application of the principles of physical organic chemistry to the exploration of its structure and function. *Acc. Chem. Res.* **1986**, *19*, 194–201. [CrossRef]
4. Esterbauer, H.; Dieber-Rotheneder, M.; Striegl, G.; Waeg, G. Role of vitamin E in preventing the oxidation of low density lipoprotein. *Am. J. Clin. Nutr.* **1991**, *53*, 314S–321S. [CrossRef] [PubMed]
5. Sheppard, A.J.; Pennington, J.A.T.; Weihrauch, J.L. Analysis and distribution of vitamin E in vegetable oils and foods. In *Vitamin E in Health and Disease*; Packer, L., Fuchs, J., Eds.; Marcel Dekker: New York, NY, USA, 1993; pp. 9–31, ISBN 0-8247-8692-0.
6. Ramaswamy, K.; Subash, C.G.; Ji, H.K.; Bharat, B.A. Tocotrienols fight cancer by targeting multiple cell signaling pathways. *Genes Nutr.* **2012**, *7*, 43–52. [CrossRef]

7. Kobayashi, H.; Kanno, C.; Yamauchi, K.; Tsugo, T. Identification of alpha-, beta-, gamma-, and delta-tocopherols and their contents in human milk. *Biochim. Biophys. Acta* **1975**, *380*, 282–290. [PubMed]
8. Nehdi, I.; Omri, S.; Khalil, M.I.; Al-Resayes, S.I. Characteristics and chemical composition of date palm (*Phoenix canariensis*) seeds and seed oil. *Ind. Crops Prod.* **2010**, *32*, 360–365. [CrossRef]
9. Tan, B. Vitamin E: Tocotrienols—The Science behind Tocotrienols. Available online: https://assets.kyani.net/documents/us/Tocotrienols_Science_White_Paper-1.12-EN-ALL.pdf (accessed on 14 August 2017).
10. Rimbach, G.; Jennifer, M.; Patricia, H.; John, K.L. Gene-Regulatory Activity of α-Tocopherol. *Molecules* **2010**, *15*, 1746–1761. [CrossRef] [PubMed]
11. IUPAC-IUB Joint Commission on Biochemical Nomenclature. Nomenclature of tocopherols and related compounds. (Recommendations 1981). *Eur. J. Biochem.* **1982**, *123*, 473–475.
12. Rimbach, G.; Minihane, A.M.; Majewicz, J.; Fischer, A.; Pallauf, J.; Virgli, F.; Weinberg, P.D. Regulation of cell signalling by vitamin E. *Proc. Nutr. Soc.* **2002**, *61*, 415–425. [CrossRef] [PubMed]
13. Pignitter, M.; Stolze, K.; Gartner, S.; Dumhart, B.; Stoll, C.; Steiger, G.; Kraemer, K.; Somoza, V. Cold fluorescent light as major inducer of lipid oxidation in soybean oil stored at household conditions for eight weeks. *J. Agric. Food Chem.* **2014**, *62*, 2297–2305. [CrossRef] [PubMed]
14. The Structure of Vitamin, E. Available online: https://www.omicsonline.org/articles-images/2155-9899-4-137-g001.html (accessed on 23 January 2018).
15. Wigle, D.T.; Arbuckle, T.E.; Turner, M.C.; Bérubé, A.; Yang, Q.; Liu, S.; Krewski, D. Epidemiologic evidence of relationships between reproductive and child health outcomes and environmental chemical contaminants. *J. Toxicol. Environ. Health B Crit. Rev.* **2008**, *11*, 373–517. [CrossRef] [PubMed]
16. Rider, C.V.; Furr, J.R.; Wilson, V.S.; Gray, L.E., Jr. Cumulative effects of in utero administration of mixtures of reproductive toxicants that disrupt common target tissues via diverse mechanisms of toxicity. *J. Androl.* **2010**, *33*, 443–462. [CrossRef] [PubMed]
17. Al-Gubory, K.H. Environmental pollutants and lifestyle factors induce oxidative stress and poor prenatal development. *Reprod. Biomed. Online* **2014**, *29*, 17–31. [CrossRef] [PubMed]
18. Kortenkamp, A. Ten years of mixing cocktails: A review of combination effects of endocrine-disrupting chemicals. *Environ. Health Perspect.* **2007**, *115* (Suppl. 1), 98–105. [CrossRef] [PubMed]
19. Luo, Z.C.; Liu, J.M.; Fraser, W.D. Large prospective birth cohort studies on environmental contaminants and child health—Goals, challenges, limitations and needs. *Med. Hypotheses* **2010**, *74*, 318–324. [CrossRef] [PubMed]
20. Ruder, E.H.; Hartman, T.J.; Blumberg, J.; Goldman, M.B. Oxidative stress and antioxidants: Exposure and impact on female fertility. *Hum. Reprod. Update* **2008**, *14*, 345–357. [CrossRef] [PubMed]
21. Wells, P.G.; McCallum, G.P.; Chen, C.S.; Henderson, J.T.; Lee, C.J.; Perstin, J.; Preston, T.J.; Wiley, M.J.; Wong, A.W. Oxidative stress in developmental origins of disease: Teratogenesis, neurodevelopmental deficits, and cancer. *Toxicol. Sci.* **2009**, *108*, 4–18. [CrossRef] [PubMed]
22. Al-Gubory, K.H.; Fowler, P.A.; Garrel, C. The roles of cellular reactive oxygen species, oxidative stress and antioxidants in pregnancy outcomes. *Int. J. Biochem. Cell Biol.* **2010**, *42*, 1634–1650. [CrossRef] [PubMed]
23. Agarwal, A.; Aponte-Mellado, A.; Premkumar, B.J.; Shaman, A.; Gupta, S. The effects of oxidative stress on female reproduction: A review. *Reprod. Biol. Endocrinol.* **2012**, *10*, 49. [CrossRef] [PubMed]
24. Anderson, K.; Nisenblat, V.; Norman, R. Lifestyle factors in people seeking infertility treatment—A review. *Aust. N. Z. J. Obstet. Gynaecol.* **2010**, *50*, 8–20. [CrossRef] [PubMed]
25. Sharma, R.; Biedenharn, K.R.; Fedor, J.M.; Agarwal, A. Lifestyle factors and reproductive health: Taking control of your fertility. *Reprod. Biol. Endocrinol.* **2013**, *11*, 66. [CrossRef] [PubMed]
26. Kovacic, P.; Somanathan, R. Mechanism of teratogenesis: Electron transfer, reactive oxygen species, and antioxidants. *Birth Defects Res. C Embryo Today* **2006**, *78*, 308–325. [CrossRef] [PubMed]
27. Rasch, V. Cigarette, alcohol, and caffeine consumption: Risk factors for spontaneous abortion. *Acta Obstet. Gynecol. Scand.* **2003**, *82*, 182–188. [CrossRef] [PubMed]
28. Weng, X.; Odouli, R.; Li, D.K. Maternal caffeine consumption during pregnancy and the risk of miscarriage: A prospective cohort study. *Am. J. Obstet. Gynecol.* **2008**, *198*, 279.e1–279.e8. [CrossRef] [PubMed]
29. Barua, S.; Junaid, M.A. Lifestyle, pregnancy and epigenetic effects. *Epigenomics* **2015**, *7*, 85–102. [CrossRef] [PubMed]

30. Dechanet, C.; Anahory, T.; Mathieu Daude, J.C.; Quantin, X.; Reyftmann, L.; Hamamah, S.; Hedon, B.; Dechaud, H. Effects of cigarette smoking on reproduction. *Hum. Reprod. Update* **2011**, *17*, 76–95. [CrossRef] [PubMed]
31. Dembele, K.; Yao, X.H.; Chen, L.; Nyomba, B.L. Intrauterine ethanol exposure results in hypothalamic oxidative stress and neuroendocrine alterations in adult rat offspring. *Am. J. Physiol. Regul. Integr. Comp. Physiol.* **2006**, *291*, R796–R802. [CrossRef] [PubMed]
32. Wentzel, P.; Eriksson, U.J. Ethanol-induced fetal dysmorphogenesis in the mouse is diminished by high antioxidative capacity of the mother. *Toxicol. Sci.* **2006**, *92*, 416–422. [CrossRef] [PubMed]
33. Wentzel, P.; Rydberg, U.; Eriksson, U.J. Antioxidative treatment diminishes ethanol-induced congenital malformations in the rat. *Alcohol. Clin. Exp. Res.* **2006**, *30*, 1752–1760. [CrossRef] [PubMed]
34. Van Gelder, M.M.; van Rooij, I.A.; Miller, R.K.; Zielhuis, G.A.; de Jong-van den Berg, L.T.; Roeleveld, N. Teratogenic mechanisms of medical drugs. *Hum. Reprod. Update* **2010**, *16*, 378–394. [CrossRef] [PubMed]
35. Deavall, D.G.; Martin, E.A.; Horner, J.M.; Roberts, R. Drug-induced oxidative stress and toxicity. *J. Toxicol.* **2012**. [CrossRef] [PubMed]
36. Liu, L.; Wells, P.G. In vivo phenytoin-initiated oxidative damage to proteins and lipids in murine maternal hepatic and embryonic tissue organelles: Potential molecular targets of chemical teratogenesis. *Toxicol. Appl. Pharmacol.* **1994**, *125*, 247–255. [CrossRef] [PubMed]
37. Hansen, J.M.; Harris, C. A novel hypothesis for thalidomide-induced limb teratogenesis: Redox misregulation of the NF-kappaB pathway. *Antioxid. Redox Signal.* **2004**, *6*, 1–14. [CrossRef] [PubMed]
38. Defoort, E.N.; Kim, P.M.; Winn, L.M. Valproic acid increases conservative homologous recombination frequency and reactive oxygen species formation: A potential mechanism for valproic acid-induced neural tube defects. *Mol. Pharmacol.* **2006**, *69*, 1304–1310. [CrossRef] [PubMed]
39. Danielsson, B.R.; Danielsson, C.; Nilsson, M.F. Embryonic cardiac arrhythmia and generation of reactive oxygen species: Common teratogenic mechanism for IKr blocking drugs. *Reprod. Toxicol.* **2007**, *24*, 42–56. [CrossRef] [PubMed]
40. Borgerding, M.; Klus, H. Analysis of complex mixtures—Cigarette smoke. *Exp. Toxicol. Pathol.* **2005**, *57*, 43–73. [CrossRef] [PubMed]
41. Feltes, B.C.; de Faria Poloni, J.; Notari, D.L.; Bonatto, D. Toxicological effects of the different substances in tobacco smoke on human embryonic development by a systems chemo-biology approach. *PLoS ONE* **2013**, *8*, e61743. [CrossRef] [PubMed]
42. George, L.; Granath, F.; Johansson, A.L.; Anneren, G.; Cnattingius, S. Environmental tobacco smoke and risk of spontaneous abortion. *Epidemiology* **2006**, *17*, 500–505. [CrossRef] [PubMed]
43. Ananth, C.V.; Smulian, J.C.; Vintzileos, A.M. Incidence of placental abruption in relation to cigarette smoking and hypertensive disorders during pregnancy: A meta-analysis of observational studies. *Obstet. Gynecol.* **1999**, *93*, 622–628. [CrossRef] [PubMed]
44. Faiz, A.S.; Ananth, C.V. Etiology and risk factors for placenta previa: An overview and meta-analysis of observational studies. *J. Matern. Fetal Neonatal Med.* **2003**, *13*, 175–190. [CrossRef] [PubMed]
45. Hung, T.H.; Hsieh, C.C.; Hsu, J.J.; Chiu, T.H.; Lo, L.M.; Hsieh, T.T. Risk factors for placenta previa in an Asian population. *Int. J. Gynaecol. Obstet.* **2007**, *97*, 26–30. [CrossRef] [PubMed]
46. Kolas, T.; Nakling, J.; Salvesen, K.A. Smoking during pregnancy increases the risk of preterm births among parous women. *Acta Obstet. Gynecol. Scand.* **2000**, *79*, 644–648. [PubMed]
47. Fantuzzi, G.; Aggazzotti, G.; Righi, E.; Facchinetti, F.; Bertucci, E.; Kanitz, S.; Barbone, F.; Sansebastiano, G.; Battaglia, M.A.; Leoni, V.; et al. Preterm delivery and exposure to active and passive smoking during pregnancy: A case-control study from Italy. *Paediatr. Perinat. Epidemiol.* **2007**, *21*, 194–200. [CrossRef] [PubMed]
48. Jaddoe, V.W.; Troe, E.J.; Hofman, A.; Mackenbach, J.P.; Moll, H.A.; Steegers, E.A.; Witteman, J.C. Active and passive maternal smoking during pregnancy and the risks of low birthweight and preterm birth: The Generation R Study. *Paediatr. Perinat. Epidemiol.* **2008**, *22*, 162–171. [CrossRef] [PubMed]
49. Wisborg, K.; Kesmodel, U.; Henriksen, T.B.; Olsen, S.F.; Secher, N.J. Exposure to tobacco smoke in utero and the risk of stillbirth and death in the first year of life. *Am. J. Epidemiol.* **2001**, *154*, 322–327. [CrossRef] [PubMed]
50. Hogberg, L.; Cnattingius, S. The influence of maternal smoking habits on the risk of subsequent stillbirth: Is there a causal relation? *BJOG* **2007**, *114*, 699–704. [CrossRef] [PubMed]

51. Mitchell, E.A.; Milerad, J. Smoking and the sudden infant death syndrome. *Rev. Environ. Health* **2006**, *21*, 81–103. [CrossRef] [PubMed]
52. Sharpe, R.M.; Franks, S. Environment, lifestyle and infertility—An inter-generational issue. *Nat. Cell Biol.* **2002**, *4*, s33–s40. [CrossRef] [PubMed]
53. Zenzes, M.T.; Krishnan, S.; Krishnan, B.; Zhang, H.; Casper, R.F. Cadmium accumulation in follicular fluid of women in in vitro fertilization-embryo transfer is higher in smokers. *Fertil. Steril.* **1995**, *64*, 599–603. [CrossRef]
54. Younglai, E.V.; Foster, W.G.; Hughes, E.G.; Trim, K.; Jarrell, J.F. Levels of environmental contaminants in human follicular fluid, serum, and seminal plasma of couples undergoing in vitro fertilization. *Arch. Environ. Contam. Toxicol.* **2002**, *43*, 121–126. [CrossRef] [PubMed]
55. Neal, M.S.; Zhu, J.; Foster, W.G. Quantification of benzo[a]pyrene and other PAHs in the serum and follicular fluid of smokers versus non-smokers. *Reprod. Toxicol.* **2008**, *25*, 100–106. [CrossRef] [PubMed]
56. Van Voorhis, B.J.; Dawson, J.D.; Stovall, D.W.; Sparks, A.E.; Syrop, C.H. The effects of smoking on ovarian function and fertility during assisted reproduction cycles. *Obstet. Gynecol.* **1996**, *88*, 785–791. [CrossRef]
57. Ness, R.B.; Grisso, J.A.; Hirschinger, N.; Markovic, N.; Shaw, L.M.; Day, N.L.; Kline, J. Cocaine and tobacco use and the risk of spontaneous abortion. *N. Engl. J. Med.* **1999**, *340*, 333–339. [CrossRef] [PubMed]
58. Huang, J.; Okuka, M.; McLean, M.; Keefe, D.L.; Liu, L. Effects of cigarette smoke on fertilization and embryo development in vivo. *Fertil. Steril.* **2009**, *92*, 1456–1465. [CrossRef] [PubMed]
59. Zhao, Z.; Reece, E.A. Nicotine-induced embryonic malformations mediated by apoptosis from increasing intracellular calcium and oxidative stress. *Birth Defects Res. B Dev. Reprod. Toxicol.* **2005**, *74*, 383–391. [CrossRef] [PubMed]
60. Holloway, A.C.; Kellenberger, L.D.; Petrik, J.J. Fetal and neonatal exposure to nicotine disrupts ovarian function and fertility in adult female rats. *Endocrine* **2006**, *30*, 213–216. [CrossRef]
61. Mokhtar, N.; Rajikin, M.H.; Zakaria, Z. Role of tocotrienol-rich palm vitamin E on pregnancy and preimplantation embryos in nicotine treated rats. *Biomed. Res.* **2008**, *19*, 181–184.
62. Rajikin, M.H.; Latif, E.S.; Mar, M.R.; Mat Top, A.G.; Mokhtar, N.M. Deleterious effects of nicotine on the ultrastructure of oocytes: Role of gamma-tocotrienol. *Med. Sci. Monit.* **2009**, *15*, BR378–BR383. [PubMed]
63. Asadi, E.; Mehrdad, J.; Mohammad, J.G. Effect of vitamin E on oocytes apoptosis in nicotine-treated mice. *Iran. J. Basic Med. Sci.* **2012**, *15*, 880–884. [PubMed]
64. Kamsani, Y.S.; Rajikin, M.H.; Nor-Ashikin, M.N.K.; Nuraliza, A.S.; Chatterjee, A. Nicotine-induced cessation of embryonic development is reversed by γ-tocotrienol in mice. *Med. Sci. Monit. Basic Res.* **2013**, *19*, 87–92. [CrossRef] [PubMed]
65. Phoebe, C.J.; Julie, A.M.; Emma, L.B.; Philip, M.H.; Keith, T.J. Increased zona pellucida thickness and meiotic spindle disruption in oocytes from cigarette smoking mice. *Hum. Reprod.* **2011**, *26*, 878–884. [CrossRef]
66. Agarwal, A.; Gupta, S.; Sekhon, L.; Shah, R. Redox considerations in female reproductive function and assisted reproduction: From molecular mechanisms to health implications. *Antioxid. Redox Signal.* **2008**, *10*, 1375–1403. [CrossRef] [PubMed]
67. Ames, B.N.; Shigenaga, M.K.; Hagen, T.M. Oxidants, antioxidants, and the degenerative diseases of aging. *Proc. Natl. Acad. Sci. USA* **1993**, *90*, 7915–7922. [CrossRef] [PubMed]
68. Puglia, C.D.; Powell, S.R. Inhibition of cellular antioxidants: A possible mechanism of toxic cell injury. *Environ. Health Perspect.* **1984**, *57*, 307–311. [CrossRef] [PubMed]
69. Evans, M.D.; Dizdaroglu, M.; Cooke, M.S. Oxidative DNA damage and disease: Induction, repair and significance. *Mutat. Res.* **2004**, *567*, 1–61. [CrossRef] [PubMed]
70. Dennery, P.A. Role of redox in fetal development and neonatal diseases. *Antioxid. Redox Signal.* **2004**, *6*, 147–153. [CrossRef] [PubMed]
71. Lee, T.H.; Wu, M.Y.; Chen, M.J.; Chao, K.H.; Ho, H.N.; Yang, Y.S. Nitric oxide is associated with poor embryo quality and pregnancy outcome in in vitro fertilization cycles. *Fertil. Steril.* **2004**, *82*, 126–131. [CrossRef] [PubMed]
72. Sharma, R.K.; Agarwal, A. Role of reactive oxygen species in gynecologic diseases. *Reprod. Med. Biol.* **2004**, *3*, 177–199. [CrossRef]
73. Guerin, P.; El Mouatassim, S.; Menezo, Y. Oxidative stress and protection against reactive oxygen species in the pre-implantation embryo and its surroundings. *Hum. Reprod. Update* **2001**, *7*, 175–189. [CrossRef] [PubMed]

74. Agarwal, A.; Saleh, R.A.; Bedaiwy, M.A. Role of reactive oxygen species in the pathophysiology of human reproduction. *Fertil. Steril.* **2003**, *79*, 829–843. [CrossRef]
75. Jurisicova, A.; Varmuza, S.; Casper, R.F. Programmed cell death and human embryo fragmentation. *Mol. Hum. Reprod.* **1996**, *2*, 93–98. [CrossRef] [PubMed]
76. Walsh, S.W.; Wang, Y. Secretion of lipid peroxides by the human placenta. *Am. J. Obstet. Gynecol.* **1993**, *169*, 1462–1466. [CrossRef]
77. Myatt, L.; Cui, X. Oxidative stress in the placenta. *Histochem. Cell Biol.* **2004**, *122*, 369–382. [CrossRef] [PubMed]
78. Poston, L.; Raijmakers, M.T. Trophoblast oxidative stress, antioxidants and pregnancy outcome—A review. *Placenta* **2004**, *25* (Suppl. A), S72–S78. [CrossRef] [PubMed]
79. Wang, Y.; Walsh, S.W. Placental mitochondria as a source of oxidative stress in pre-eclampsia. *Placenta* **1998**, *19*, 581–586. [CrossRef]
80. Jauniaux, E.; Watson, A.L.; Hempstock, J.; Bao, Y.; Skepper, J.N.; Burton, G.J. Onset of maternal arterial blood flow and placental oxidative stress: A possible factor in human early pregnancy failure. *Am. J. Pathol.* **2000**, *157*, 2111–2122. [CrossRef]
81. Parman, T.; Wiley, M.J.; Wells, P.G. Free radical-mediated oxidative DNA damage in the mechanism of thalidomide teratogenicity. *Nat. Med.* **1999**, *5*, 582–585. [PubMed]
82. Burton, G.J.; Hempstock, J.; Jauniaux, E. Oxygen, early embryonic metabolism and free radical-mediated embryopathies. *Reprod. Biomed. Online* **2003**, *6*, 84–96. [CrossRef]
83. Nicol, C.J.; Zielenski, J.; Tsui, L.C.; Wells, P.G. An embryoprotective role for glucose-6-phosphate dehydrogenase in developmental oxidative stress and chemical teratogenesis. *FASEB J.* **2000**, *14*, 111–127. [CrossRef] [PubMed]
84. Murphy, A.A.; Santanam, N.; Parthasarathy, S. Endometriosis: A disease of oxidative stress? *Semin. Reprod. Endocrinol.* **1998**, *16*, 263–273. [CrossRef] [PubMed]
85. Rong, R.; Ramachandran, S.; Santanam, N.; Murphy, A.A.; Parthasarathy, S. Induction of monocyte chemotactic protein-1 in peritoneal mesothelial and endometrial cells by oxidized low-density lipoprotein and peritoneal fluid from women with endometriosis. *Fertil. Steril.* **2002**, *78*, 843–848. [CrossRef]
86. Szczepanska, M.; Kozlik, J.; Skrzypczak, J.; Mikolajczyk, M. Oxidative stress may be a piece in the endometriosis puzzle. *Fertil. Steril.* **2003**, *79*, 1288–1293. [CrossRef]
87. Bedaiwy, M.A.; Falcone, T. Peritoneal fluid environment in endometriosis. Clinicopathological implications. *Minerva Ginecol.* **2003**, *55*, 333–345. [PubMed]
88. Jackson, L.W.; Schisterman, E.F.; Dey-Rao, R.; Browne, R.; Armstrong, D. Oxidative stress and endometriosis. *Hum. Reprod.* **2005**, *20*, 2014–2020. [CrossRef] [PubMed]
89. Mier-Cabrera, M.; Jimenez-Zamudio, L.; Garcia-Latorre, E.; Cruz-Orozco, O.; Hernandez-Guerrero, C. Quantitative and qualitative peritoneal immune profiles, T-cell apoptosis and oxidative stress-associated characteristics in women with minimal and mild endometriosis. *BJOG* **2011**, *118*, 6–16. [CrossRef] [PubMed]
90. Sharma, I.; Dhaliwal, L.K.; Saha, S.C.; Sangwan, S.; Dhawan, V. Role of 8-iso-prostaglandin F 2alpha and 25-hydroxycholesterol in the pathophysiology of endometriosis. *Fertil. Steril.* **2010**, *94*, 63–70. [CrossRef] [PubMed]
91. Gupta, S.; Agarwal, A.; Banerjee, J.; Alvarez, J.G. The role of oxidative stress in spontaneous abortion and recurrent pregnancy loss: A systematic review. *Obstet. Gynecol. Surv.* **2007**, *62*, 335–347. [CrossRef] [PubMed]
92. Polak, G.; Rola, R.; Gogacz, M.; Koziol-Montewka, M.; Kotarski, J. Malonyldialdehyde and total antioxidant status in the peritoneal fluid of infertile women. *Ginekol. Pol.* **1999**, *70*, 135–140. [PubMed]
93. Polak, G.; Koziol-Montewka, M.; Tarkowski, R.; Kotarski, J. Peritoneal fluid and plasma 4-hydroxynonenal and malonyldialdehyde concentrations in infertile women. *Ginekol. Pol.* **2011**, *72*, 1316–1320.
94. Agarwal, A.; Gupta, S.; Sikka, S. The role of free radicals and antioxidants in reproduction. *Curr. Opin. Obstet. Gynecol.* **2006**, *18*, 325–332. [CrossRef] [PubMed]
95. Burton, G.J.; Jauniaux, E. Placental oxidative stress: From miscarriage to preeclampsia. *J. Soc. Gynecol. Investig.* **2004**, *11*, 342–352. [CrossRef] [PubMed]
96. Redman, C.W.; Sargent, I.L. Placental stress and pre-eclampsia: A revised view. *Placenta* **2009**, *30* (Suppl. A), S38–S42. [CrossRef] [PubMed]
97. Burton, G.J.; Yung, H.W.; Cindrova-Davies, T.; Charnock-Jones, D.S. Placental endoplasmic reticulum stress and oxidative stress in the pathophysiology of unexplained intrauterine growth restriction and early onset preeclampsia. *Placenta* **2009**, *30* (Suppl. A), S43–S48. [CrossRef] [PubMed]

98. Karowicz-Bilinska, A. Lipid peroxides concentration in women with intrauterine growth restriction. *Ginekol. Pol.* **2004**, *75*, 6–9. [PubMed]
99. Biri, A.; Bozkurt, N.; Turp, A.; Kavutcu, M.; Himmetoglu, O.; Durak, I. Role of oxidative stress in intrauterine growth restriction. *Gynecol. Obstet. Investig.* **2007**, *64*, 187–192. [CrossRef] [PubMed]
100. Hong, Y.C.; Lee, K.H.; Yi, C.H.; Ha, E.H.; Christiani, D.C. Genetic susceptibility of term pregnant women to oxidative damage. *Toxicol. Lett.* **2002**, *129*, 255–262. [CrossRef]
101. Frosali, S.; DiSimplicio, P.; Perrone, S.; DiGiuseppe, D.; Longini, M.; Tanganelli, D.; Buonocore, G. Glutathione recycling and antioxidant enzyme activities in erythrocytes of term and preterm newborns at birth. *Neonatology* **2004**, *85*, 188–194. [CrossRef] [PubMed]
102. Mustafa, M.D.; Pathak, R.; Ahmed, T.; Ahmed, R.S.; Tripathi, A.K.; Guleria, K.; Banerjee, B.D. Association of glutathione S-transferase M1 and T1 gene polymorphisms and oxidative stress markers in preterm labor. *Clin. Biochem.* **2010**, *43*, 1124–1128. [CrossRef] [PubMed]
103. Pathak, R.; Suke, S.G.; Ahmed, T.; Ahmed, R.S.; Tripathi, A.K.; Guleria, K.; Sharma, C.S.; Makhijani, S.D.; Banerjee, B.D. Organochlorine pesticide residue levels and oxidative stress in preterm delivery cases. *Hum. Exp. Toxicol.* **2010**, *29*, 351–358. [CrossRef] [PubMed]
104. Perkins, A.V. Anti-oxidants in pregnancy Endogenous anti-oxidants in pregnancy and preeclampsia. *Aust. N. Z. J. Obstet. Gynaecol.* **2006**, *46*, 77–83. [CrossRef] [PubMed]
105. Mustacich, D.; Powis, G. Thioredoxin reductase. *Biochem. J.* **2000**, *346*, 1–8. [CrossRef] [PubMed]
106. Rhee, S.G.; Chae, H.Z.; Kim, K. Peroxiredoxins: A historical overview and speculative preview of novel mechanisms and emerging concepts in cell signaling. *Free Radic. Biol. Med.* **2005**, *38*, 1543–1552. [CrossRef] [PubMed]
107. Gasdaska, J.R.; Berggren, M.; Powis, G. Cell growth stimulation by the redox protein thioredoxin occurs by a novel helper mechanism. *Cell Growth Differ.* **1995**, *6*, 1643–1650. [PubMed]
108. Saitoh, M.; Nishitoh, H.; Fujii, M.; Takeda, K.; Tobiume, K.; Sawada, Y.; Kawabata, M.; Miyazono, K.; Ichijo, H. Mammalian thioredoxin is a direct inhibitor of apoptosis signal-regulating kinase (ASK) 1. *EMBO J.* **1998**, *17*, 2596–2606. [CrossRef] [PubMed]
109. Nordberg, J.; Arner, E.S.J. Reactive oxygen species, antioxidants, and the mammalian thioredoxin system. *Free Radic. Biol. Med.* **2001**, *31*, 1287–1312. [CrossRef]
110. Aerts, L.; Van, A.F.A. Taurine and taurine-deficiency in the perinatal period. *J. Perinat. Med.* **2002**, *30*, 281–286. [CrossRef] [PubMed]
111. Uriu-Adams, J.Y.; Keen, C.L. Zinc and reproduction: Effects of zinc deficiency on prenatal and early postnatal development. *Birth Defects Res. B. Dev. Reprod. Toxicol.* **2010**, *89*, 313–325. [CrossRef] [PubMed]
112. Silvia, I.A.; Castañón, S.G.; Ruata, M.L.; Aragüés, E.F.; Terraz, P.B.; Irazabal, Y.G.; González, E.G.; Rodríguez, B.G. Updating of normal levels of copper, zinc and selenium in serum of pregnant women. *J. Trace Elem. Med. Biol.* **2007**, *21* (Suppl. 1), 49–52. [CrossRef]
113. Hess, S.Y.; King, J.C. Effects of maternal zinc supplementation on pregnancy and lactation outcomes. *Food Nutr. Bull.* **2009**, *30* (Suppl. 1), S60–S78. [CrossRef] [PubMed]
114. Levine, M.; Katz, A.; Padayatty, S.J.; Vitamin, C. *Modern Nutrition in Health and Disease*; Shils, M.E., Shike, M., Ross, A.C., Caballero, B., Cousins, R.J., Eds.; Lippincott Williams & Wilkins: Philadelphia, PA, USA, 2006; pp. 507–524.
115. Zhang, C.; Williams, M.A.; King, I.B.; Dashow, E.E.; Sorensen, T.K.; Frederick, I.O.; Thompson, M.L.; Luthy, D.A. Vitamin C and the risk of preeclampsia—Results from dietary questionnaire and plasma assay. *Epidemiology* **2002**, *13*, 409–416. [CrossRef] [PubMed]
116. Henmi, H.; Endo, T.; Kitajima, Y.; Manase, K.; Hata, H.; Kudo, R. Effects of ascorbic acid supplementation on serum progesterone levels in patients with a luteal phase defect. *Fertil. Steril.* **2003**, *80*, 459–461. [CrossRef]
117. Westphal, L.M.; Polan, M.L.; Trant, A.S.; Mooney, S.B. A nutritional supplement for improving fertility in women: A pilot study. *J. Reprod. Med.* **2004**, *49*, 289–293. [PubMed]
118. Rumiris, D.; Purwosunu, Y.; Wibowo, N.; Farina, A.; Sekizawa, A. Lower rate of preeclampsia after antioxidant supplementation in pregnant women with low antioxidant status. *Hypertens. Pregnancy* **2006**, *25*, 241–253. [CrossRef] [PubMed]
119. Traber, M.G.; Jeffrey, A. Vitamin E, antioxidant and nothing more. *Free Radic. Biol. Med.* **2007**, *43*, 4–15. [CrossRef] [PubMed]

120. Fraser, W.D.; Audibert, F.; Bujold, E.; Leduc, L.; Xu, H.; Boulvain, M.; Julien, P. The Vitamin E debate: Implications for ongoing trials of pre-eclampsia prevention. *BJOG* **2005**, *112*, 684–688. [CrossRef] [PubMed]
121. Parvin, B.; Kobra, H.; Fatemeh, A.; Nazli, N. Effects of vitamin E supplementation on some pregnancy health indices: A randomized clinical trial. *Int. J. Gen. Med.* **2011**, *4*, 461–464. [CrossRef]
122. De Vriese, S.R.; Dhont, M.; Christophe, A.B. Oxidative stability of low density lipoproteins and vitamin E levels increase in maternal blood during normal pregnancy. *Lipids* **2001**, *36*, 361–366. [CrossRef] [PubMed]
123. Chelchowska, M.; Laskowska-Klita, T.; Leibschang, J. The effect of tobacco smoking during pregnancy on concentration of vitamin E in blood of mothers and their newborns in umbilical cord blood. *Ginekol. Pol.* **2006**, *77*, 263–268. [PubMed]
124. Von Mandach, U.; Huch, R.; Huch, A. Maternal and cord serum vitamin E levels in normal and abnormal pregnancy. *Int. J. Vitam. Nutr. Res.* **1994**, *64*, 26–32. [PubMed]
125. Tamura, T.; Goldenberg, R.L.; Johnston, K.E.; Cliver, S.P.; Hoffman, H.J. Serum concentrations of zinc, folate, vitamins A and E, and proteins, and their relationships to pregnancy outcome. *Acta Obstet. Gynecol. Scand. Suppl.* **1997**, *165*, 63–70. [PubMed]
126. Cicek, N.; Eryilmaz, O.G.; Sarikaya, E.; Gulerman, C.; Genc, Y. Vitamin E effect on controlled ovarian stimulation of unexplained infertile women. *J. Assist. Reprod. Genet.* **2012**, *29*, 325–328. [CrossRef] [PubMed]
127. Traber, G.M. Vitamin E Inadequacy in Humans: Causes and Consequences. *Adv. Nutr.* **2014**, *5*, 503–514. [CrossRef] [PubMed]
128. Barrie, M.M. Vitamin E deficiency in rats: Fertility in the female. *Biochem. J.* **1938**, *32*, 2134–2137. [CrossRef] [PubMed]
129. Simsek, M.; Naziroglu, M.; Simsek, H.; Cay, M.; Aksakal, M.; Kumru, S. Blood plasma levels of lipoperoxides, glutathione peroxidase, beta carotene, vitamin A and E in women with habitual abortion. *Cell Biochem. Funct.* **1998**, *16*, 227–231. [CrossRef]
130. Ibrahim, S.A.; Abd el-Maksoud, A.; Nassar, M.F. Nutritional stunting in Egypt: Which nutrient is responsible? *East. Mediterr. Health J.* **2002**, *8*, 272–280. [PubMed]
131. Fares, S.; Sethom, M.M.; Khouaja-Mokrani, C.; Jabnoun, S.; Feki, M.; Kaabachi, N. Vitamin A, E, and D deficiencies in Tunisian very low birth weight neonates: Prevalence and risk factors. *Pediatr. Neonatol.* **2014**, *55*, 196–201. [CrossRef] [PubMed]
132. Saleh, H.; Omar, E.; Froemming, G.; Said, R. Tocotrienol rich fraction supplementation confers protection on the ovary from cyclophasphamide induced apoptosis. *Asian Pac. J. Trop. Dis.* **2014**, *4*, 234. [CrossRef]
133. Saleh, H.; Omar, E.; Froemming, G.; Said, R. Tocotrienol preserves ovarian function in cyclophosphamide therapy. *Hum. Exp. Toxicol.* **2015**, *34*, 946–952. [CrossRef] [PubMed]
134. Nasibah, A.; Rajikin, M.H.; Nor-Ashikin, M.N.K.; Nuraliza, A.S. Tocotrienol improves the quality of impaired mouse embryos induced by corticosterone. In Proceedings of the Symposium on Humanities, Science and Engineering Research (SHUSER2012), Kuala Lumpur, Malaysia, 24–27 June 2012; pp. 135–138.
135. Lee, E.; Min, S.-H.; Song, B.-S.; Yeon, J.-Y.; Kim, J.-W.; Bae, J.-H.; Park, S.-Y.; Lee, Y.-H.; Kim, S.-U.; Lee, D.-S.; et al. Exogenous γ-tocotrienol promotes preimplantation development and improves the quality of porcine embryos. *Reprod. Fertil. Dev.* **2014**. [CrossRef] [PubMed]
136. Paumgartten, F.J.R.; De-Carvalho, R.R.; Araujo, I.B.; Pinto, F.M.; Borges, O.O.; Souza, C.A.M.; Kuriyama, S.M. Evaluation of the developmental toxicity of annatto in the rat. *Food Chem. Toxicol.* **2002**, *40*, 1595–1601. [CrossRef]
137. Syairah, S.M.M.; Rajikin, M.H.; Sharaniza, A.-R.; Nor-Ashikin, M.N.K.; Anne, T.; Barrie, T. Annatto (*Bixa orellana*) derived δ-tocotrienol supplementation suppresses PIK3CA oncogene expression in 2- and 4-cell embryos of nicotine-induced mice. *Anticancer Res.* **2014**, *34*, 6064.
138. Syairah, S.M.M.; Rajikin, M.H.; Sharaniza, A.-R. Supplementation of annatto (*Bixa orellana*)-derived δ-tocotrienol produced high number of morula through increased expression of 3-phosphoinositide dependent protein kinase-1 (PDK1) in mice. *Int. J. Biol. Biomol. Agric. Food Biotechnol. Eng.* **2015**, *9*, 741–745.
139. Syairah, S.M.M.; Rajikin, M.H.; Sharaniza, A.R.; Nor-Ashikin, N.K.; Kamsani, Y.S. Chromosomal status in murine preimplantation 2-cell embryos following annatto (*Bixa orellana*)-derived pure delta-tocotrienol supplementation in normal and nicotine-treated mice. *WASJ* **2016**, *34*, 1855–1859. [CrossRef]
140. Syairah, S.M.M.; Rajikin, M.H.; Sharaniza, A.R.; Nor-Ashikin, M.N.K. Annatto (*Bixa orellana*) δ-TCT supplementation protected against embryonic DNA damages through alterations in PI3K/Akt-Cyclin D1 pathway. *Int. J. Vitam. Nutr. Res.* **2017**, accepted.

141. Sugahara, R.; Sato, A.; Uchida, A.; Shiozawa, S.; Sato, C.; Virgona, N.; Yano, T. Annatto tocotrienol induces a cytotoxic effect on human prostate cancer PC3 cells via the simultaneous inhibition of Src and Stat3. *J. Nutr. Sci. Vitaminol.* **2015**, *61*, 497–501. [CrossRef] [PubMed]
142. Olson, S.E.; Seidel, G.E., Jr. Culture of in vitro-produced bovine embryos with vitamin E improves development in vitro and after transfer to recipients. *Biol. Reprod.* **2000**, *62*, 248–252. [CrossRef] [PubMed]
143. Kitagawa, Y.; Suzuki, K.; Yoneda, A.; Watanabe, T. Effects of oxygen concentration and antioxidants on the *in vitro* developmental ability, production of reactive oxygen species (ROS), and DNA fragmentation in porcine embryos. *Theriogenology* **2004**, *62*, 1186–1197. [CrossRef] [PubMed]
144. Thiyagarajan, B.; Valivittan, K. Ameliorating effect of vitamin E on in vitro development of preimplantation buffalo embryos. *J. Assist. Reprod. Genet.* **2009**, *26*, 217–225. [CrossRef] [PubMed]
145. Natarajan, R.; Shankar, M.B.; Munuswamy, D. Effect of α-tocopherol supplementation on in vitro maturation of sheep oocytes and in vitro development of preimplantation sheep embryos to the blastocyst stage. *J. Assist. Reprod. Genet.* **2010**, *27*, 483–490. [CrossRef] [PubMed]

12

The Subcellular Distribution of Alpha-Tocopherol in the Adult Primate Brain and its Relationship with Membrane Arachidonic Acid and Its Oxidation Products

Emily S. Mohn [1,*], Matthew J. Kuchan [2], John W. Erdman Jr. [3], Martha Neuringer [4], Nirupa R. Matthan [1], Chung-Yen Oliver Chen [1] and Elizabeth J. Johnson [1]

1 Jean Mayer US Department of Agriculture Human Nutrition Research Center on Aging, Tufts University, Boston, MA 02111, USA; Nirupa.Matthan@tufts.edu (N.R.M.); Oliver.Chen@tufts.edu (C.-Y.O.C.); Elizabeth.Johnson@tufts.edu (E.J.J.)
2 Discovery Research, Abbott Nutrition, Columbus, OH 43229, USA; Matthew.Kuchan@abbott.com
3 Department of Food Science and Human Nutrition, University of Illinois at Urbana-Champaign, Urbana, IL 61802, USA; jwerdman@illinois.edu
4 Oregon National Primate Research Center, Oregon Health and Science University, Beaverton, OR 97006, USA; neuringe@ohsu.edu
* Correspondence: Emily.Mohn@tufts.edu

Abstract: The relationship between α-tocopherol, a known antioxidant, and polyunsaturated fatty acid (PUFA) oxidation, has not been directly investigated in the primate brain. This study characterized the membrane distribution of α-tocopherol in brain regions and investigated the association between membrane α-tocopherol and PUFA content, as well as brain PUFA oxidation products. Nuclear, myelin, mitochondrial, and neuronal membranes were isolated using a density gradient from the prefrontal cortex (PFC), cerebellum (CER), striatum (ST), and hippocampus (HC) of adult rhesus monkeys ($n = 9$), fed a stock diet containing vitamin E (α-, γ-tocopherol intake: ~0.7 μmol/kg body weight/day, ~5 μmol/kg body weight/day, respectively). α-tocopherol, PUFAs, and PUFA oxidation products were measured using high performance liquid chromatography (HPLC), gas chromatography (GC) and liquid chromatography-gas chromatography/mass spectrometry (LC-GC/MS) respectively. α-Tocopherol (ng/mg protein) was highest in nuclear membranes ($p < 0.05$) for all regions except HC. In PFC and ST, arachidonic acid (AA, μg/mg protein) had a similar membrane distribution to α-tocopherol. Total α-tocopherol concentrations were inversely associated with AA oxidation products (isoprostanes) ($p < 0.05$), but not docosahexaenoic acid oxidation products (neuroprostanes). This study reports novel data on α-tocopherol accumulation in primate brain regions and membranes and provides evidence that α-tocopherol and AA are similarly distributed in PFC and ST membranes, which may reflect a protective effect of α-tocopherol against AA oxidation.

Keywords: α-tocopherol; brain; membranes; arachidonic acid; isoprostanes; rhesus monkey

1. Introduction

Vitamin E is an essential, fat-soluble nutrient, obtained from nuts, oils, and green leafy vegetables [1]. Vitamin E has eight structural isomers: 4 (α-, β-, γ- and δ-)tocopherols and 4 (α-, β-, γ- and δ-)tocotrienols; however, mammals preferentially take up and use α-tocopherol [2,3]. α-Tocopherol is crucial for proper brain function, and deficiency can result in a number of neurologic symptoms, such as ataxia, peripheral neuropathy, myopathy, and retinopathy, which can be reversed with supplementation [1]. Although deficiency is rare, there is considerable evidence linking lower α-tocopherol intake levels with cognitive decline and neurodegenerative disease. Epidemiological studies have reported that lower tocopherol intake is associated with poorer cognitive function, compared to individuals with higher intakes [4], and reduced levels of α-tocopherol in plasma [5,6] and cerebrospinal fluid [7,8] have been reported in patients with mild cognitive impairment and Alzheimer's Disease (AD), the most common form of dementia. Post-mortem brain concentrations of α-tocopherol have also been shown to be positively related to cognitive test scores in a centenarian population [6].

The brain is one of the most metabolically active organs in the body, which causes the production of reactive oxygen species (ROS). As a result, it is highly susceptible to ROS attacks on lipid, protein, and DNA [9]. This susceptibility is accentuated by the high concentrations of polyunsaturated fatty acids (PUFA) found in brain cell membranes. Enhanced oxidative stress is thought to contribute to the pathogenesis of cognitive impairment and dementia [10]. α-Tocopherol's function as a lipid antioxidant may underlie its association with cognition. Therefore, it is possible that α-tocopherol maintains the integrity of cell membranes through inhibiting oxidation of PUFAs [11], particularly arachidonic acid (AA) and docosahexaenoic acid (DHA), the two major PUFAs found in the brain [12], and thereby combats the cell damage and neurodegeneration underlying cognitive impairment. In addition, emerging evidence indicates this vitamin may also possess non-antioxidant functions, including the regulation of gene expression [13,14]. In vitro and ex vivo studies have reported that treatment with α-tocopherol can down-regulate the expression of pro-inflammatory genes [15,16] and modulate the expression of several cell signaling and cell cycle genes [15–18]. Thus, the mechanism of action underlying the inverse association between α-tocopherol and cognitive impairment/dementia in humans is of considerable interest.

It is well established that α-tocopherol accumulates within membranes [19], and its subcellular distribution has been investigated in rat brains [20,21]. However, its distribution among different types of membranes and its direct association with membrane PUFA content and brain PUFA oxidation products have not been determined in primates. Determining the subcellular localization of α-tocopherol in brain tissue may provide insight into understanding its potential function(s). The objective of the present study was to determine the distribution of α-tocopherol in membranes from different brain regions and to characterize the relationship between membrane-specific α-tocopherol, membrane PUFA content, and brain PUFA oxidation products (isoprostanes [IsoP] and neuroprostanes [NP]) in primates. This study was performed in rhesus monkeys because they are a well-accepted model for human brain physiology [22].

2. Materials and Methods

2.1. Animals and Diet

Rhesus monkey (*Macaca mulatta*) brains, analyzed in the present study, were from a subgroup of a larger parent study sample, which investigated the effect of lutein supplementation on lutein accumulation in brain regions and membranes of primates [23]. Our study samples included serum and brain tissue from 6 female and 3 male adult monkeys (mean age: 11.7 ± 3.3 years; mean body weight: 7.87 ± 2.24 kg) that were obtained through the Oregon National Primate Research Center (ONPRC) (Beaverton, Oregon) Tissue Distribution Program; animals were not euthanized specifically for this study, but were euthanized for other projects or for veterinary reasons. All animals had consumed a standard stock diet (Monkey Diet Jumbo 5037, Lab Diet, St. Louis, MO, USA) at least twice a day, along with daily supplements of a variety of fruits and vegetables. The stock diet was measured for vitamin E (α- and γ-tocopherol), using previously reported methods [24]. The n-6 PUFA content of the diet was predominantly linoleic acid (1.7% of ration), with less than 0.01% of each ration being arachidonic acid (AA). The n-3 PUFA content was 0.13% of ration, mainly contributed by linolenic acid (0.10% of ration), but also containing DHA (~0.01% of ration). Our previous study [23] also included tissue from 4 monkeys receiving lutein supplementation, but these animals were not included in the current study, due to potential confounding effects on measures of oxidation.

The study was in compliance with all institutional and federal regulations on the use of laboratory animals as well as the Guide for the Care and Use of Laboratory Animals [25]. Procedures were approved by the Institutional Animal Care and Use Committee (IACUC) of Oregon Health and Science University (Protocol IS00003766). Professional care was provided by the ONPRC Division of Comparative Medicine and all animals were observed at least twice a day by trained veterinary technicians. In addition to rotating dietary supplements of fruits and vegetables, animals were provided with environmental enrichments, including a changing variety of toys. Euthanasia was conducted by a veterinary pathologist; animals were sedated with ketamine, and then deeply anesthetized with sodium pentobarbital, according to the Guidelines of the American Veterinary Medical Association. IACUC approval from Tufts University was also obtained for biological sample receipt, storage, and analysis.

2.2. Serum and Brain Collection

Fasting blood was drawn from the saphenous vein at the time of euthanasia. Because the monkeys were not euthanized exclusively for this study, blood samples were not collected in every case but were available for 7 out of 9 animals. Blood was processed for serum (1000× *g*, 10 min, 4 °C) and then stored at −80 °C prior to analysis.

Brains were removed immediately after euthanasia and the prefrontal cortex (PFC), cerebellum (CER), striatum (ST), and hippocampus (HC) were dissected from the right and left hemispheres. The regions consisted of both gray and white matter but excluded major white matter tracts. The dissected regions were immediately placed on dry ice and then stored at −80 °C. The right and left hemispheres of each region were pooled, pulverized in liquid nitrogen, aliquoted, and stored at −80 °C.

2.3. Preparation of Brain Membranes

Nuclear, myelin, mitochondrial, and neuronal plasma membranes were isolated from the PFC, CER, ST, and HC, using differential centrifugation with a Ficoll density gradient [26,27]. Pulverized brain samples were homogenized in aqueous buffer (10 mM hydroxyethyl piperazineethanesulfonic acid (HEPES), 0.25 mM ethylenediaminetetraacetic acid EDTA, 0.32 M sucrose, pH 7.2), containing protease inhibitors (cOmpleteTM protease inhibitor cocktail, Roche, Basel, Switzerland). The homogenates were subsequently subjected to low-speed centrifugation (1000× *g*, 4 °C) to isolate the crude nuclear membrane pellet. The resulting supernatant was removed to a new tube and the protocol was repeated with the pellet. Supernatant from the second low-speed centrifugation was combined with the first. The combined supernatants were then centrifuged (17,000× *g*, 4 °C) to obtain the "crude membrane pellet", containing myelin, mitochondrial, and neuronal plasma membranes. The crude membrane pellet was re-homogenized in buffer containing protease inhibitors but no sucrose (10 mM HEPES, 0.25 mM EDTA, pH 7.2) and was applied to a Ficoll density gradient (consisting of 14% and 7% Ficoll solutions). The homogenate was then subjected to high-speed centrifugation (87,000× *g*, 4 °C), to separate myelin, mitochondrial, and neuronal plasma membranes. All membranes, including the crude nuclear membrane, were purified via centrifugation at 17,000× *g*, 4 °C. Pure membranes were aliquoted and stored at −80 °C for tocopherol and fatty acid analyses. Membrane recovery was 76 ± 1%, as determined by measuring the sum of α-tocopherol levels in all membranes and supernatants and comparing this to total α-tocopherol in each brain region.

2.4. α-Tocopherol Extraction from Brain Regions, Membranes, and Serum

The process for the extraction of α- and γ-tocopherol from brain regions and membranes was adapted from Park et al. [28] and has been previously described in detail [29]. Briefly, after the additions of an internal standard (echinenone) and antioxidant (sodium ascorbate), samples were saponified with 5% sodium hydroxide and α-tocopherol was extracted using hexane. Extracts were then injected into a reverse-phase HPLC system to separate and quantify α- and γ-tocopherol.

Both α- and γ-tocopherol were extracted and analyzed from serum, using a previously published Folch method [30]. The lower limit of detection was 2.7 pmol, and the interassay coefficient of variation (CV) was 4%. Concentrations are expressed as ng/mg protein.

2.5. Fatty Acid Extraction and Protein Determination in Brain Regions and Membranes

Lipids were extracted overnight from homogenates of brain regions and membranes using a modified Folch method [31]. Fatty acids were analyzed using an established gas chromatography method [32]. Peaks of interest were identified by comparison with authentic fatty acid standards (Nu-Chek Prep, Inc., Elysian, MN, USA) and expressed as μg/mg protein and mole percent (%). The interassay CV ranged from 0.5 to 4.3% for fatty acids present at levels >5% of total fatty acids (TFAs), 1.8–10.1% for fatty acids present at levels between 1–5% TFAs, and 9.8–25.1% for fatty acids present at levels <1% TFAs. For the present analysis, we focused on the content of total PUFA, total n-6, total n-3, AA, and DHA.

Delipidated brain tissue and membranes from the overnight lipid extraction were digested in 1N sodium hydroxide for the determination of protein, using the bicinchoninic acid (BCA) assay, as per the manufacturer's instructions (Pierce Inc., Rockford, IL, USA). Brain regions and membranes were digested for 8 and 5 days, respectively.

2.6. PUFA Oxidation Determination in Brain Tissue

Total NP and IsoP, formed from the oxidation of DHA and AA, respectively, were extracted from the PFC, CER and ST, and quantified using published methods [33,34] with modifications. Due to the small size of HC, the amount of tissue from this region was insufficient for analysis. Briefly, lipids were extracted from homogenized brain samples using the Folch method. The lipid extract was then saponified to release esterified NP and IsoP. Neutral lipids were removed from the resulting mixture, using hexane, and samples were acidified to pH 3 to protonate NP and IsoP carboxylic acid groups. An internal standard, [$^2H_4$] 15-F_{2t}-IsoP (Cayman Chemicals, Ann Arbor, MI, USA), was added prior to extraction with ethyl acetate. NP and IsoP were then derivatized to form pentafluorobenzyl (PFB) esters and subjected to HPLC (Agilent 1050, Santa Clara, CA, USA), using the method described by Walter et al. [33]. NP and IsoP fractions were collected, converted to trimethylsilyl ether derivatives, and quantified using GC/MS [33]. Selective ion monitoring was used for analysis at m/z 593 for NP, m/z 569 for IsoP and m/z 573 for the internal standard, [$^2H_4$] 15-F_{2t}-IsoP. The inter-assay CV was 10%.

2.7. Statistical Analysis

α- and γ-tocopherol and fatty acid data are expressed as mean ± standard deviation. A one-way analysis of variance (ANOVA) with Tukey's honest significant difference (HSD) was performed to determine differences in tocopherol concentrations across brain regions. Due to significant differences in brain region tocopherol concentrations ($p < 0.05$), membrane data from each region was analyzed separately. A one-way ANOVA with Tukey's HSD was performed for α- and γ-tocopherol as well as PUFAs (total, n-6, n-3, AA, and DHA), to determine their membrane distributions within each region. Pearson correlations were performed to determine whether region and membrane-specific α-tocopherol, membrane PUFAs, and brain region PUFA oxidation products were related, adjusting for age. We considered r = 0.30–0.49 to be a weak correlation, r = 0.50–0.69, a moderate correlation and r = 0.70–0.99 a strong correlation [35]. All analyses were performed using Statistical Analysis Software, SAS 9.4, with significance set at the 0.05 level.

3. Results

3.1. Tocopherol Concentrations in Rhesus Monkey Stock Diet and Serum

Tocopherol concentrations in the monkey diet and serum are presented in Table 1. In the stock diet, γ-tocopherol concentrations were ~7.5 times greater than the α-tocopherol content. The average amount of α-tocopherol consumed from the stock diet was ~2 mg/day or 0.70 μmol/kg body weight, while average γ-tocopherol intakes were ~16 mg/day or 5.3 μmol/kg body weight. Conversely, concentrations of α-tocopherol in serum were ~8 times greater than γ-tocopherol concentrations.

Table 1. Tocopherol Concentrations (mean ± SD) in Monkey Stock Diet * and Serum (n = 7).

	α-Tocopherol	γ-Tocopherol
Stock Diet (μmol/kg)	23 ± 1.2	171 ± 34
Serum (μmol/L)	20.8 ± 8.3	2.5 ± 0.6

* Sample run in triplicate.

3.2. Distribution of α-Tocopherol in Brain Regions and Membranes of Adult Rhesus Monkeys

The α-tocopherol contents in the PFC, CER, ST, and HC of rhesus monkeys are presented in Figure 1. Concentrations of α-tocopherol were significantly lower in the PFC, CER and ST than in HC (p = 0.02), and also significantly lower in the CER than in the ST ($p < 0.05$). α-Tocopherol concentrations did not significantly differ between the ST and PFC. Concentrations of γ-tocopherol in the HC were significantly greater than in all other regions ($p < 0.05$, Figure S1). As in serum, α-tocopherol concentrations were 7–10 times greater than γ-tocopherol concentrations in the brain regions (Figure S2).

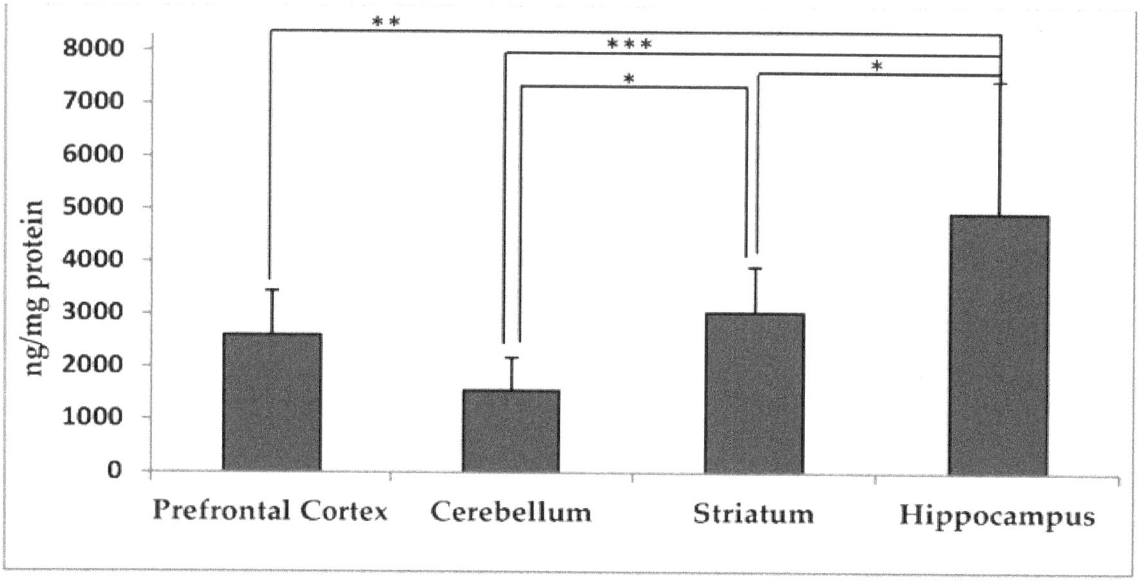

Figure 1. α-Tocopherol concentrations (ng/mg protein, mean ± SD) in different regions of the brain from adult rhesus macaques (n = 9). Asterisks indicate significant differences between brain regions according to one-way analysis of variance (ANOVA) followed by Tukey's honest significance difference (HSD) test; * $p < 0.05$, ** $p < 0.01$, *** $p < 0.001$.

Membrane concentrations of α-tocopherol in the PFC, CER, ST, and HC of rhesus monkeys are presented in Figure 2A–D. The distribution of α-tocopherol among membrane types differed in a region-specific manner. In the PFC, α-tocopherol concentrations were significantly greater in nuclear membranes than in mitochondrial membranes ($p < 0.05$). In the CER, α-tocopherol concentrations were significantly greater in nuclear membranes than in all other membranes, and significantly greater in myelin than in mitochondrial membranes ($p < 0.05$). In the ST, α-tocopherol was again significantly greater in nuclear membranes than in all other membrane types ($p < 0.05$). In the HC, however, there were no significant differences in α-tocopherol concentrations across membrane types. Membrane concentrations of γ-tocopherol in brain regions were considerably lower than α-tocopherol (Figure S3A–D), and there were no significant differences among membrane types in the PFC and HC. However, in the CER and ST, γ-tocopherol concentrations were significantly greater in nuclear membranes than in all other membrane types ($p \leq 0.02$).

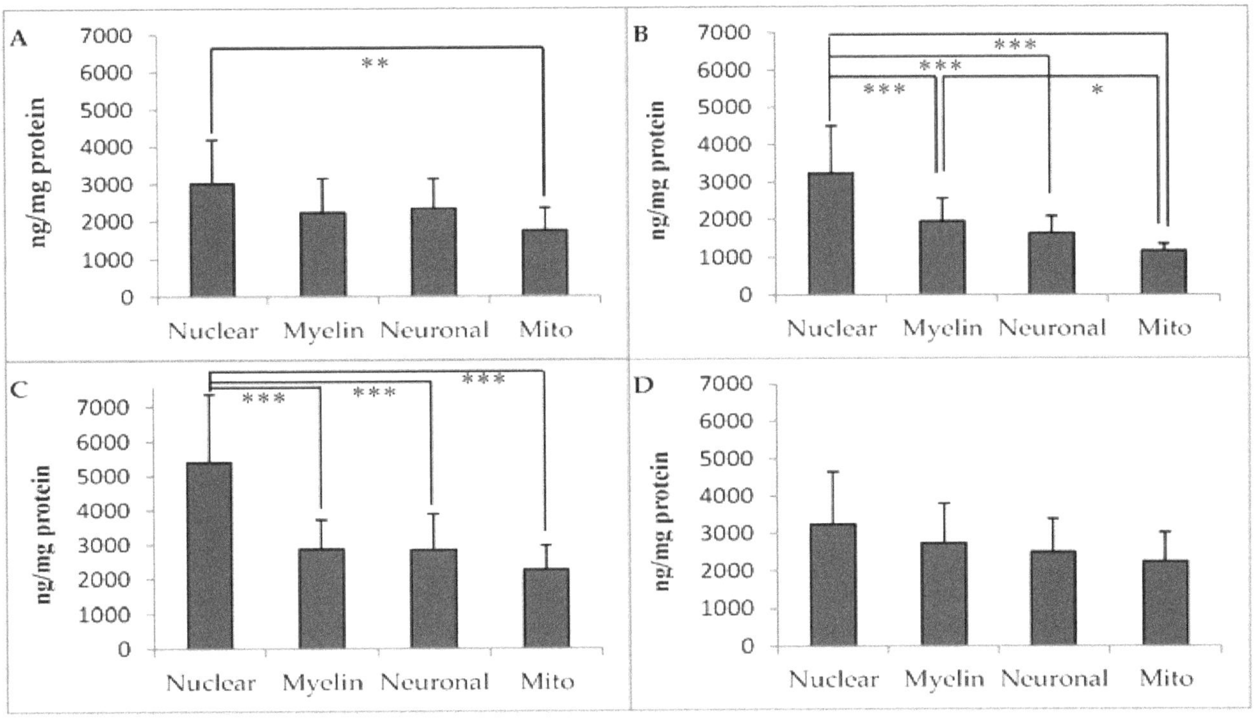

Figure 2. Membrane α-tocopherol concentrations (ng/mg protein, mean ± SD) in the (**A**) prefrontal cortex; (**B**) cerebellum; (**C**) striatum; and (**D**) hippocampus of adult rhesus macaques (n = 9). Asterisks indicate significant differences between brain regions according to one-way analysis of variance (ANOVA) followed by Tukey's honest significant difference (HSD) test; * $p < 0.05$, ** $p < 0.01$, *** $p < 0.001$. Nuclear: nuclear membrane; myelin: myelin membranes; Neuronal: neuronal plasma membrane; Mito: mitochondrial membranes.

3.3. Distribution of Membrane PUFAs in Different Brain Regions of Adult Rhesus Macaques

Membrane concentrations of total PUFA, n-6, n-3, AA, and DHA in the PFC, CER, ST, and HC of rhesus monkeys are presented in Table 2. In the PFC and ST, AA and total n-6 PUFA concentrations were highest in nuclear membranes, intermediate in myelin and neuronal membranes, and lowest in mitochondrial membranes ($p < 0.05$). However, in the CER, AA was similar among all membranes, except mitochondrial membranes, where concentrations were lower than in all other membrane fractions. In the HC, mean values were highest in myelin and nuclear membranes, followed by neuronal and mitochondrial membranes ($p < 0.05$).

Table 2. Membrane polyunsaturated fatty acid concentration (μg/mg protein, mean ± SD) in the prefrontal cortex, cerebellum, striatum, and hippocampus of adult rhesus macaques ($n = 9$).

Region		Nuclear	Myelin	Neuronal	Mitochondrial
Prefrontal Cortex	Arachidonic Acid	123.5 ± 30.0 [a]	99.3 ± 30.5 [b]	96.44 ± 20.0 [b]	28.0 ± 16.3 [c]
	PUFA n-6	291.7 ± 77.5 [a]	204.9 ± 48.9 [b]	201.6 ± 63.5 [b]	49.2 ± 27.6 [c]
	Docosahexaenoic acid	151.9 ± 37.2 [a]	180.6 ± 48.9 [a]	175.8 ± 54.8 [a]	35.3 ± 19.2 [b]
	PUFA n-3	164.2 ± 44.6 [a]	187.6 ± 51.7 [a]	182.9 ± 56.8 [a]	36.2 ± 19.8 [b]
	Total PUFA	455.9 ± 120.6 [a]	392.4 ± 99.9 [a]	384.5 ± 120.1 [a]	85.4 ± 47.1 [b]
Cerebellum	Arachidonic Acid	91.4 ± 19.1 [a]	84.4 ± 32.8 [a]	95.9 ± 20.4 [a]	15.1 ± 5.8 [b]
	PUFAn-6	213.0 ± 40.2 [a]	166.1 ± 59.3 [b]	187.6 ± 38.0 [a,b]	30.3 ± 11.4 [c]
	Docosahexaenoic acid	136.0 ± 26.5 [a]	178.2 ± 59.9 [b]	199.8 ± 39.7 [b]	27.8 ± 10.2 [c]
	PUFA n-3	148.8 ± 30.0 [a]	185.9 ± 63.3 [b]	207.3 ± 40.9 [b]	28.7 ± 10.5 [c]
	Total PUFA	361.8 ± 69.4 [a]	352.0 ± 121.4 [a]	394.9 ± 76.7 [a]	59.0 ± 21.9 [b]
Striatum	Arachidonic Acid	221.5 ± 65.4 [a]	156.2 ± 20.5 [b]	143.9 ± 26.5 [b]	30.5 ± 13.3 [c]
	PUFA n-6	525.2 ± 177.7 [a]	315.5 ± 46.4 [b]	289.0 ± 47.6 [b]	52.9 ± 22.1 [c]
	Docosahexaenoic acid	196.9 ± 36.1 [a]	257.7 ± 35.0 [b]	201.0 ± 37.2 [a]	37.3 ± 17.4 [c]
	PUFA n-3	224.0 ± 43.9 [a]	268.7 ± 36.7 [b]	211.7 ± 38.5 [a]	38.4 ± 17.8 [c]
	Total PUFA	749.2 ± 217.5 [a]	584.2 ± 81.6 [b]	500.7 ± 85.1 [c]	91.4 ± 39.6 [d]
Hippocampus	Arachidonic Acid	208.0 ± 54.6 [a,b]	247.1 ± 119.7 [a]	170.6 ± 50.4 [b]	21.6 ± 6.6 [c]
	PUFA n-6	452.0 ± 126.0 [a]	519.7 ± 226.7 [a]	340.0 ± 104.9 [b]	37.0 ± 10.9 [c]
	Docosahexaenoic acid	144.2 ± 40.9 [a]	325.2 ± 118.7 [b]	201.5 ± 63.4 [c]	16.7 ± 5.5 [d]
	PUFA n-3	191.6 ± 54.2 [a]	347.7 ± 127.5 [b]	219.4 ± 69.7 [a]	18.2 ± 5.5 [c]
	Total PUFA	643.6 ± 177.5 [a,b]	867.5 ± 351.2 [a]	559.5 ± 173.8 [b]	55.2 ± 16.1 [c]

Means with different superscripts (a, b, c, d) in each row are significantly different, according to one-way analysis of variance (ANOVA) followed by Tukey's honest significance difference (HSD) test ($p < 0.05$). PUFA: polyunsaturated fatty acids.

In the PFC, DHA, n-3 PUFAs, and the total PUFA concentration were lowest in mitochondrial membranes ($p < 0.05$), but did not differ in the other membranes. In the CER, DHA and n-3 PUFAs were highest in neuronal membranes and myelin, followed by nuclear membranes, and lowest in mitochondrial membranes ($p < 0.05$). In this region, the total PUFA content was lowest in mitochondrial membranes compared to the other membranes ($p < 0.05$). In both the ST and HC, PUFA n-3 and DHA were highest in myelin membranes, intermediate in neuronal and nuclear membranes, and lowest in mitochondrial membranes ($p < 0.05$). In the ST, total PUFA concentrations differed across all membranes (nuclear > myelin > neuronal > mitochondrial, $p < 0.05$). In the HC, total PUFAs were highest in myelin, intermediate in neuronal and nuclear membranes, and lowest in mitochondrial membranes ($p < 0.05$).

While the absolute concentration of fatty acids provides a measurement of the amount of each fatty acid, independent of other fatty acids, mole % data measures the relative importance of a fatty acid against the total fatty acid concentration. Thus, the membrane distribution of fatty acids differs, depending on whether fatty acids are expressed as mole % or μg/mg protein. Membrane fatty acid profiles among brain regions, expressed as mole %, are reported in the supplementary material (Tables S1–S4). Briefly, in the PFC, CER and ST, the mole % AA was highest in mitochondrial membranes, intermediate in neuronal and myelin membranes, and lowest in nuclear membranes (Tables S1–S3, $p < 0.05$). In the PFC, DHA was distributed similarly to AA among membranes (Table S1, $p < 0.05$). In the CER, the mole % DHA was highest in mitochondrial membranes, followed by neuronal membranes, followed by myelin membranes, and lowest in nuclear membranes (Table S2, $p < 0.05$). In the ST, the mole % DHA was highest in mitochondrial and myelin membranes, intermediate in neuronal membranes, and lowest in nuclear membranes (Table S3, $p < 0.05$). In the HC, the mole % AA was highest in mitochondrial membranes, but did not differ among the other membranes (Table S4, $p < 0.05$). The mole % DHA in this region was lowest in nuclear membranes but did not differ among other membrane types ($p < 0.05$).

3.4. Relationship between Membrane α-Tocopherol and PUFA Concentrations in Brain Regions

The association between the membrane-specific α-tocopherol and PUFA concentrations in the PFC, CER, ST, and HC is presented in Table 3. In all regions, except the HC, α-tocopherol concentrations were positively associated with all PUFA concentrations—including AA, DHA, n-6 and n-3 PUFA and total PUFA—in nuclear membranes ($p < 0.05$), with the single exception of DHA in the CER. No other significant associations were observed in the CER. In the PFC, α-tocopherol concentrations were also associated with all PUFAs in neuronal plasma membranes ($p < 0.05$). In the ST, α-tocopherol was significantly associated with all PUFAs in all membrane types ($p < 0.05$). In the HC, α-tocopherol was associated with all PUFAs in myelin, but only DHA and total PUFA n–3 in mitochondrial membranes ($p < 0.05$). No significant associations were observed in nuclear and neuronal plasma membranes from this region.

Table 3. Partial correlations between membrane α-tocopherol (ng/mg protein) and PUFA concentrations (μg/mg protein) from different brain regions of rhesus macaques ($n = 9$).

Region		Nuclear	Myelin	Neuronal	Mitochondrial
Prefrontal Cortex	Arachidonic acid	0.68 **	0.69 **	0.78 **	–
	PUFA n-6	0.70 **	0.61	0.82 **	–
	Docosahexaenoic acid	0.70 **	0.55	0.94 ***	–
	PUFA n-3	0.71 **	0.54	0.94 ***	–
	Total PUFA	0.71 **	0.58	0.91 ***	–
Cerebellum	Arachidonic acid	0.78 **	0.43	0.52	0.53
	PUFA n-6	0.85 ***	0.47	0.58	0.57
	Docosahexaenoic acid	0.61	0.40	0.63	0.56
	PUFA n-3	0.70 **	0.41	0.62	0.56
	Total PUFA	0.76 **	0.44	0.60	0.57
Striatum	Arachidonic acid	0.89 ***	0.81 **	0.86 ***	0.80 **
	PUFA n-6	0.81 **	0.76 **	0.84 ***	0.75 **
	Docosahexaenoic acid	0.89 ***	0.81 **	0.80 **	0.80 **
	PUFA n-3	0.91 ***	0.80 **	0.79 **	0.79 **
	Total PUFA	0.85 ***	0.79 **	0.83 **	0.77 **
Hippocampus	Arachidonic acid	0.60	0.71 **	0.48	0.61
	PUFA n-6	0.64	0.79 **	0.50	0.58
	Docosahexaenoic acid	0.61	0.70 **	0.57	0.79 **
	PUFA n-3	0.67	0.70 **	0.56	0.77 **
	Total PUFA	0.66	0.76 **	0.53	0.66

Values are partial correlation coefficients (r values) adjusted for age; ** $p < 0.05$, *** $p < 0.01$. –: r values below 0.40 are not shown.

3.5. Relationship between Membrane α-Tocopherol and PUFA Oxidation Products in Brain Regions

Concentrations of DHA oxidation products (NP) and AA oxidation products (IsoP) among the PFC, CER, and ST are presented in Figure 3. NP and IsoP were significantly lower in the CER compared to both the PFC and ST ($p < 0.01$). The ratio of IsoP/NP was also significantly lower in the CER, compared to the other two regions ($p < 0.05$). NP, IsoP, and the ratio of IsoP/NP did not differ between the PFC and ST.

The cross-sectional relationship between region and membrane-specific α-tocopherol concentrations and brain PUFA oxidation products in the PFC, CER, and ST is presented in Table 4. NP concentrations (pg/μg DHA), measured in whole tissue, were not significantly associated with α-tocopherol concentrations (ng/μg DHA) in any membrane type or brain region. Similarly, IsoP concentrations (pg/μg AA) were not associated with α-tocopherol (ng/μg AA) in any individual membrane type. However, AA oxidation products were inversely associated with concentrations of α-tocopherol in whole tissue, in both the PFC and ST ($p < 0.05$). PUFA oxidation products were not associated with γ-tocopherol concentrations in any membrane or region (data not shown).

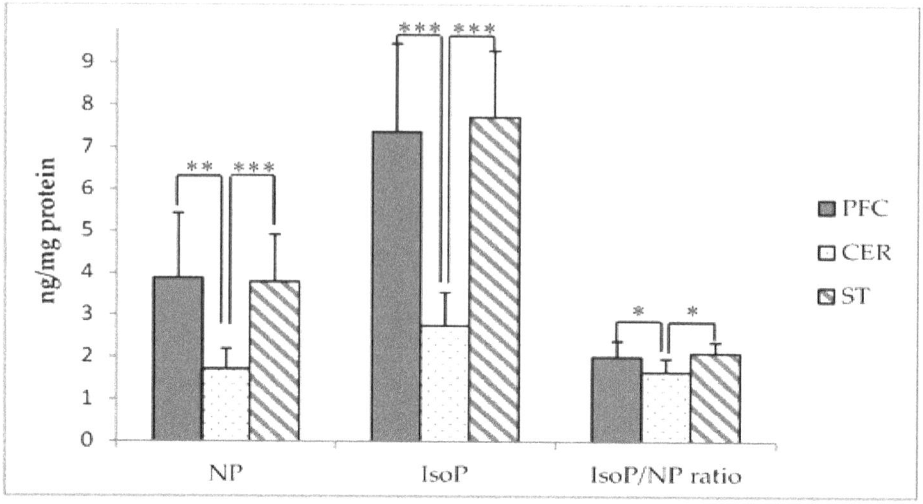

Figure 3. Neuroprostane (NP) and isoprostane (IsoP) concentrations (ng/mg protein) in the prefrontal cortex (PFC), cerebellum (CER), and striatum (ST) of adult rhesus macaques ($n = 9$). Asterisks indicate significant differences between brain regions according to one-way ANOVA followed by Tukey's HSD test; * $p < 0.05$, ** $p < 0.01$, *** $p < 0.001$.

Table 4. Partial correlations between membrane α-tocopherol and neuroprostanes and isoprostanes from different brain regions of rhesus macaques ($n = 9$).

	Total	Nuclear	Myelin	Neuronal	Mitochondrial
		Neuroprostanes			
Prefrontal Cortex	−0.66 *	–	–	–	–
Cerebellum	–	–	–	–	–
Striatum	−0.43	−0.62 *	–	–	–
		Isoprostanes			
Prefrontal Cortex	−0.74 **	−0.47	–	–	–
Cerebellum	–	−0.66 *	–	–	−0.61 *
Striatum	−0.73 **	–	−0.64 *	-0.50	–

Values are partial correlation coefficients (r values) adjusted for age; ** $p < 0.05$, * $p < 0.1$. –: r values below 0.40 are not shown.

4. Discussion

This study is the first to report the distribution of α-tocopherol and γ-tocopherol in multiple subcellular membrane types (nuclear, myelin, neuronal, and mitochondrial) for multiple brain regions in the primate brain. We also directly investigated the relationship between membrane α-tocopherol concentration and both membrane PUFA content and brain PUFA oxidation. We report that α-tocopherol was differentially distributed among the membranes, with the highest concentrations found in nuclear membranes for all regions tested, except the HC. In the PFC and ST, AA and total n-6 PUFA distribution among membrane types were similar to that of α-tocopherol, and total α-tocopherol concentrations in these regions were inversely related to AA oxidation products.

4.1. α-Tocopherol Distribution in Brain Regions of Adult Rhesus Monkeys

Although no other studies have reported on the concentration of α-tocopherol in monkey brain regions, our results are similar to α-tocopherol concentrations reported in different regions of the adult human brain [6,36], but slightly greater than those reported for human infants [37] and rats [20]. In the current study, the CER had the lowest α-tocopherol concentrations among the brain regions analyzed. This is consistent with previous findings in brain tissue from human adults and centenarians [6,36] as well as rats [20]. In the rat brain, researchers have also observed that the uptake of α-tocopherol is greatest in the CER, despite this region having the lowest steady-state amounts of α-tocopherol, suggesting a more rapid turnover of α-tocopherol in the CER, compared to other regions [20]. Alternatively, this observation in primates may be due to differences in α-tocopherol transfer protein (α-TTP) and/or tocopherol-associated protein (TAP) expression among brain regions [38,39]. In human infants, there were no differences in α-tocopherol concentrations across brain regions tested [37], suggesting that α-tocopherol distribution in the brain might differ across the lifespan. However, that study did not analyze the CER. Future studies investigating the mechanisms underlying the differential distribution of α-tocopherol across the brain tissue of adult primates are warranted.

Our detection of γ-tocopherol at significantly lower concentrations than α-tocopherol is also consistent with findings from studies in human brain tissue [36,37], but differs from rodent studies, in which only α-tocopherol has been detected [20,40]. The distribution pattern of γ-tocopherol among brain regions and membrane fractions was similar to that of α-tocopherol, indicating that tocopherol delivery to brain regions may depend on both serum levels and brain region-specific factors.

4.2. Accumulation of α-Tocopherol in Brain Membranes of Adult Rhesus Monkeys

The distribution of α-tocopherol among membrane types differed in a region-specific manner. However, α-tocopherol concentrations were generally greater in nuclear membranes, compared to other membranes, in each region, except for the HC. The enrichment of α-tocopherol in nuclear membranes suggests that α-tocopherol may play a role in nuclear-associated functions in the brain. This role may be particularly important in the ST and CER, where preferential accumulation of α-tocopherol in the nuclear membrane was most apparent. Accumulating evidence from a number of in vitro and ex vivo studies indicates that α-tocopherol can modulate the expression of cell signaling, cell cycle regulation, and pro-inflammatory genes [15–18,41]. In mice and rats, dietary and supplemental α-tocopherol or the combination of α- and γ-tocopherol has been shown to modulate the expression of genes involved in apoptosis, lipid biosynthesis, adenosine triphosphate (ATP) biosynthesis, and immune/inflammatory responses in the aging brain [42,43]. Additionally, the expression of genes encoding synaptic proteins, protein kinase C family members, and myelin proteins were decreased in transgenic mice deficient in α-TTP [44]. These results may have important implications for the potential role of α-tocopherol in protecting against cognitive impairment and dementia, given that microarray studies have demonstrated that dysregulation of genes involved in inflammation, synaptic signaling, and neuronal apoptosis alter brain cell function and contribute to the pathogenesis of these conditions [45–47]. Future studies investigating the effect of α-tocopherol enrichment in nuclear membranes and changes in gene expression in the primate brain are needed to gain a better understanding of why α-tocopherol may accumulate in this membrane.

Membrane α-tocopherol and PUFA concentrations were found to be positively associated with one another, particularly in the PFC and ST, and to a lesser extent in the CER and HC. This finding is consistent with previous studies, which demonstrated that α-tocopherol accumulates in PUFA-rich membrane domains [48,49]. No significant relationship was observed between α-tocopherol and brain PUFA oxidation products in individual membrane fractions. However, concentrations of both DHA and AA oxidation products (as measured by NP and IsoP, respectively), as well as the relative amount of AA oxidation products to DHA oxidation products (IsoP/NP ratio) were lower in the CER compared to other brain regions, similar to α-tocopherol. Additionally, α-tocopherol concentrations in whole tissue were inversely associated with AA oxidation products (IsoP) in both the PFC and ST. These are the only two brain regions where concentrations of both α-tocopherol and AA were highest in nuclear membranes, intermediate in myelin and neuronal membranes, and lowest in mitochondrial membranes. In contrast, α-tocopherol concentrations were not correlated with DHA oxidation products, as measured by NP levels. These results suggest that (1) α-tocopherol may accumulate in regions with higher PUFA oxidation, particularly AA oxidation relative to DHA oxidation; and (2) α-tocopherol concentrations within these regions of relative higher accumulation may be associated with lower AA oxidation. This is consistent with previous rodent studies, which demonstrated that supplementation with α-tocopherol is more effective at decreasing AA oxidation than DHA oxidation [50,51]. Taken together, our findings indicate that, although α-tocopherol accumulates in membranes, rich in both n-6 and n-3 PUFAs, it may be associated with preferentially protecting AA from oxidative damage. Our observation that only concentrations of α-tocopherol in whole tissue were associated with AA oxidation suggests that the free-radical scavenging function of this nutrient may not be specific to a particular membrane type. Therefore, the contribution of total α-tocopherol concentrations within regions may have the strongest relationship to total AA oxidation in brain regions compared to individual membranes. However, only whole tissue concentrations of AA and DHA oxidation products were determined in these studies as it is currently not feasible to measure membrane-specific concentrations, due to limitations in methodology. Therefore, the relationship between α-tocopherol and PUFA oxidation products within each membrane type remains unknown. Our α-tocopherol result differs from our previous findings that membrane-specific concentrations of the antioxidant, lutein, are associated with total DHA oxidation products, but not total AA oxidation products in rhesus monkey brains [23]. One limitation of both studies is that neither accounts for the potential synergistic effects of other antioxidants present in the brain and their influence on DHA and AA oxidation. Therefore, future studies measuring a more comprehensive profile of antioxidants in the brain and their associations with PUFA oxidation, are needed. Another limitation of this study is the small sample size. Our results need to be replicated in a larger sample population. However, our study provides an important first step in characterizing previously unknown relationships between membrane-associated antioxidants and PUFA oxidation in the primate brain and can guide future investigations into the antioxidant functions of α- and γ-tocopherol in the brain.

Our findings support an antioxidant-associated function of α-tocopherol towards AA, but we cannot rule out the possibility that non-antioxidant functions underlie the association between these two nutrients. Previous studies have demonstrated that α-tocopherol can significantly inhibit the activity of phospholipase A2 [41,52], which is primarily responsible for cleavage and release of AA from membrane phospholipids. Therefore, it is possible that the similarity in membrane distribution between α-tocopherol and AA may reflect not only a role of α-tocopherol in inhibiting AA oxidation, but also a role in the modulation of AA cleavage and release from membranes. Future studies, investigating the relationship between membrane α-tocopherol levels and phospholipase A2 activity in regions of the primate brain, are needed, to better understand the contribution of this potential mechanism to the overall function of α-tocopherol in the primate brain.

5. Conclusions

In conclusion, we found that dietary α-tocopherol was higher in the HC than in the PFC, CER or ST in the non-human primate brain. Within membrane types, α-tocopherol showed preferential accumulation in nuclear membranes compared to other membrane types, except in the HC. We speculate that this observation may be indicative of a role of α-tocopherol in nuclear functions in brain cells. Additionally, we observed that α-tocopherol is positively related to PUFA concentrations in membranes, but only concentrations of AA were distributed similarly to α-tocopherol among membrane types. Finally, whole tissue, but not membrane, α-tocopherol concentrations were significantly associated with AA oxidation products, in both the PFC and ST. Thus, correlations between α-tocopherol and PUFA concentrations may be associated with a protective role of α-tocopherol against AA oxidation, but may also reflect a role of α-tocopherol in inhibiting AA release from membrane phospholipids. Collectively, our study provides insight into the accumulation of dietary α-tocopherol in the primate brain, which may have important implications regarding its functions in this tissue.

Acknowledgments: Emily E. Johnson and the ONPRC Veterinary Pathology Service assisted with brain tissue collection. Jean Gallucio, Audrey Goldbaum, and Kathryn Baldyga at Tufts University performed brain region and membrane fatty acid and protein analysis. This work was supported by a grant from Abbott Nutrition through the Center for Nutrition, Learning, and Memory (CNLM) at the University of Illinois at Urbana-Champaign, DSM Nutritional Products, and USDA under grant 8050-51000-095-01S.

Author Contributions: John W. Erdman Jr, Elizabeth J. Johnson, Matthew J. Kuchan, and Martha Neuringer conceived and designed the experiments; Emily S. Mohn, Nirupa R. Matthan, and Martha Neuringer performed the experiments; Emily S. Mohn analyzed the data; Elizabeth J. Johnson, Nirupa R. Matthan, Martha Neuringer, Chun-Yen. Oliver Chen contributed reagents/materials/analysis tools; Emily S. Mohn wrote the paper; all authors edited the paper.

References

1. Institute of Medicine (US) Panel on Dietary Antioxidants and Related Compounds. *Dietary Reference Intakes for Vitamin C, Vitamin E, Selenium, and Carotenoids*; National Academies Press (US): Washington, DC, USA, 2000; Available online: http://www.ncbi.nlm.nih.gov/books/NBK225483/ (accessed on 1 February 2017).
2. Traber, M.G.; Arai, H. Molecular mechanisms of vitamin E transport. *Annu. Rev. Nutr.* **1999**, *19*, 343–355. [CrossRef] [PubMed]
3. Rigotti, A. Absorption, transport, and tissue delivery of vitamin E. *Mol. Asp. Med.* **2007**, *28*, 423–436. [CrossRef] [PubMed]
4. Grodstein, F.; Chen, J.; Willett, W.C. High-dose antioxidant supplements and cognitive function in community-dwelling elderly women. *Am. J. Clin. Nutr.* **2003**, *77*, 975–984. [PubMed]
5. Mangialasche, F.; Xu, W.; Kivipelto, M.; Costanzi, E.; Ercolani, S.; Pigliautile, M.; Cecchetti, R.; Baglioni, M.; Simmons, A.; Soininen, H.; et al. Tocopherols and tocotrienols plasma levels are associated with cognitive impairment. *Neurobiol. Aging* **2012**, *33*, 2282–2290. [CrossRef] [PubMed]
6. Johnson, E.J.; Vishwanathan, R.; Johnson, M.A.; Hausman, D.B.; Davey, A.; Scott, T.M.; Green, R.C.; Miller, L.S.; Gearing, M.; Woodard, J.; et al. Relationship between Serum and Brain Carotenoids, α-Tocopherol, and Retinol Concentrations and Cognitive Performance in the Oldest Old from the Georgia Centenarian Study. *J. Aging Res.* **2013**, *2013*, 951786. [CrossRef] [PubMed]
7. Hensley, K.; Barnes, L.L.; Christov, A.; Tangney, C.; Honer, W.G.; Schneider, J.A.; Bennett, D.A.; Morris, M.C. Analysis of Postmortem Ventricular Cerebrospinal Fluid from Patients with and without Dementia Indicates Association of Vitamin E with Neuritic Plaques and Specific Measures of Cognitive Performance. *J. Alzheimers Dis.* **2011**, *24*, 767–774. [CrossRef] [PubMed]
8. Jiménez-Jiménez, F.J.; de Bustos, F.; Molina, J.A.; Benito-León, J.; Tallón-Barranco, A.; Gasalla, T.; Ortí-Pareja, M.; Guillamón, F.; Rubio, J.C.; Arenas, J.; et al. Cerebrospinal fluid levels of alpha-tocopherol (vitamin E) in Alzheimer's disease. *J. Neural Transm.* **1997**, *104*, 703–710. [CrossRef] [PubMed]
9. Uttara, B.; Singh, A.V.; Zamboni, P.; Mahajan, R. Oxidative Stress and Neurodegenerative Diseases: A Review of Upstream and Downstream Antioxidant Therapeutic Options. *Curr. Neuropharmacol.* **2009**, *7*, 65–74. [CrossRef] [PubMed]
10. Kim, G.H.; Kim, J.E.; Rhie, S.J.; Yoon, S. The Role of Oxidative Stress in Neurodegenerative Diseases. *Exp. Neurobiol.* **2015**, *24*, 325–340. [CrossRef] [PubMed]
11. Traber, M.G.; Atkinson, J. Vitamin E, antioxidant and nothing more. *Free Radic. Biol. Med.* **2007**, *43*, 4–15. [CrossRef] [PubMed]
12. Qi, K.; Hall, M.; Deckelbaum, R.J. Long-chain polyunsaturated fatty acid accretion in brain. *Curr. Opin. Clin. Nutr. Metab. Care* **2002**, *5*, 133–138. [CrossRef] [PubMed]
13. Engin, K.N. Alpha-tocopherol: Looking beyond an antioxidant. *Mol. Vis.* **2009**, *15*, 855–860. [PubMed]
14. Quinn, P.J. Is the distribution of alpha-tocopherol in membranes consistent with its putative functions? *Biochemistry* **2004**, *69*, 58–66. [PubMed]
15. Azzi, A.; Gysin, R.; Kempná, P.; Munteanu, A.; Negis, Y.; Villacorta, L.; Visarius, T.; Zingg, J.M. Vitamin E Mediates Cell Signaling and Regulation of Gene Expression. *Ann. N. Y. Acad. Sci.* **2004**, *1031*, 86–95. [CrossRef] [PubMed]
16. Han, S.N.; Pang, E.; Zingg, J.-M.; Meydani, S.N.; Meydani, M.; Azzi, A. Differential effects of natural and synthetic vitamin E on gene transcription in murine T lymphocytes. *Arch. Biochem. Biophys.* **2010**, *495*, 49–55. [CrossRef] [PubMed]

17. Han, S.N.; Adolfsson, O.; Lee, C.-K.; Prolla, T.A.; Ordovas, J.; Meydani, S.N. Age and vitamin E-induced changes in gene expression profiles of T cells. *J. Immunol.* **2006**, *177*, 6052–6061. [CrossRef] [PubMed]
18. Han, S.N.; Adolfsson, O.; Lee, C.-K.; Prolla, T.A.; Ordovas, J.; Meydani, S.N. Vitamin E and gene expression in immune cells. *Ann. N. Y. Acad. Sci.* **2004**, *1031*, 96–101. [CrossRef] [PubMed]
19. Wang, X.; Quinn, P.J. Vitamin E and its function in membranes. *Prog. Lipid Res.* **1999**, *38*, 309–336. [CrossRef]
20. Vatassery, G.T.; Angerhofer, C.K.; Knox, C.A.; Deshmukh, D.S. Concentrations of vitamin E in various neuroanatomical regions and subcellular fractions, and the uptake of vitamin E by specific areas, of rat brain. *Biochim. Biophys. Acta* **1984**, *792*, 118–122. [CrossRef]
21. Vatassery, G.T.; Smith, W.E.; Quach, H.T. α-Tocopherol in Rat Brain Subcellular Fractions Is Oxidized Rapidly during Incubations with Low Concentrations of Peroxynitrite. *J. Nutr.* **1998**, *128*, 152–157. [PubMed]
22. Perretta, G. Non-Human Primate Models in Neuroscience Research. *Scand. J. Lab. Anim. Sci.* **2009**, *36*, 77–85.
23. Mohn, E.S.; Erdman, J.W.; Kuchan, M.J.; Neuringer, M.; Johnson, E.J. Lutein accumulates in subcellular membranes of brain regions in adult rhesus macaques: Relationship to DHA oxidation products. *PLoS ONE* **2017**, *12*, e0186767. [CrossRef] [PubMed]
24. Muzhingi, T.; Yeum, K.-J.; Russell, R.M.; Johnson, E.J.; Qin, J.; Tang, G. Determination of carotenoids in yellow maize, the effects of saponification and food preparations. *Int. J. Vitam. Nutr. Res.* **2008**, *78*, 112–120. [CrossRef] [PubMed]
25. National Research Council (US) Committee for the Update of the Guide for the Care and Use of Laboratory Animals. *Guide for the Care and Use of Laboratory Animal*, 8th ed.; National Academies Press (US): Washington, DC, USA, 2011; Available online: http://www.ncbi.nlm.nih.gov/books/NBK54050/ (accessed on 15 February 2017).
26. Sun, G.Y.; Sun, Y. Phospholipids and acyl groups of synaptosomal and myelin membranes isolated from the cerebral cortex of squirrel monkey (*Saimiri sciureus*). *Biochim. Biophys. Acta* **1972**, *280*, 306–315. [CrossRef]
27. Sun, G.Y. Phospholipids and acyl groups in subcellular fractions from human cerebral cortex. *J. Lipid Res.* **1973**, *14*, 656–663. [PubMed]
28. Park, J.; Hwang, H.; Kim, M.; Lee-Kim, Y. Effects of dietary fatty acids and vitamin E supplementation on antioxidant vitamin status of the second generation rat brain sections. *Korean J. Nutr.* **2001**, *34*, 754–761.
29. Vishwanathan, R.; Neuringer, M.; Snodderly, D.M.; Schalch, W.; Johnson, E.J. Macular lutein and zeaxanthin are related to brain lutein and zeaxanthin in primates. *Nutr. Neurosci.* **2013**, *16*, 21–29. [CrossRef] [PubMed]
30. Johnson, E.J.; Neuringer, M.; Russell, R.M.; Schalch, W.; Snodderly, D.M. Nutritional manipulation of primate retinas, III: Effects of lutein or zeaxanthin supplementation on adipose tissue and retina of xanthophyll-free monkeys. *Investig. Ophthalmol. Vis. Sci.* **2005**, *46*, 692–702. [CrossRef] [PubMed]
31. Folch, J.; Lees, M.; Sloane Stanley, G.H. A simple method for the isolation and purification of total lipides from animal tissues. *J. Biol. Chem.* **1957**, *226*, 497–509. [PubMed]
32. Lichtenstein, A.H.; Matthan, N.R.; Jalbert, S.M.; Resteghini, N.A.; Schaefer, E.J.; Ausman, L.M. Novel soybean oils with different fatty acid profiles alter cardiovascular disease risk factors in moderately hyperlipidemic subjects. *Am. J. Clin. Nutr.* **2006**, *84*, 497–504. [PubMed]
33. Walter, M.F.; Blumberg, J.B.; Dolnikowski, G.G.; Handelman, G.J. Streamlined F2-isoprostane analysis in plasma and urine with high-performance liquid chromatography and gas chromatography/mass spectroscopy. *Anal. Biochem.* **2000**, *280*, 73–79. [CrossRef] [PubMed]
34. Arneson, K.O.; Roberts, L.J., 2nd. Measurement of products of docosahexaenoic acid peroxidation, neuroprostanes, and neurofurans. *Methods Enzymol.* **2007**, *433*, 127–143. [CrossRef] [PubMed]
35. Mukaka, M. A guide to appropriate use of Correlation coefficient in medical research. *Malawi Med. J.* **2012**, *24*, 69–71. [PubMed]
36. Craft, N.E.; Haitema, T.B.; Garnett, K.M.; Fitch, K.A.; Dorey, C.K. Carotenoid, tocopherol, and retinol concentrations in elderly human brain. *J. Nutr. Health Aging* **2004**, *8*, 156–162. [PubMed]
37. Kuchan, M.J.; Jensen, S.K.; Johnson, E.J.; Lieblein-Boff, J.C. The naturally occurring α-tocopherol stereoisomer RRR-α-tocopherol is predominant in the human infant brain. *Br. J. Nutr.* **2016**, *116*, 126–131. [CrossRef] [PubMed]
38. Copp, R.P.; Wisniewski, T.; Hentati, F.; Larnaout, A.; Ben Hamida, M.; Kayden, H.J. Localization of alpha-tocopherol transfer protein in the brains of patients with ataxia with vitamin E deficiency and other oxidative stress related neurodegenerative disorders. *Brain Res.* **1999**, *822*, 80–87. [CrossRef]

39. Zimmer, S.; Stocker, A.; Sarbolouki, M.N.; Spycher, S.E.; Sassoon, J.; Azzi, A. A novel human tocopherol-associated protein: cloning, in vitro expression, and characterization. *J. Biol. Chem.* **2000**, *275*, 25672–25680. [CrossRef] [PubMed]
40. Podda, M.; Weber, C.; Traber, M.G.; Packer, L. Simultaneous determination of tissue tocopherols, tocotrienols, ubiquinols, and ubiquinones. *J. Lipid Res.* **1996**, *37*, 893–901. [PubMed]
41. Zingg, J.-M.; Azzi, A. Non-antioxidant activities of vitamin E. *Curr. Med. Chem.* **2004**, *11*, 1113–1133. [CrossRef] [PubMed]
42. Rota, C.; Rimbach, G.; Minihane, A.M.; Stoecklin, E.; Barella, L. Dietary vitamin E modulates differential gene expression in the rat hippocampus: potential implications for its neuroprotective properties. *Nutr. Neurosci.* **2005**, *8*, 21–29. [CrossRef] [PubMed]
43. Park, S.-K.; Page, G.P.; Kim, K. Differential effect of α- and γ-tocopherol supplementation in age-related transcriptional alterations in heart and brain of B6/C3H F1 mice. *J. Nutr.* **2008**, *138*, 1010–1018. [PubMed]
44. Gohil, K.; Schock, B.C.; Chakraborty, A.A.; Terasawa, Y.; Raber, J.; Farese, R.V., Jr.; Packer, L.; Cross, C.E.; Traber, M.G. Gene expression profile of oxidant stress and neurodegeneration in transgenic mice deficient in alpha-tocopherol transfer protein. *Free Radic. Biol. Med.* **2003**, *35*, 1343–1354. [CrossRef]
45. Berchtold, N.C.; Coleman, P.D.; Cribbs, D.H.; Rogers, J.; Gillen, D.L.; Cotman, C.W. Synaptic genes are extensively downregulated across multiple brain regions in normal human aging and Alzheimer's disease. *Neurobiol. Aging* **2013**, *34*, 1653–1661. [CrossRef] [PubMed]
46. Berchtold, N.C.; Sabbagh, M.N.; Beach, T.G.; Kim, R.C.; Cribbs, D.H.; Cotman, C.W. Brain gene expression patterns differentiate Mild Cognitive Impairment from normal Aged and Alzheimer Disease. *Neurobiol. Aging* **2014**, *35*, 1961–1972. [CrossRef] [PubMed]
47. Simen, A.A.; Bordner, K.A.; Martin, M.P.; Moy, L.A.; Barry, L.C. Cognitive Dysfunction with Aging and the Role of Inflammation. *Ther. Adv. Chronic Dis.* **2011**, *2*, 175–195. [CrossRef] [PubMed]
48. Atkinson, J.; Harroun, T.; Wassall, S.R.; Stillwell, W.; Katsaras, J. The location and behavior of alpha-tocopherol in membranes. *Mol. Nutr. Food Res.* **2010**, *54*, 641–651. [CrossRef] [PubMed]
49. Raederstorff, D.; Wyss, A.; Calder, P.C.; Weber, P.; Eggersdorfer, M. Vitamin E function and requirements in relation to PUFA. *Br. J. Nutr.* **2015**, *114*, 1113–1122. [CrossRef] [PubMed]
50. Montine, T.J.; Montine, K.S.; Reich, E.E.; Terry, E.S.; Porter, N.A.; Morrow, J.D. Antioxidants significantly affect the formation of different classes of isoprostanes and neuroprostanes in rat cerebral synaptosomes. *Biochem. Pharmacol.* **2003**, *65*, 611–617. [CrossRef]
51. Reich, E.E.; Montine, K.S.; Gross, M.D.; Roberts, L.J., 2nd; Swift, L.L.; Morrow, J.D.; Montine, T.J. Interactions between Apolipoprotein E Gene and Dietary α-Tocopherol Influence Cerebral Oxidative Damage in Aged Mice. *J. Neurosci.* **2001**, *21*, 5993–5999. [PubMed]
52. Lebold, K.M.; Traber, M.G. Interactions between alpha-tocopherol, polyunsaturated fatty acids, and lipoxygenases during embryogenesis. *Free Radic. Biol. Med.* **2014**, *66*, 13–19. [CrossRef] [PubMed]

13

Phylogeny of the Vitamin K 2,3-Epoxide Reductase (VKOR) Family and Evolutionary Relationship to the Disulfide Bond Formation Protein B (DsbB) Family

Carville G. Bevans [1], Christoph Krettler [2], Christoph Reinhart [2], Matthias Watzka [3] and Johannes Oldenburg [3,*]

[1] Im Hermeshain 6, 60388 Frankfurt am Main, Germany; E-Mail: bevans@jhu.edu
[2] Department of Molecular Membrane Biology, Max Planck Institute of Biophysics, 60388 Frankfurt am Main, Germany; E-Mails: christoph.krettler@biophys.mpg.de (C.K.); christoph.reinhart@biophys.mpg.de (C.R.)
[3] Institute of Experimental Haematology and Transfusion Medicine, University Clinic Bonn, 53105 Bonn, Germany; E-Mail: matthias.watzka@ukb.uni-bonn.de
* Author to whom correspondence should be addressed; E-Mail: johannes.oldenburg@ukb.uni-bonn.de

Abstract: In humans and other vertebrate animals, vitamin K 2,3-epoxide reductase (VKOR) family enzymes are the gatekeepers between nutritionally acquired K vitamins and the vitamin K cycle responsible for posttranslational modifications that confer biological activity upon vitamin K-dependent proteins with crucial roles in hemostasis, bone development and homeostasis, hormonal carbohydrate regulation and fertility. We report a phylogenetic analysis of the VKOR family that identifies five major clades. Combined phylogenetic and site-specific conservation analyses point to clade-specific similarities and differences in structure and function. We discovered a single-site determinant uniquely identifying VKOR homologs belonging to human pathogenic, obligate intracellular prokaryotes and protists. Building on previous work by Sevier *et al.* (*Protein Science* 14:1630), we analyzed structural data from both VKOR and prokaryotic disulfide bond formation protein B (DsbB) families and hypothesize an ancient evolutionary relationship between the two families where one family arose from the other through a gene duplication/deletion event. This has resulted in circular permutation of primary sequence threading through the four-helical bundle protein folds of both families. This is the first report of circular permutation relating distant α-helical membrane protein sequences and folds. In conclusion, we suggest a chronology for the evolution of the five extant VKOR clades.

Keywords: cyclic permutation; DsbB; homology modeling; phylogeny; sequence conservation; vitamin K; vitamin K 2,3-epoxide; VKOR; VKORC1; VKORC1L1

---

1. Introduction

In humans and other animals, vitamin K 2,3-epoxide complex subunit 1 (VKORC1) is the primary oxidoreductase enzyme that reduces vitamin K quinone (K), acquired in trace amounts by dietary uptake, to the hydroquinone (KH_2) form, functioning as the point of entry for vitamin K into the vitamin K cycle [1–3]. Subsequently, vitamin K hydroquinone is oxidized to vitamin K 2,3-epoxide (K>O) during the posttranslational activation of vitamin K-dependent (VKD) proteins involving enzymatic conversion of specific glutamate (Glu) residues to γ-carboxyglutamate (Gla) residues. To complete the cycle, VKORC1 sequentially reduces K>O to K and KH_2, ensuring that the limiting trace amounts of vitamin K are efficiently recycled to drive further rounds of γ-glutamyl carboxylation.

VKORC1 has been demonstrated to be essential to the production of VKD blood clotting factors which takes place in liver hepatocytes [4]. Suboptimal availability of K from dietary sources can eventually result in interruption of vitamin K cycle turnover and lead to pathophysiological anticoagulation and, in the extreme case, uncontrollable bleeding [3,5]. In the case of pathological hypercoagulative conditions such as thrombosis and embolism, 4-hydroxycoumarin based oral anticoagulants, including warfarin as a well-known example, are administered to block the enzymatic function of VKORC1, effectively diminishing turnover of the vitamin K cycle [6]. This results in induction of a controlled hypocoagulative state to counteract the tendency towards clot formation. Thus, the biological action of vitamin K on hemostasis, mediated by function of the VKORC1 enzyme, is entirely dependent on vitamin K nutritional status and, occasionally, on treatment with oral anticoagulant drugs. Very recently, evidence has been presented that a second VKOR enzyme, VKORC1-like 1 (VKORC1L1), is responsible for extrahepatic VKOR activity crucial to bone growth and homeostasis [7,8]. Interestingly, although VKORC1L1 carries out the same two enzymatic steps of the vitamin K cycle as does VKORC1, it appears to be far less sensitive to oral anticoagulant drugs, suggesting that its biological activity may not be substantially reduced when oral anticoagulants are administered at levels that effectively modulate hemostasis and reduce coagulation tendency [7,9].

To date, homologous VKOR enzymes have been detected in hundreds of prokaryotic and eukaryotic species through whole genome sequencing efforts. A number of representative VKOR enzymes from bacteria, plants and animals have been cloned and studied [7,9–16]. Surprisingly, bacterial and plant VKOR homologs studied so far have been shown to not possess K>O de-epoxidase (VKOR) activity and do not use K>O as a substrate. Alternatively, these enzymes possess only quinone reductase activity which reduces ubiquinone or K substrates to the respective hydroquinone forms. Thus, an updated analysis of VKOR oxidoreductase family phylogenetics and associated review of functional and structural similarities and differences is warranted.

Structural and functional similarities among prokaryotic periplasmic and eukaryotic ER-resident oxidoreductase families involved in oxidative protein folding have been previously suggested, although lack of significant sequence homology suggests these families arose independently during evolution [17]. Specifically, these include Endopasmic Reticulum Oxidoreductin 1 (ERO1, PFAM PF04137, common to all eukaryotes), Augmenter of Liver Regeneration (Erv1/Alr, PFAM PF04777, common to all eukaryotes, some proteobacteria, cyanobacteria and all known cytoplasmic DNA virus taxa), and Disulfide Bond-forming protein B (DsbB, PFAM PF02600, common only to prokaryotes) families that share similar pairs of redox-active disulfide motifs [18]. Recently, studies confirmed a direct role for VKORC1 in oxidative protein folding in addition to its classically reported role in the vitamin K cycle which enables post-translational γ-glutamyl carboxylation of vitamin K-dependent proteins including a number of blood clotting factors [19,20]. VKORC1 is a representative of the vitamin K epoxide reductase family (VKOR, PFAM PF07884), named for the enzymatic function first identified in humans and rodents, namely, vitamin K 2,3-epoxide reductase (VKOR) activity, which is potently inhibited by warfarin and other 4-hydroxycoumarin derivatives [10,11]. Since the 1950s, warfarin and homologous 4-hydroxycoumarins have been the most widely prescribed oral anticoagulants to treat thromboembolitic diseases in humans and, at much higher, lethal dosages as rodenticides [21]. VKOR family sequences also possess two redox-active cysteine pairs and have been detected in taxa from the entire Tree of Life except for yeasts and fungi [22,23]. In prokaryotes, either VKOR or DsbB homologs are required for oxidative protein folding (Figure 1) [24,25]. Both DsbB and VKOR enzymes receive reducing equivalents via thioredoxin-like (Trx-like) oxidoreductases from pairs of redox-active cysteines during oxidative protein folding, ultimately passing the reducing equivalents to diffusible quinone cofactors. DsbB cofactors include ubiquinones (UQ) principally for aerobically respiring taxa and menaquinones (MK, K_2 vitamins) for anaerobic respirants [26]. With the exception of only a very few obligate intracellular prokaryotic pathogens, all prokaryotic VKOR homologs apparently use UQ or MK, while plant VKORs use phylloquinone (PK, vitamin K_1) as the sole electron accepting cofactor. All other eukaryote genomes from single-celled protists through higher invertebrates and vertebrates, but not those of fungi, encode VKOR homologs that can use MK or PK as cofactors, while jawed vertebrates (gnathostomes) can additionally use the more highly oxidized 2,3-epoxides of K vitamins which are naturally produced only in taxa possessing genomically encoded-glutamyl carboxlase homologs. While menaquinone 2,3-epoxides have been found in vertebrates, they are not known to exist in any prokaryotes [27,28].

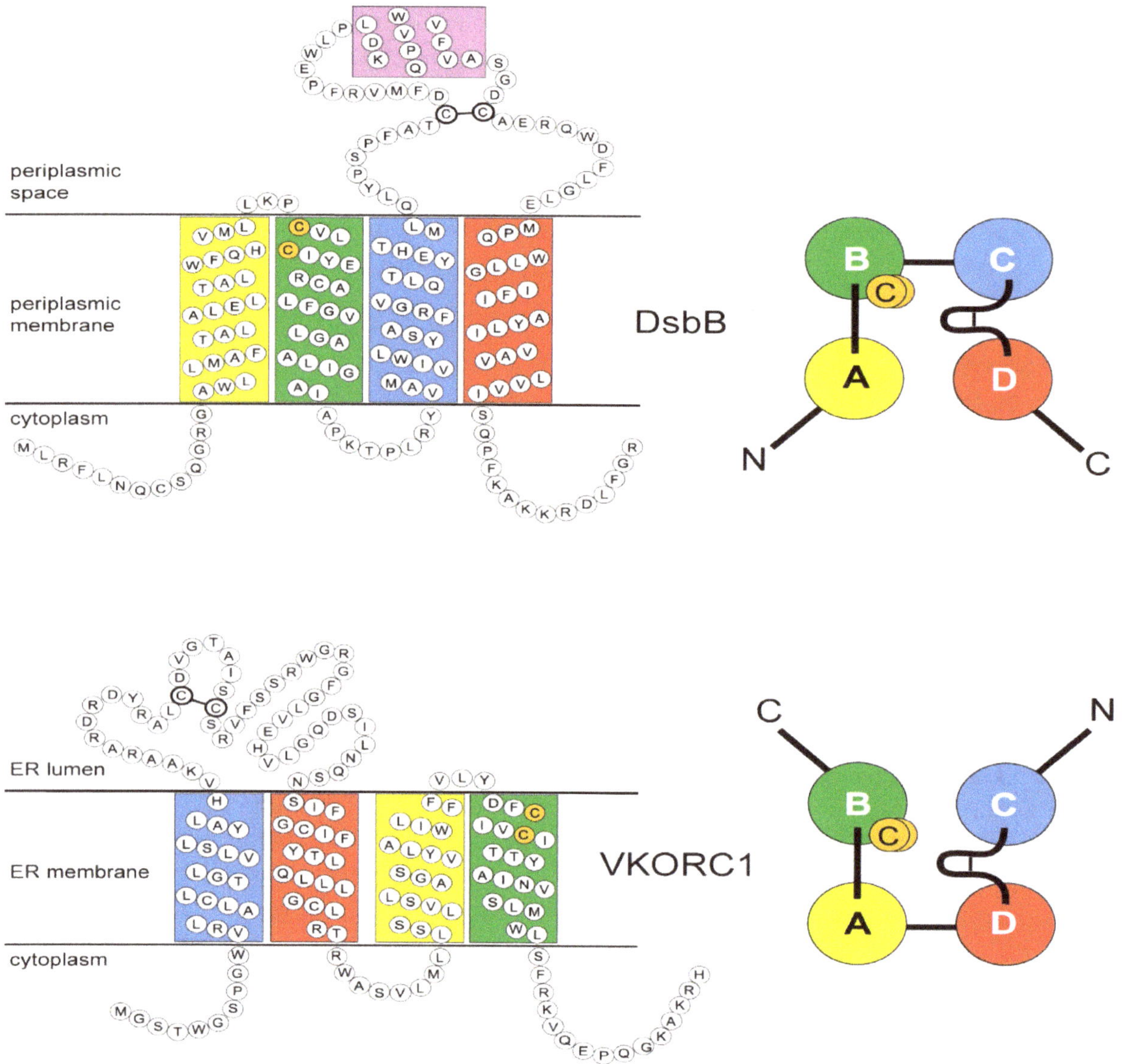

Figure 1. Relationship of structural elements for *E. coli* DsbB and human VKORC1. Single-letter amino acids (circles); transmembrane helices (four colored rectangles; coloring scheme according to [17]); two active site cysteines (orange circles); DsbB (top left) short helix (purple rectangle); two redox-active cysteines in DsbB large periplasmic loop (thick connected circles); Human VKORC1 (bottom left), transmembrane helix colors for homologous positions relative to DsbB. Transmembrane helical bundle organization and primary sequence threading (N, N-terminus; C, C-terminus) for DsbB (top right, view from periplasm) and VKORC1 (bottom right, view from ER lumen) are shown based on X-ray crystallographic structures. Letters A–D on the right side indicate helix designations used throughout the text. N- to C-terminus direction threading of the primary sequence through DsbB is "ABCD", but "CDAB" for VKORC1; thus, both threadings are related to each other by circular permutation (CP). Structural elements for DsbB from PDB entry 2HI7 [29], for VKORC1 from PDB entry 3KP9 [14].

Five studies have previously explored VKOR family phylogeny. Rost *et al.* (2004) reported cloning paralogous pairs of VKOR genes in human, rat, mouse and the fish Takifugu ruprides and identified VKOR homologs by gene annotations in the mosquito Anopheles gambiae, but not in the fruit fly Drosophila melangaster, suggesting that evolution of VKOR family proteins was later than the evolution of carboxylase enzymes for which *Drosophila* is known to possess a homologous gene [10]. They also noted the existence of two human VKORC1 retropseudogenes that arose independently. Goodstadt & Ponting (2004) presented a multiple sequence alignment analysis identifying VKOR homologs in 37 species of archaea, eubacteria, plants, invertebrates and vertebrates [22]. They further identified four conserved cysteines and a conserved serine/threonine as residues likely required for enzymatic function. Additionally, they noted that many plant and prokaryote VKOR homologs are multidomain proteins that often include a C-terminal thioredoxin-like domain in addition to the core VKOR domain. Using prediction algorithms, they also identified four putative transmembrane helices in the VKOR core domain. Indeed, a four-helical bundle organization of the VKOR domain was recently confirmed for a prokaryotic VKOR homolog by X-ray crystallographic analysis [14,30]. A study by Robertson (2004) confirmed that, while vertebrate genomes encode two VKOR paralogs, only single VKOR homologs are present in invertebrates, basal deuterostomes, protists and plants with no VKOR homologs detected in fungal taxa [23]. He also identified additional VKOR family retropseudogenes—three similar to human VKORC1L1, five similar to VKORC1L1 in mouse and three with VKORC1L1 similarity in rat. In contrast to the report by Rost *et al.*, Robertson was able to detect a VKOR homolog sequence in *Drosophila melanogaster* [10]. Robertson calculated an inferred phylogenetic tree with low bootstrap support using trypanosome protists as an outgroup, representing the most highly divergent homologs from higher animals. His results suggest that a gene duplication occurred resulting in VKORC1 and VKORC1L1 clades after vertebrates diverged from non-chordates. Schwarz *et al.* (2009) used profile hidden Markov models derived from multiple sequence alignments and correspondence analysis to distinguish between evolutionary and functional site-specific signals for VKORC1/VKORC1L1 paralog pairs of twelve vertebrate species [31]. Their analytical methods were able to distinguish functionally conserved and variable sites, detect clade-specific sequence clustering and revealed specific sites associated with clade splittings. Importantly, they identified the timing of the duplication event leading to VKORC1 and VKORC1L1 paralogs as occurring at the base of the vertebrate split from other metazoans. Finally, a recent study by Wan *et al.* (2014) that identified and characterized a VKOR family homolog in the tomato plant, presented evidence suggesting that all plant VKOR homologs possess an N-terminal signal peptide responsible for transit of the protein to inner thylakoid membranes and a C-terminal thioredoxin-like domain with four conserved cysteines [16]. They constructed a phylogenetic tree with 41 species that include plants, algae, photosynthetic bacteria and vertebrate animals. Vertebrates, monocot and dicot plants were segregated into three distinct clades, while conifers, mosses, cyanobacteria and green algae formed a weak clade with low branch support. Highest branch supports were for monocots and vertebrates.

In the present study, we reconstruct a comprehensive phylogeny for the VKOR family that includes 327 sequences from major representative phyla of the Kingdoms of Life and use the results to define major clades, explore clade-specific sequence differences that correlate with structural and functional differences of the clades, and propose an evolutionary scenario for the VKOR family that suggests an ancient common ancestor shared with the DsbB family.

2. Experimental Section

2.1. Protein Sequences and Multiple Sequence Alignments

Protein sequences were obtained from the NCBI Conserved Domain Database (http://www.ncbi.nlm.nih.gov/cdd/) and from the PFAM database (http://pfam.xfam.org) for VKOR (CDD: cl01729, VKOR Superfamily, 3748 raw sequences; PFAM: PF07884, VKOR family, 864 raw sequences) and DsbB (CDD: cl00649, DsbB Superfamily, 6673 raw sequences; PFAM:

PF02600, DsbB family, 2959 raw sequences) families [32,33]. For each family, sequences were initially aligned using the MAFFT fast algorithm (FFT-NS-1 option) implemented in JalView2.8 by masking non-core domain sequence segments (core domains defined as DsbB (*E. coli*): Trp15-Ile162 and VKOR (*Synechococcus* sp.): Ile22-Val148 including first residue of first transmembrane helix to last residue of fourth transmembrane helix based on X-ray crystallographic data from PDB entries 2HI7 and 3KP9, respectively) [34,35]. Identical sequences from redundant species, partial or unrelated sequences not fully encompassing the core domain lengths, and sequences lacking known conserved residues were manually culled. Further reduction of sequences in over-represented phyla and classes resulted in final data sets of 327 non-redundant VKOR and 514 non-redundant DsbB sequences for phylogenetic analysis. The DsbB family multiple sequence alignment (MSA) was not subjected to further phylogenetic analysis. For the full-length (multidomain) MSA for the VKOR family, N- and C-terminal non-core domains were aligned independently of the core domain. Core domain alignment was iteratively refined based on WSP and consistency scores using MAFFT (G-INS-i option) and manually adjusted to align any obvious positionally conserved residues while minimizing the number of gapped segments. Additional sequence-truncated versions of each MSA included either only the core domains (defined above) or a 44 residue subsequence comprising the large loop joining the 1st and 2nd transmembrane helices of the VKOR core domain ("VKORloop"—delimited by VKORC1(*H. sapiens*): Asp36-Ser79). All multiple sequence alignment and tree files are included with the online Supplementary Materials and Research Data.

2.2. Phylogenetic Analyses

Maximum Likelihood (ML) analyses were conducted using the TOPALi2 ver2.5 (http://www.topali.org/index.shtml) and IQ-TREE ver1.2.3 (http://www.cibiv.at/software/iqtree/) server-based phylogenetic packages [36,37]. Phylogenetic model testing and selection included 40 distinct models by TOPALi2 and 150 models by IQ-TREE. Model evaluation was based on standard Akaike infomation criterion (AIC), corrected AIC (cAIC) and Bayesian information criterion (BIC) scores, where best models correlate with minimized scores. Preliminary ML phylogenetic tree reconstructions were estimated using either PhyML3.0 [38] or RaxML8.0.0 [39] with branch supports for 1000 bootstrap replicates calculated by the rapid UFBoot method [40]. The final VKORloop consensus tree was constructed from 1000 bootstrap trees using the IQ-TREE1.0 tree search algorithm [37]. Branch lengths were optimized by maximum likelihood on original alignment and bootstrap branch support calculated. To simplify visual presentation, the consensus tree was further pruned to 310 sequences using IQ-TREE1.0 and graphically rendered using the Interactive Tree of Life (iTOL) server (http://itol.embl.de) [41].

2.3. Assessment of Residue-Specific Evolutionary Conservation and Structural Correlates

For determination of residue-specific sequence conservation from VKOR and DsbB family MSAs, we used the ConSurf server (http://consurf.tau.ac.il) [42,43]. Briefly, ConSurf computes position-specific evolutionary rate inferences as continuous-variable conservation scores using the empirical Bayesian algorithm. The server creates an output text file where the continuous conservation scores are binned into nine grades for visualization, from the most variable positions (grade 1, colored turquoise), through intermediately conserved positions (grade 5, colored white), to the most conserved positions (grade 9, colored maroon). We mapped these conservation grades onto MSAs using JalView2.8 for analysis and graphical rendering. We further explored structural features corresponding to the conservation data revealed by ConSurf analysis by using the TMPad server (http://bio-cluster.iis.sinica.edu.tw/TMPad/) to visualize and determine residues involved in direct interhelical contacts from the representative X-ray crystallographic structures (PDB entries 2HI7 and 3KP9) [44].

2.4. Homology Modeling of Human VKORC1 and VKORC1L1 Paralogs Using a Cyclic Permutation of E. coli DsbB as the Target Structure

Homology models of human VKORC1 and VKORC1L1 were created using template sequences from the NCBI Protein database (Accession: Q9BQB6.1 GI: 62511226 and Accession: Q8N0U8.2 GI: 62511214, respectively) and *E. coli* DsbB (PDB entry 2K74, model 1 [45]) as template structure. The nearly identical lengths of DsbB (176 aa), VKORC1 (163 aa) and VKORC1L1 (176 aa) suggested to us that indels would not be a major concern in modeling. Briefly, we swapped the first and second halves of the VKORC1 and VKORC1L1 primary sequences in order to create an optimized alignment to the DsbB sequence (see Figures S1–S4 and detailed methods in the online Supplementary Materials and Research Data) and generated initial models using MODELLER 9v7 [46]. In order to restore the native primary sequences and threading, the best quality initial models were edited to join the N- and C-termini and create new termini at the loop between the second and third transmembrane helices (TMHs) using Coot 0.6-pre-1 [47]. The 50 residue loops between the first and second TMHs of the edited models were replaced with same-sequence loops *de novo* modeled using the I-TASSER server [48]. Addition of hydrogen atoms and quality assessment of final models was performed using the MolProbity server [49]. Final models were submitted to the Protein Model DataBase (VKORC1: PMDB entry PM0075969, VKORC1L1: PM007970; both models deposited 21 September 2009, public release 1 September 2010).

3. Results

3.1. Multiple Sequence Alignments Reveal Greater Inhomogeneity in Indels for the VKOR Family Core Domain Relative to the DsbB Family

Initial inspection of high quality multiple sequence alignments for the core domains of the VKOR family (327 sequences, truncated to residues corresponding to human VKORC1: Leu13-Phe150 in order to remove highly variable N- and C-terminal sequences) and DsbB family (514 sequences, truncated to residues corresponding to *E. coli* DsbB: Gly13-Pro165 in order to remove highly variable N- and C-terminal sequences) revealed a larger heterogeneity in indel sizes and locations for the VKOR core domain (10 major indels for >1 sequences, ranging 2–27 residues in length) relative to the DsbB core domain (5 major indels for >1 sequences, ranging 2–11 residues in length) (see online Supplementary Materials Figures S5 and S6 and Research Data for FASTA-formatted MSA and graphical summary files; only non-terminal indels were counted in order to avoid possible incomplete sequencing reads in the original data; minor indels comprising single residues were not included.) Thus, the greater overall sequence diversity for the VKOR family core domain suggests greater overall evolutionary diversity, relative to the DsbB core domain. This is consistent with the evolutionary limitation of DsbB family taxa to prokaryotes *versus* the expansion of the VKOR family taxa into all major Kingdoms of Life.

3.2. VKOR Family Phylogeny is Organized into Five Principal Clades

Testing of standard phylogenetic amino acid substitution models using both TOPALi2 and IQ-TREE for the VKOR family MSA using 327 non-redundant full-length sequences resulted in the Whelan & Goldman rate heterogeneity model with invariant sites as the best model (see online Supplementary Materials and Research Data for sequences, MSAs and substitution model statistics). Subsequent phylogeny reconstruction using PhyML or RaxML revealed unrooted trees with five large cladistic groupings, although two clades included mixed prokaryotic, invertebrate and vertebrate VKOR homologs and animal sequences were found among the predominantly bacterial and plant clades. Similar results were obtained, with increased mingling of prokaryotic sequences among the predominantly invertebrate and vertebrate clades, when we truncated the MSA to include only the VKOR core domain (defined in Section 2.1). Previous reports have suggested that TMHs considerably contribute to phylogenetic noise, due to high frequency of occurrance and degeneracy among nonpolar residues in the hydrophobic membrane core and a relatively low selection pressure on residues that face into the lipid bilayer [50,51]. Also, a phylogenetic study of DsbB family homologs reported difficulties in automated sequence alignments due to amino acid compositional bias in the transmembrane region [52]. Accordingly, to enhance phylogenetic signal-to-noise levels for the VKOR family, we chose to further truncate the MSA to the large loop segment between the first two TMHs for two principal reasons: (1) the loop includes three out of five conserved residues known to be essential to VKOR enzymatic activity and other residues in this segment may also contribute to substrate specificity and/or catalysis; and (2) the loop is known to bind to and accept reducing equivalents from species-specific partner oxidoreductases essential for VKOR enzymatic function *in vivo* [53]. Thus, the loop-specific sequences (50 residues) encode a large amount of evolutionary information pertinent to enzyme function. Indeed, phylogeny reconstruction using the VKORloop sequences (corresponding to human VKORC1: Asp36-Ser79) and the best model (WAG + I + G) yielded a consensus tree with well-defined clades consistent with proposed versions of the Tree of Life based on, for example, ribosomal protein or tRNA synthase phylogeny (Figure 2) [54–57].

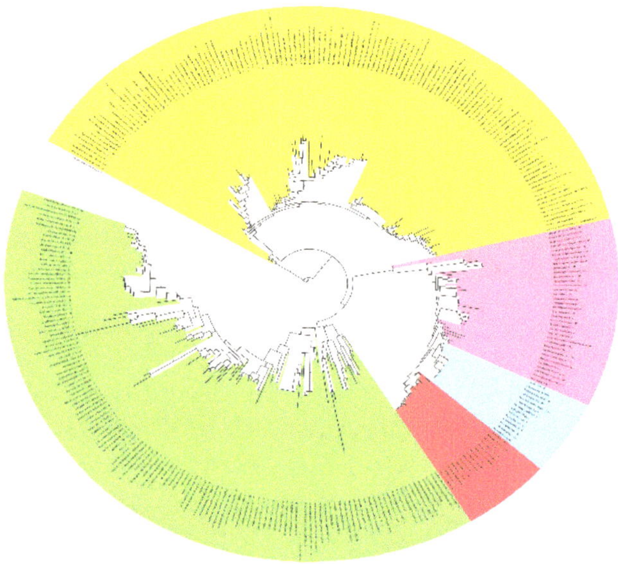

Figure 2. Maximum likelihood-estimated phylogeny for VKOR family based on VKORloop sequences for 327 non-redundant sequences (pruned to 310 sequences). Five major clades are shown in color (yellow, non-photosynthetic prokaryotes; green, photosynthetic prokaryotes and plants; magenta, primitive single-celled animals and invertebrates; blue, vertebrate VKORC1L1 homologs; red, vertebrate VKORC1 homologs. Tree is rooted using the archaeon *Caldivirga maquilingensis* as outgroup (single uncolored branch between yellow and green clades). Numbers at branches (see online Supplementary Materials and Research Data; visible when enlarged in PDF reader) indicate bootstrap supports (%). Accurate inclusion of all sequences in the VKORC1 and VKORC1L1 clades was manually verified despite incorrect annotations in some sequence database entries that led to false name assignments (e.g., where C1 and L1, representing VKORC1 and VKORC1L1, respectively, are indicated after the genus/species names). A PDF file of this figure is included with online supplementary data for enlarged viewing.

Figure 3 summarizes the major taxonomic classes and phyla comprising the five clades for the 327 non-redundant sequences. Clade 1 (Figure 2, colored yellow) is polyphyletic and includes non-photosynthetic archea and eubacteria. Actinobacteria, one of the three major Gram-positive phyla, comprise the major grouping along with acidobacteria, crenarchaeota (including species of the *Caldivirga*, *Pyrobaculum* and *Thermoproteus* genera grouped together in a discrete subclade), proteobacteria and spirochete representatives. All actinobacteria possess a predicted fifth transmembrane helix (TMH), but no C-terminal Trx-like domain, whereas proteobacteria and spirochetes possess both a fifth TMH and C-terminal Trx-like domain. Clades 2 and 3 (Figure 2, blue and red, respectively) are both individually and together monophyletic and include members of the vertebrate VKORC1 and VKORC1L1 paralogs, respectively, as single VKOR domains. Clade 4 (Figure 2, magenta) is paraphyletic and comprises single-domain VKOR homologs encoded in genomes of non-vertebrate animals including amoebazoans, choanoflagellates and lower metazoans through invertebrates. Clade 5 (Figure 2, green) is polyphyletic and comprises archaea, eubacteria and eukaryotes capable of various forms of photosynthesis from green sulfur-metabolizing hyperthermophilic prokaryotes through algae and higher plants. Bacteriodetes, Chloroflexus and Roseiflexus taxa all have additional N-terminal domains. Trx-like CXXC signature motifs are found in only the Chloroflexus and Roseiflexus N-terminal domains and these taxa lack C-terminal Trx-like domains. All other clade 5 taxa possess C-terminal Trx-like domains except for Archaea and Gemmatimonadetes. Interestingly, Clade 5 includes intermingled archaeal and eukaryotic taxa, suggesting horizontal gene transfer (HGT): a cluster of three archaeal *Pyrobaculum* species, all different from those in Clade 1, appear along with a single Verrucomicrobia representative (genus *Chthoniobacter*), the only non-photosynth grouping in Clade 5 (there are, however, other single Verrucomicrobia sequences intermingled among various Clade 5 branches, further suggesting HGT); a single Rhizaria eukaryote, *Paulinella chromatophora*, is found on a Clade 5 branch between branches bearing *Synechococcus* species. *P. chromatophora* is a freshwater amoeboid widely noted for its very recently acquired cyanobacterial symbiont previously believed to stem from an ancestor of either *Synechococcus* or *Prochlorococcus* genera [58]. Compared to free living *Synechococcus* species, the *P. chromatophora* plastid has retained ~26% of the original genome (*i.e.*, retained 867 protein-coding genes), although the VKOR family homolog (NCBI Protein: YP_002048937.1) was previously transferred, along with most of the plastid genes, to the *P. chromatophora* nuclear genome [59]. Thus, our reconstruction of the VKORloop phylogeny strongly suggests that the *P. chromatophora* chloroplast evolved from an acquired *Synechococcus* endosymbiont, further resolving the uncertainty of a phylogenetic reconstruction study by Marin *et al.*, based on analysis of concatenated rDNA operon or rRNA sequences, to determine if the ancestral endosymbiont was an ancestor of *Synechococcus* or *Prochlorococcus* [60].

3.3. Similarities and Differences among Sequence Position-Specific Substitutions Reveal VKOR Family Clade-Specific Structural and Functional Residues

In order to explore VKOR family clade-dependent and clade-independent sequence conservation, and to assess if conserved sites might have functional or structural correlates, we performed site-specific conservational analyses on the complete MSA as well as on the aligned sequences for each of the five identified VKOR family clades. Figure 4 graphically summarizes the conservation analysis results.

We identified 22 residue positions (Figure 4, bold black letters **s**, **f**, **x** below the Clade 1 line) that are highly conserved across all VKOR clades. We have assigned structural and functional roles to these positions as follows:

(1) The five fully conserved VKOR signature residue positions (Figure 4, marked **f**) are functional, playing direct roles in vitamin K 2,3-epoxide to vitamin K quinone and vitamin K quinone to vitamin K quinol reduction (Cys43, Cys51, Ser57, Cys132, Cys135 according to human VKORC1 numbering);
(2) Nine highly conserved positions (Figure 4, marked **s**) represent residues that form putative helix-helix structural contacts identified by visual inspection of the X-ray crystallographic structure for the prokaryotic VKOR homolog (PDB entry 3KP9, residue numbering corresponds to human VKORC1 sequence in Figure 4). On TMH1, Cys16, Gly19, Ser23 and Ala26 pack against TMH2, TMH2 and TMH4, TMH2, TMH2 and TMH3, respectively. On TMH2, Ser81 and Gly84 both pack against TMH1. On TMH3, Ser117 packs against TMH4, while Leu124 packs against only residues on the same helix (TMH3). On TMH4, Thr138 packs against TMH1;

(3) Eight highly conserved positions (Figure 4, marked **x**) may be putative functional residues either essential for quinone substrate reduction or involved in substrate binding and specificity (Asp44, Gly80, Gly84, Asn80, Tyr88, Gly95, Leu120, Leu128).

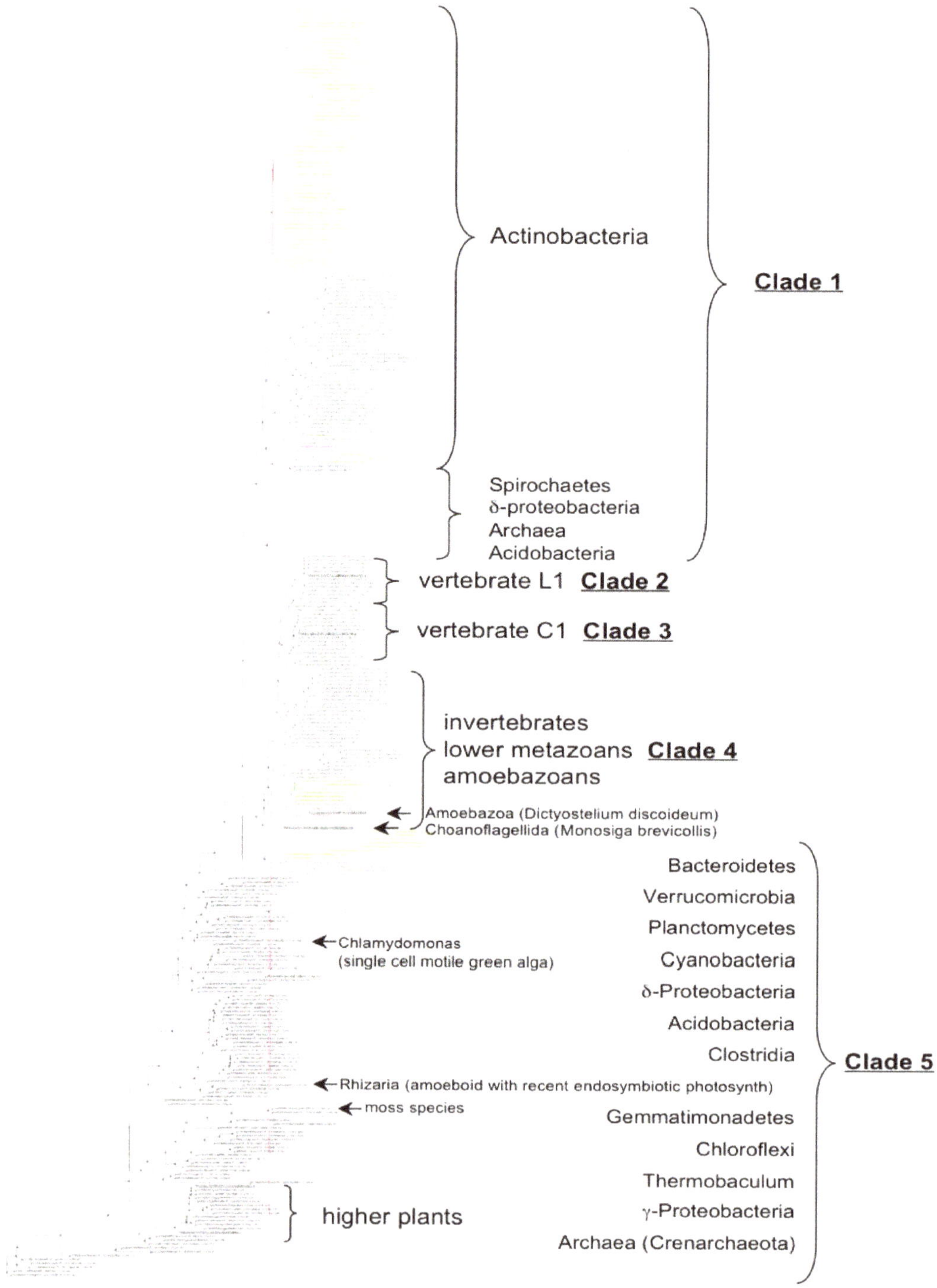

Figure 3. Cladogram (unrooted tree) of VKORloop sequences identifying groupings into highest common Linnaean taxonomic ranks. (See online supplemental data for a complete listing of protein identifiers in the FASTA-formatted MSA file; also, Figure S7 of the online Supplementary Materials and Research Data shows the full-length aligned sequences, including non-VKOR domains, corresponding to the cladogram in this figure).

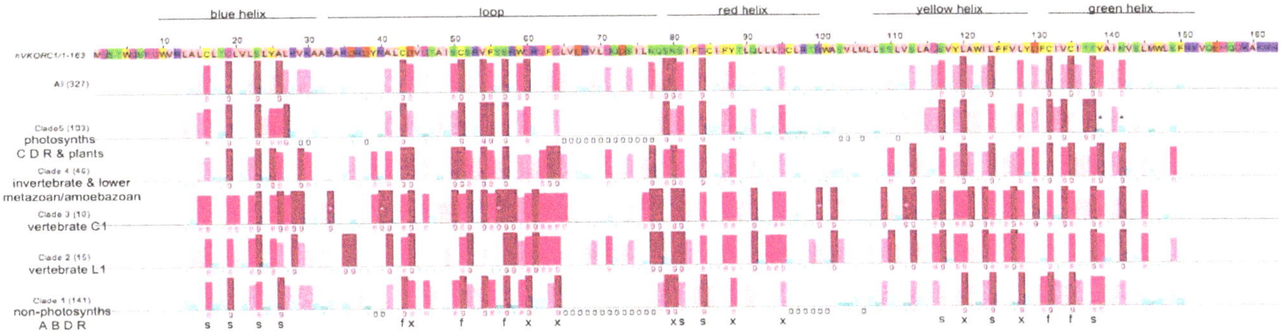

Figure 4. Comparison of Consurf conservational scoring for combined VKOR family sequences and the five individual VKOR clades. Human VKORC1 primary sequence is with relative postions of transmembrane helices (indicated using color scheme from [17]) and large loop as line segments (top); calculated Consurf conservation scores on lines below the sequence (six lines, top to bottom): All 327 VKOR sequences; Clade 5, 103 photosynthetic prokaryotes of the super-taxa C, D and R (prokaryotic super-taxa: A = Actinobacteria, B = Bacilli an related, C = Clostridia and related, D = double membrane Gram-negative bacteria, R = Archaea [56]); Clade 4, 46 invertebrates, lower metazoans, euglenozoans and mycetozoans; Clade 3, 10 vertebrate VKORC1 orthologs; Clade 2, 15 vertebrate VKORC1L1 orthologs; Clade 1, 141 non-photosynthetic prokaryotes of the super-taxa A, B, D and R. Darker red bars indicate greater positional conservation, darker blue bars indicate greater positional non-conservation (conservation scores below bars; lowest score 1 to highest score 9). Systematically absent from the prokaryotic sequences (clades 1 and 5) indicated with black zeros in place of Consurf scores. Fully conserved vertebrate VKORC1 residues (white asterisks superimposed upon dark red bars); Clade 5-specific absences of conserved Tyr139 and Asn142 (black asterisks above dark blue bars, human VKORC1 numbering). Letters and symbols (bottom) for positions highly conserved across all five major clades: s = structural residue contributing to helix-helix packing interactions; f = residues full conserved across all species and presumed to be catalytically active (Cys43, Cys51, Ser57, Cys132, Cys135); x = residues that are highly conserved, but presently lacking assignment as to structural or functional importance.

Notable differences in position-specific conservation between VKOR family clades include:

(1) Compared to non-animal VKOR homologs, there are conserved sequence insertions among animal VKOR homologs (clades 2–4; Figure 4, absence of animal-specific sequences indicated as conservation scores "0" for clades 1 and 5). A few of these insertions are individual or adjacent pairs of residues located in two groupings—one at the margin including the C-terminal portion of TMH1 and the large loop joining TMH1 and TMH2, and the other in the C-terminal margin of TMH2 and the variable-sized loop connecting TMH2 and TMH3. The largest insertion is a linear sequence of 13–14 residues that comprise and extension at the C-terminal end of the large loop which joins TMH1 and TMH2. Thus, these animal insertions positively correlate with the representative homologs possessing VKOR (*i.e.*, phyloquinone- and menaquinone-2,3-epoxidase) catalytic activity in addition to general quinone (*i.e.*, menaquinone, phyloquinone or ubiquinone) reductase activity common to all VKOR family members. To-date, with only the exception of demonstrated *in vitro* VKOR activity for two obligate intracellular bacteria that are pathogenic in eukaryotes (*M. tuberculosis*, *Corynebacterium jeikeium*) [13], all representative non-animal VKOR enzymes for which quinone substrate usage has been biochemically characterized were found to lack VKOR activity (eubacteria: *Synechococcus* species [14]; *Synechocystis* sp. PCC6803 [61]; *Roseiflexus* sp. RS-1, *Salinispora tropica* CNB-440 [13]; plants: *Arabidopsis thaliana* [15], *Solanum lycopersicum* [16]).

(2) A site-directed mutagenesis study by Matagrin *et al.* (2013) of rat VKORC1 revealed Tyr139 (homologous residue for human VKORC1 is also Tyr139) to be critical to VKOR catalysis in that removal of a 3-hydroxy group from vitamin K, once the epoxide oxirane ring has been opened, is apparently hindered by substitution of the tyrosine by cysteine, phenylalanine or serine as in naturally occurring warfarin resistant VKORC1 variants in rats [62]. In agreement with their results, a previous study also reported the production of a proposed VKOR catalytic intermediate product, 3-hydroxyvitamin K, by liver microsomes from a homozygous warfarin-resistant HW Welsh rat strain later genotyped as VKORC1:Tyr139Ser [63,64]. We find that tyrosine is completely conserved at the primary sequence position homologous to human and rat Tyr139 among all metazoan VKOR family homologs belonging to Clades 2, 3 and 4. Alternative substitutions at this positions include chiefly tryptophan (infrequently, methionine or threonine) among Clade 1 homologs, while Clade 5 substitutions include chiefly residues with aliphatic side-chains (*i.e.*, Ala, Leu, Ile). Interestingly, the only Clade 1 or 5 homologs with Tyr at this position include prokaryotes of the genera *Leptospira* (spirochetes) and *Streptomyces* (filamentous soil bacteria), *Leishmania* (a genus of trypanosomatid protozoa) and *Trypanosoma* (a genus of kinetoplastid protozoa), all obligate intracellular pathogens in vertebrates, suggesting that these VKOR family homologs might catalyze VKOR activity. At least nine *Streptomyces* species have been reported to be pathogenic in humans (55) [65]. Also, *Leptospira interrogans* is known to possess a gene for a glutamyl carboxylase homolog presumed to have been obtained through HGT, lending support to the possibility that the genomically encoded VKOR family homolog enables production of vitamin K-dependent proteins involved in pathogenesis (56) [66]. For identification purposes, we name this the *LSLT* group of pathogenic organisms.

(3) We identified a covariant site for the *LSLT* pathogenic group at the residue homologous to human VKORC1: Ile136 immediately following the conserved active site CXXC motif. Species in the *LSLT* group possess a cysteine at this position homologous to the human sequence numbering VKORC1: Ile136Cys and include *T. brucei*, *L.* major strain Friedlin, *L. infantum*, and *Streptomyces* species (*coelicolor A3(2)*, *griseus* sub.sp. *griseus*, *sviceus*, sp. SPB74, and two distinctly non-identical VKOR family homologs for sp. Mg1) from our MSA data set. We could not identify any additional position-specific markers in the VKOR core domain for this group.

A notable, distinguishing feature of all vertebrate VKORC1 and VKORC1L1 sequences (clades 2 and 3) is the systematic absence of segments of the large loop region from the prokaryotic sequences (Figure 4; clades 1 and 5, indicated with black zeros among the Consurf scores). Thus, both prokaryotic clades are missing the equivalent of human VKORC1 sequence residues Leu65 through Asn77 that comprise the distal C-terminal residues of the large loops in clade 2, 3 and 4 sequences. Differential clade-specific absences of additional sequence segments occur in the N-terminal portion of the loop as well as in regions comprising portions of the red and yellow helices and adjoining small cytoplasmic loop for the prokaryotes (Figure 4; clades 1 and 5, indicated by black zeros). Vertebrate VKORC1 (clade 3-specific) full conservation is indicated in Figure 4 by white asterisks superimposed upon the highest conservation score bars (dark red) at Arg33, Arg40, Ser56, Arg100 and Val112 (human VKORC1 numbering). Interestingly, lack of clade 5-specific conservation at Tyr139 (human VKORC1 numbering), as well as at Asn142 (one helical turn away from Tyr139) indicates non-conservation at these positions, in striking contrast to conservation at these positions in the other four clades.

3.4. Evidence for an Evolutionary Relationship between VKOR and DsbB Families

In order to investigate our hypothesis that the VKOR and DsbB families may have evolved from a common ancestor, we explored sequence similarity and conservation by creating aligned

Consurf profiles for homologous structural elements from each family based on the availability of high-resolution X-ray crystallographic structures for the representative *Synechococcus* sp. VKOR and *E. coli* DsbB homologs. Specifically, we aligned two different conservation profiles representing helix pair-loop modules. The first (AB) module encompasses the primary sequences including the first two TMHs of VKOR and the last two TMHs for DsbB and including the intervening large loops (Figure 5, upper half). Accordingly, the second (CD) module encompasses the last two TMHs of VKOR and the first two TMHs of DsbB, together with the respective short connecting loops (Figure 5, lower half). As individual sequences among the VKOR and DsbB families have variable lengths due to species-specific indels, we truncated the family MSAs to include only sites of the primary sequences of the human VKORC1 and VKORC1L1 paralogs and *E. coli* DsbB homolog. To align the VKOR and DsbB family conservation profiles for each module, the representative human and prokaryotic index sequences were translated relative to each other until the invariant CXXC motifs were aligned for the AB module; the CD module was aligned by assessing pairwise identity between the VKORC1 and DsbB index sequences and between the VKORC1L1 and DsbB index sequences (Figure 5, black bars). Altogether, the best AB module alignment resulted in a maximum of five identity sites among the three index sequences; the best CD module alignment resulted in a maximum of four identity sites among the three index sequences (Figure 5, for each upper and lower figure halves, compare black bars on both pairwise identity lines). Inspection of the aligned positional conservation scores representing 327 VKOR homologs and 514 DsbB homologs reveals a very strong correlation in position specific conservation (compare patterns of dark red bars representing high Consurf scores).

In addition to the interfamily conservation of the active site CXXC motifs in the AB module for both families, we could assign conserved interhelical contact residues for the DsbB family: five helix-helix contacts (HHCs) for the A helices, three HHCs for the B helices (by inspection of the best high-resolution NMR structure; PDB entry 2K74). Of these DsbB family AB module HHCs, there is a perfect match (Figure 5, top half, AB module alignment position 26) corresponding to an HHC with a Consurf score of 8 at the corresponding human VKORC1:S117 position in the A helix (see Figure 4) representing an HHC also common to all VKOR family members. Similarly, at AB module position 33, the DsbB family conserved HHC matches a VKOR family conserved HHC with a Consurf score of 9 at the corresponding human VKORC1: Leu124 position in the A helix. For the B helices of both families, a conserved HHC at VKORC1: Thr138 with Consurf score 9 matches a similar highly conserved HHC in the DsbB family (Figure 5, upper half, AB module position 47).

For the CD module, the C helix of the DsbB family has five conserved HHCs, of which four VKOR family conserved HHCs including VKORC1: Cys16 (CD module position 23), VKORC1: Gly19 (CD module position 26), VKORC1: Ser23 (CD module position 30) and VKORC1: Ala26 (CD module postion 33) are perfect matches. The DsbB family D helix has three conserved HHCs, for which one VKOR family conserved HHC (VKORC1: Ser81, CD module position 88) is a perfect match.

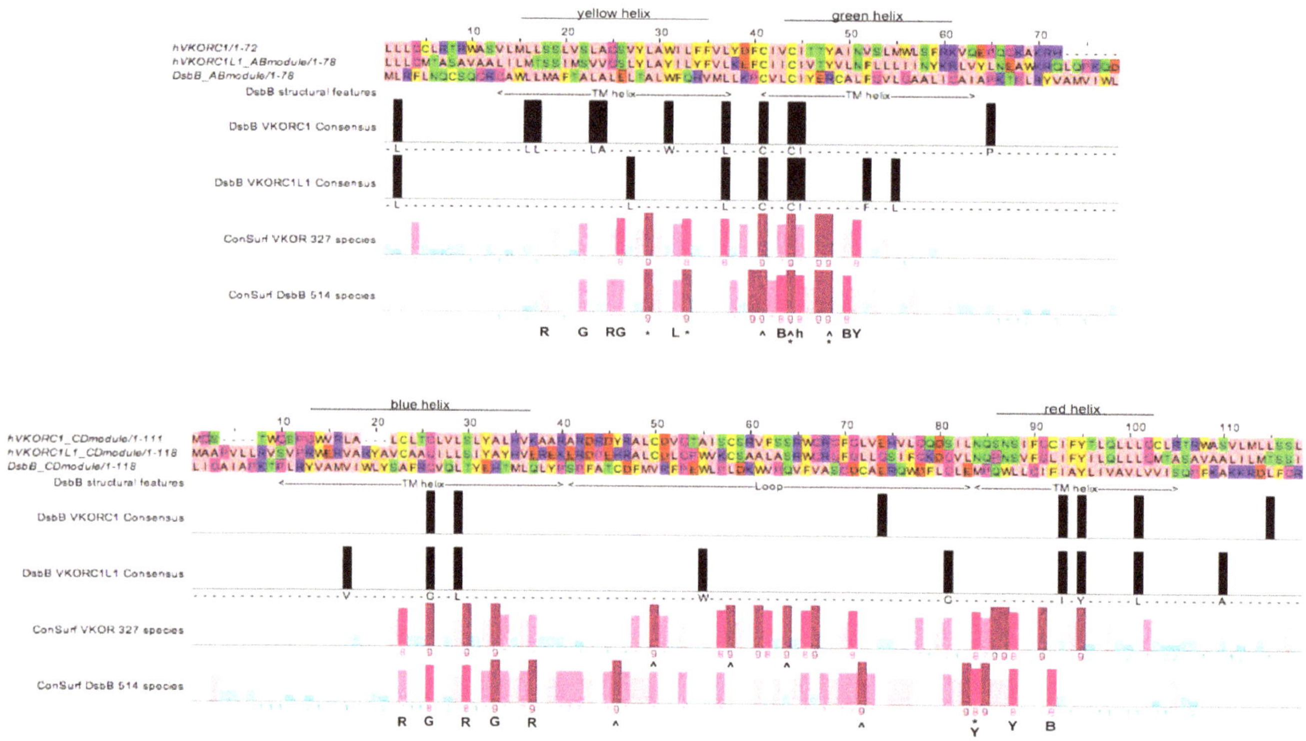

Figure 5. Alignment of helix pair-loop module sequences of VKORC1, VKORC1L1 and DsbB showing pairwise identity, Consurf conservational scoring and known DsbB secondary structure elements and interhelical packing residues (Note 1 [67]). ClustalW2 alignments for AB (top) and CD (bottom) modules. Positions of transmembrane helices for DsbB are indicated below alignment, helix color indicated above alignment. Vertical black bars, sequence identity between DsbB and VKOR proteins; bottom two lines, Consurf conservation scores for VKOR multiple sequence alignment (second from bottom line) and DsbB multiple sequence alignment (bottom line). Vertical colored bars, positional conservation as described in Figure 4—Letters and symbols below conservation score lines: R = interhelical contact to red helix, G = interhelical contact to green helix, B = interhelical contact to blue helix, Y = interhelical contact to yellow helix, * = residue making contact with quinone cofactor, L = residue mediating hydrophobic packing against a C-terminal segment of the large loop, ^ = residues completely conserved in all species, h = residue making hydrophobic contact with the small amphipathic helix of the large loop.

Thus, independent of different threading of primary sequences through the helical bundle for each family (*i.e.*, N- to C-terminus threading comprises helices ordered ABCD for the DsbB family, but CDAB for the VKOR family), a highly conserved network of altogether 8 interhelical structural contacts (3 AB module and 5 CD module HHCs) is shared by both VKOR and DsbB family protein folds.

Similarly, when we surveyed the available high-resolution structural data for position-specific matches between VKOR and DsbB residues interacting with bound ubiquinone substrates, out of a total of 9 DsbB residues contacting a bound ubiquinone-2 and 18 VKOR residues contacting a bound ubiquinone-4, we found conserved matches at AB module positions 25, 29, 33, 44 for both VKOR and DsbB families. The greater number of ubiquinone contacts for *Synechococcus* sp. VKOR compared to those for *E. coli* DsbB is primarily due to the longer isoprenoid chain length of ubiquinone-4 *versus* that of ubiquinone-2. Of the four positions common to ubiquinone binding for both representative high-resolution structures, position 44 represents one of the conserved active site cysteines in the CXXC motif (homologous to human VKORC1: Cys135) located on helix B, while positions 25 (Consurf scores 6 and 7), 29 (Consurf scores both 6) and 33 (Consurf scores 8 and 9) represent conserved residues on the adjacent helix A. We interpret these findings to be highly supportive for conservation of key homologous substrate binding site residues among VKOR and DsbB families. Taken together, we believe these results constitute substantial evidence for structural feature conservation for both VKOR and DsbB families in support of our hypothesis that both families share a common ancestor.

3.5. Identification of Transmembrane-Helical Bundle Protein Families Related by Cyclical Permuted Primary Sequences Can Extend Homology Modeling into the "Twilight Zone" (<30% Sequence Homology between Target and Template)

Figure 6 shows the human VKORC1 and VKORC1L1 models we produced along with the NMR structure of the DsbB template and the X-ray crystallographic structure of the prokaryotic VKOR family homolog (proVKOR) by Li *et al.* (2010) [14]. Stereochemical validation performed on both models indicated overall quality similar to that of the X-ray crystallographic and NMR structures (see online Supplementary Material & Experimental Data). Overall organization of the transmembrane helical bundles is quite similar between the DsbB and proVKOR experimentally determined structures, although the large loops (at the top of each structure) exhibit major structural differences. For DsbB, the loop extends across the bundle and is thought to be anchored in the lipid membrane by a short amphipathic helix (shown in purple). In contrast, for proVKOR, the loop is positioned entirely above the bundle (note that several short segments of the loop were not resolved in the crystallographic structure and are shown as dashed grey lines in Figure 6) with a short helix serving as a cap centered directly over the bundle (shown in magenta). The VKORC1 and VKORC1L1 models have transmembrane helical bundles organized very similarly to those of proVKOR and DsbB. Noticeably, the large loops of the models do not appear structurally homologous to that of DsbB because they were modeled separately using *de novo* modeling methods in order to avoid bias favoring structural features of the DsbB template loop region. The *de novo* modeling methods we used (see Section 2.4) identify pieces of structures from the PDB to use as templates for building up a realistic protein structure based on threading short segments of the target sequence. The resulting loop models were computationally annealed as small globular domains and could be easily fit to the respective helical bundles using standard X-ray crystallographic model building software. Interestingly, the *de novo* modeled loops for VKORC1 and VKORC1L1 prominently exhibit short helices located at nearly the same position in the final models as the short capping helix of the experimentally determined proVKOR structure (Figure 6, purple helix shown in the loop for VKORC1, for VKORC1L1 the helix is visible, but not colored, at the equivalent position). Taken together, the similarity between the experimental proVKOR loop and our modeled loops for VKORC1 and VKORC1L1 suggested to us that the large VKOR loops, in general, are likely to behave more like well-folded, small globular protein domains than the extended loop observed for the DsbB structure. Another potentially realistic feature of our modeled loops is that, for both VKORC1 and VKORC1L1, the loop cysteines appear to be within disulfide bonding distance from each other and, additionally, located at the very top periphery of the protein where they would theoretically be accessible for binding to, and for reduction by, ER lumenal partner oxidoreductases.

4. Discussion

Reconstruction of VKOR family phylogeny by standard ML methods revealed five distinct clades that follow a rationale consistent with evolution based on standard Tree of Life models. Analysis of overall VKOR family-specific and individual clade-specific sequence variability further revealed conserved sequence motifs and individual residue positions that suggest a possible evolutionary relationship with the DsbB family. Accordingly, results from our analysis of interhelical packing residues for representative experimentally determined structures from both families lends support to this hypothesis. Furthermore, differences in sequence conservation between VKOR clades have provided useful information for deducing a plausible evolutionary chronology for the VKOR family (Figure 7).

Of potentially broader implication to the structural biology of membrane proteins is the first discovery of cyclic permutation of sequence threading through seemingly unrelated protein folds for helical transmembrane proteins. In the case of the VKOR and DsbB families, there has been enough preservation of common structural elements for both protein fold and substrate binding, as well as preservation of enzymatic function, substrate class and functional partner proteins, to reveal a plausible underlying evolutionary relationship. Using phylogenetic conservation data from large multiple sequence alignments for both families, despite only 12.0%–13.6% shared primary sequence identity between the human VKOR paralogs and *E. coli* DsbB, we have presented the first evidence for evolutionary relatedness between these families.

Overall, polytopic membrane protein structures solved by X-ray and electron crystallographic and NMR methods account for <1% of Protein Data Bank entries [68], yet represent up to an estimated 30% of genomic proteins and include upwards of 70% of known or potential therapeutic drug targets [69, 70]. Identifying distant sequence homology targets for polytopic membrane protein templates with solved, high-resolution structures would prove beneficial to modeling efforts aimed at increasing structural coverage and would aid in defining functions for the rapidly growing number of new gene sequences from large-scale genomics efforts. Structural genomics aims to generate a minimum number of experimental structures to encompass all structural folds, including the subset of an estimated 550 (90% coverage) unique polytopic membrane protein folds [71]. Template-based models (TBMs) can be routinely constructed for target sequences sharing greater than 30% identity with an identified structural template [72] and used to guide hypothesis-driven experimentation [73] to study function [74] as well as to aid model building for crystallographic [75] and NMR data [76,77]. However, target sequences with less than 30% identity to any known template are considered to be in the "twilight zone" of template-based modeling [72,78], the case being exacerbated for membrane proteins where there are relatively few high-resolution structures [79].

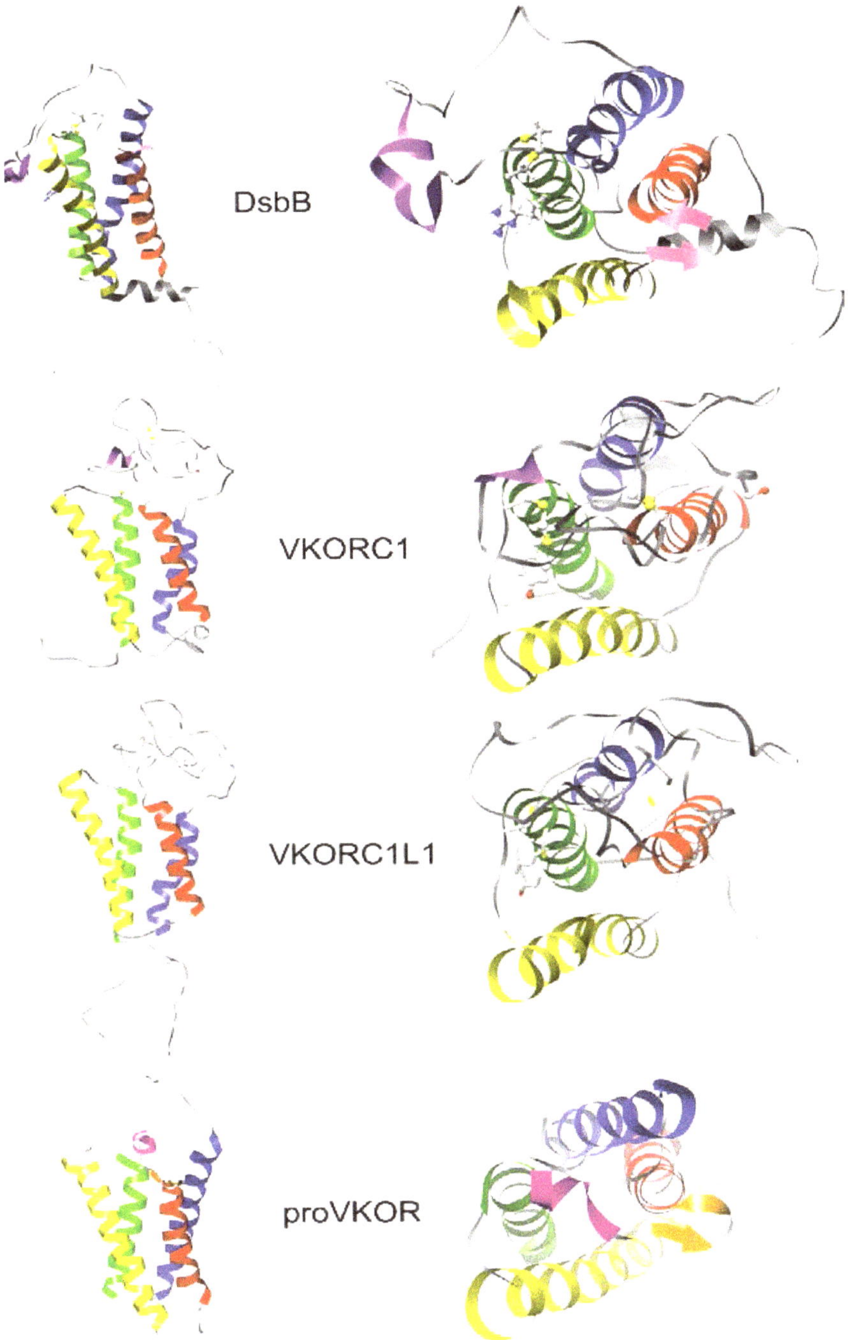

Figure 6. Backbone ribbon renderings of DsbB (PDB entry 2K74, model 1) [45], homology models of human VKORC1 and VKORC1L1 (Note 1 [67]), and Synechococcus sp. VKOR (proVKOR; PDB entry 3KP9) [14]. Views in the plane of the lipid bilayer (left) and normal (right) to the membrane plane from the ER lumenal (for VKORC1, VKORC1L1, proVKOR) or periplasmic (for DsbB) side. Transmembrane helices are colored (from N- to C-terminus) blue, red, yellow, green (designated as A, B, C and D, respectively, throughout the article text). Short loop helices for DsbB and VKORC1 (purple), for proVKOR (magenta); short β-sheet are regions (magenta or orange arrows); loop cysteines (ball and stick side-chains with yellow sulfur atoms).

E. coli DsbB and human VKORC1, for which experimental structures have been solved [14,29,30,45,80,81], share strikingly similar size, topology, two completely conserved functional cysteine pairs, lipidic quinone cofactors and oxidoreductase binding partners [19]. Moreover, primary sequence threading through the transmembrane α-helical secondary structural elements of both proteins is related by circular permutation (CP). Since 1979, there have been reports of CP relating the structural organization of naturally occurring soluble proteins (for a recent review see [82]) and underlying genetic principles leading to such permutations have been studied in the context of protein fold evolution [83]. We performed a literature-based survey of all published reports of CP in proteins and found examples for soluble protein domains, soluble domains of monotopic membrane proteins, sandwich transmembrane toxins, and a surprising number of engineered proteins including soluble domains as well as barrel transmembrane proteins occasionally genetically engineered to overcome crystallization problems for X-ray structural determinations. However, we could not identify any reports of CP for polytopic helical membrane proteins.

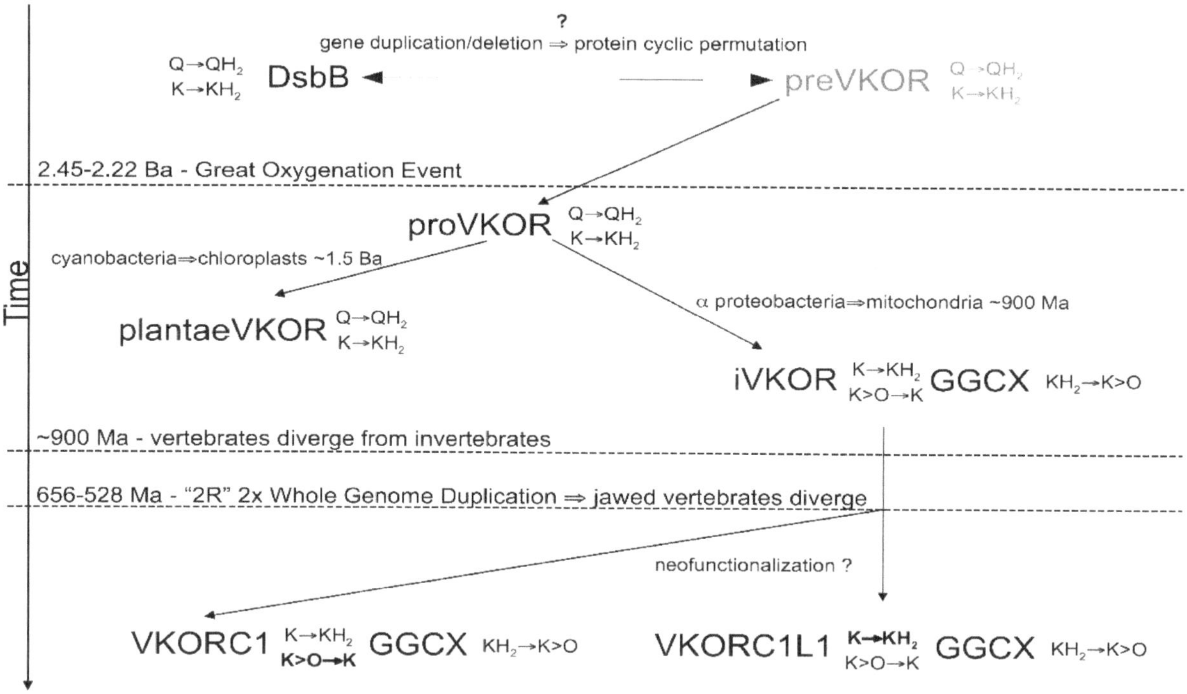

Figure 7. A comprehensive model for the evolution of the VKOR family and its hypothesized relationship to the DsbB family, suggested by the close relationship between the structure of the present reconstructed VKOR family phylogeny and that of the current consensus for the Tree of Life. Abbreviations and symbols (except if previously introduced): Ma, million years ago; Ba, billion years ago; Q, ubiquinone; QH_2, ubiquinol; K>O, vitamin K 2,3-epoxide; K, vitamin K quinone; KH_2, vitamin K hydroquinone; preVKOR, last universal common ancestral VKOR; proVKOR, prokaryotic VKOR; iVKOR, invertebrate VKOR; plantaeVKOR, plant VKOR; GGCX, γ-glutamyl carboxylase.

We advance the hypothesis and provide supporting evidence that both VKORC1 and DsbB families are evolutionarily divergent members of a single lipidic quinone:disulfide oxidoreductase superfamily (we suggest the nomenclature "LQOR superfamily") structurally related by CP threading homology that likely arose from an ancient gene duplication/deletion event. This event apparently occurred before eukaryotes evolved. It is likely that both families arose from a common ancestor in prokaryotes from a whole gene (ABCD) duplication that resulted in a concatenated linear tandem repeat (ABCDABCD), followed by deletions of the outer flanking helix pairs (~~AB~~CDAB~~CD~~) to yield the CP-related secondary structure threading (CDAB). Unfortunately, this scenario confronts us with essentially another version of the "chicken or the egg" causality dilemma—we have no way of currently deducing which permutation, and hence which family, predates the CP event. However, considering cumulative results from genetic and biochemical studies to date, we may deduce that, whereas the enzymatic function of DsbB family members has remained rather constant over long evolutionary timescales and has remained exclusively restricted to prokaryotes, multiple *de novo* enzymatic functions have arisen for members of the VKOR family since the divergence of eukaryotes and prokaryotes (Figure 7). Furthermore, it seems reasonable that neofunctionalization of VKOR family enzymes to catalyze de-epoxidation likely did not first arise before the onset of the Great Oxygenation Event.

5. Conclusions

In the present report, we have updated the phylogenetic characterization of VKOR family proteins to include broader representative taxa from the entire Tree of Life than was possible only a few years ago. We hope these results will serve as a basis to further explore fundamental relationships between available genetic data and structure/function correlates for the VKOR family.

Moreover, our results suggest a generalized approach for detecting further distant protein homologs related by cyclic permutation of a primary sequence. Our results also suggest that pairs of transmembrane helices (TMHs) together with the connecting loop may form key minimal modular building blocks that enable such evolutionary fold changes for helical intrinsic membrane proteins.

We hope our results will encourage more researchers to strive to better understand the molecular-level function of the modern VKOR enzymes from each of the major clades and what roles they play in development, growth and homeostasis. Advances on these fronts will further help to understand the evolution of these only recently discovered enzymes.

Acknowledgments: This work was supported, in part, by funding from the Deutsche Forschungsgemeinschaft (DFG) grant Ol100 5-1 (to MW and JO), from DFG grant Mi236 6-1 (to Prof. Hartmut Michel, Director, Department of Molecular Membrane Biology, Max Planck Institute of Biophysics; support for CK), and from Baxter Germany GmbH (to JO).

Author Contributions: CGB and JO conceived and drafted the article and discussed and edited it with CK, CR and MW. CGB collected and analyzed data.

References

1. Oldenburg, J.; Bevans, C.G.; Müller, C.R.; Watzka, M. Vitamin K epoxide reductase complex subunit 1 (VKORC1): The key protein of the vitamin K cycle. *Antioxid. Redox Signal.* **2006**, *8*, 347–353. [CrossRef] [PubMed]
2. Shearer, M.J.; Fu, X.; Booth, S.L. Vitamin K nutrition, metabolism, and requirements: Current concepts and future research. *Adv. Nutr.* **2012**, *3*, 182–195. [CrossRef] [PubMed]
3. Shearer, M.J.; Newman, P. Recent trends in the metabolism and cell biology of vitamin K with special reference to vitamin K cycling and MK-4 biosynthesis. *J. Lipid Res.* **2014**, *55*, 345–362. [CrossRef] [PubMed]
4. Spohn, G.; Kleinridders, A.; Wunderlich, F.T.; Watzka, M.; Zaucke, F.; Blumbach, K.; Geisen, C.; Seifried, E.; Müller, C.; Paulsson, M.; *et al.* VKORC1 deficiency in mice causes early postnatal lethality due to severe bleeding. *Thromb. Haemost.* **2009**, *101*, 1044–1050. [CrossRef] [PubMed]
5. Dam, H. The antihaemorrhagic vitamin of the chick. *Biochem. J.* **1935**, *29*, 1273–1285. [PubMed]
6. Watzka, M.; Geisen, C.; Bevans, C.G.; Sittinger, K.; Spohn, G.; Rost, S.; Seifried, E.; Müller, C.R.; Oldenburg, J. Thirteen novel VKORC1 mutations associated with oral anticoagulant resistance: Insights into improved patient diagnosis and treatment. *J. Thromb. Haemost.* **2011**, *9*, 109–118. [CrossRef] [PubMed]
7. Hammed, A.; Matagrin, B.; Spohn, G.; Prouillac, C.; Benoit, E.; Lattard, V. VKORC1L1, an enzyme rescuing the vitamin K 2,3-epoxide reductase activity in some extrahepatic tissues during anticoagulation therapy. *J. Biol. Chem.* **2013**, *288*, 28733–28742. [CrossRef] [PubMed]
8. Caspers, M.; Czogalla, K.J.; Liphardt, K.; Müller, J.; Westhofen, P.; Watzka, M.; Oldenburg, J. Two enzymes catalyze vitamin K 2,3-epoxide reductase activity in mouse: VKORC1 is highly expressed in exocrine tissues while VKORC1L1 is highly expressed in brain. *Thromb. Res.* **2015**, *135*, 977–983. [CrossRef] [PubMed]
9. Westhofen, P.; Watzka, M.; Marinova, M.; Hass, M.; Kirfel, G.; Müller, J.; Bevans, C.G.; Müller, C.R.; Oldenburg, J. Human vitamin K 2,3-epoxide reductase complex subunit 1-like 1 (VKORC1L1) mediates vitamin K-dependent intracellular antioxidant function. *J. Biol. Chem.* **2011**, *286*, 15085–15094. [CrossRef] [PubMed]

10. Rost, S.; Fregin, A.; Ivaskevicius, V.; Conzelmann, E.; Hörtnagel, K.; Pelz, H.-J.; Lappegard, K.; Seifried, E.; Scharrer, I.; Tuddenham, E.G.D.; *et al.* Mutations in VKORC1 cause warfarin resistance and multiple coagulation factor deficiency type 2. *Nature* **2004**, *427*, 537–541. [CrossRef] [PubMed]
11. Li, T.; Chang, C.-Y.; Jin, D.-Y.; Lin, P.-J.; Khvorova, A.; Stafford, D.W. Identification of the gene for vitamin K epoxide reductase. *Nature* **2004**, *427*, 541–544. [CrossRef] [PubMed]
12. Tie, J.-K.; Jin, D.-Y.; Stafford, D.W. Conserved loop cysteines of vitamin K epoxide reductase complex subunit 1-like 1 (VKORC1L1) are involved in its active site regeneration. *J. Biol. Chem.* **2014**, *289*, 9396–9407. [CrossRef] [PubMed]
13. Tie, J.-K.; Jin, D.-Y.; Stafford, D.W. Mycobacterium tuberculosis vitamin K epoxide reductase homologue supports vitamin K-dependent carboxylation in mammalian cells. *Antioxid. Redox Signal.* **2012**, *16*, 329–338. [CrossRef] [PubMed]
14. Li, W.; Schulman, S.; Dutton, R.J.; Boyd, D.; Beckwith, J.; Rapoport, T.A. Structure of a bacterial homologue of vitamin K epoxide reductase. *Nature* **2010**, *463*, 507–512. [CrossRef] [PubMed]
15. Furt, F.; van Oostende, C.; Widhalm, J.R.; Dale, M.A.; Wertz, J.; Basset, G.J.C. A bimodular oxidoreductase mediates the specific reduction of phylloquinone (vitamin K1) in chloroplasts. *Plant J. Cell Mol. Biol.* **2010**, *64*, 38–46. [CrossRef] [PubMed]
16. Wan, C.-M.; Yang, X.-J.; Du, J.-J.; Lu, Y.; Yu, Z.-B.; Feng, Y.-G.; Wang, X.-Y. Identification and characterization of SlVKOR, a disulfide bond formation protein from Solanum lycopersicum, and bioinformatic analysis of plant VKORs. *Biochem.* **2014**, *79*, 440–449. [CrossRef] [PubMed]
17. Sevier, C.S.; Kadokura, H.; Tam, V.C.; Beckwith, J.; Fass, D.; Kaiser, C.A. The prokaryotic enzyme DsbB may share key structural features with eukaryotic disulfide bond forming oxidoreductases. *Protein Sci. Publ. Protein Soc.* **2005**, *14*, 1630–1642. [CrossRef] [PubMed]
18. Sevier, C.S.; Kaiser, C.A. Conservation and diversity of the cellular disulfide bond formation pathways. *Antioxid. Redox Signal.* **2006**, *8*, 797–811. [CrossRef] [PubMed]
19. Wajih, N.; Hutson, S.M.; Wallin, R. Disulfide-dependent protein folding is linked to operation of the vitamin K cycle in the endoplasmic reticulum: A protein disulfide isomerase-VKORC1 redox enzyme complex appears to be responsible for vitamin K1 2,3-epoxide reduction. *J. Biol. Chem.* **2007**, *282*, 2626–2635. [CrossRef] [PubMed]
20. Rutkevich, L.A.; Williams, D.B. Vitamin K epoxide reductase contributes to protein disulfide formation and redox homeostasis within the endoplasmic reticulum. *Mol. Biol. Cell* **2012**, *23*, 2017–2027. [CrossRef] [PubMed]
21. Oldenburg, J.; Müller, C.R.; Rost, S.; Watzka, M.; Bevans, C.G. Comparative genetics of warfarin resistance. *Hamostaseologie* **2014**, *34*, 143–159. [CrossRef] [PubMed]
22. Goodstadt, L.; Ponting, C.P. Vitamin K epoxide reductase: homology, active site and catalytic mechanism. *Trends Biochem. Sci.* **2004**, *29*, 289–292. [CrossRef] [PubMed]
23. Robertson, H.M. Genes encoding vitamin-K epoxide reductase are present in Drosophila and trypanosomatid protists. *Genetics* **2004**, *168*, 1077–1080. [CrossRef] [PubMed]
24. Dutton, R.J.; Boyd, D.; Berkmen, M.; Beckwith, J. Bacterial species exhibit diversity in their mechanisms and capacity for protein disulfide bond formation. *Proc. Natl. Acad. Sci. USA* **2008**, *105*, 11933–11938. [CrossRef] [PubMed]
25. Heras, B.; Shouldice, S.R.; Totsika, M.; Scanlon, M.J.; Schembri, M.A.; Martin, J.L. DSB proteins and bacterial pathogenicity. *Nat. Rev. Microbiol.* **2009**, *7*, 215–225. [CrossRef] [PubMed]
26. Bader, M.; Muse, W.; Ballou, D.P.; Gassner, C.; Bardwell, J.C. Oxidative protein folding is driven by the electron transport system. *Cell* **1999**, *98*, 217–227. [CrossRef]
27. Reedstrom, C.K.; Suttie, J.W. Comparative distribution, metabolism, and utilization of phylloquinone and menaquinone-9 in rat liver. *Biol. Med.* **1995**, *209*, 403–409. [CrossRef]
28. Collins, M.D.; Jones, D. Distribution of isoprenoid quinone structural types in bacteria and their taxonomic implication. *Microbiol. Rev.* **1981**, *45*, 316–354. [PubMed]
29. Inaba, K.; Murakami, S.; Suzuki, M.; Nakagawa, A.; Yamashita, E.; Okada, K.; Ito, K. Crystal structure of the DsbB-DsbA complex reveals a mechanism of disulfide bond generation. *Cell* **2006**, *127*, 789–801. [CrossRef] [PubMed]
30. Shixuan, L.; Wei, C.; Fowle Grider, R.; Guomin, S.; Weikai, L. Structures of an intramembrane vitamin K epoxide reductase homolog reveal control mechanisms for electron transfer. *Nat. Commun.* **2014**, *5*, 3110.

31. Schwarz, R.; Seibel, P.N.; Rahmann, S.; Schoen, C.; Huenerberg, M.; Müller-Reible, C.; Dandekar, T.; Karchin, R.; Schultz, J.; Müller, T. Detecting species-site dependencies in large multiple sequence alignments. *Nucleic Acids Res.* **2009**, *37*, 5959–5968. [CrossRef] [PubMed]
32. Geer, L.Y.; Domrachev, M.; Lipman, D.J.; Bryant, S.H. CDART: Protein homology by domain architecture. *Genome Res.* **2002**, *12*, 1619–1623. [CrossRef] [PubMed]
33. Finn, R.D.; Bateman, A.; Clements, J.; Coggill, P.; Eberhardt, R.Y.; Eddy, S.R.; Heger, A.; Hetherington, K.; Holm, L.; Mistry, J.; *et al.* Pfam: The protein families database. *Nucleic Acids Res.* **2014**, *42*, D222–D230. [CrossRef] [PubMed]
34. Katoh, K.; Standley, D.M. MAFFT multiple sequence alignment software version 7: Improvements in performance and usability. *Mol. Biol. Evol.* **2013**, *30*, 772–780. [CrossRef] [PubMed]
35. Waterhouse, A.M.; Procter, J.B.; Martin, D.M.; Clamp, M.; Barton, G.J. Jalview Version 2—A multiple sequence alignment editor and analysis workbench. *Bioinformatics* **2009**, *25*, 1189–1191. [CrossRef] [PubMed]
36. Milne, I.; Lindner, D.; Bayer, M.; Husmeier, D.; McGuire, G.; Marshall, D.F.; Wright, F. TOPALi v2: A rich graphical interface for evolutionary analyses of multiple alignments on HPC clusters and multi-core desktops. *Bioinforma. Oxf. Engl.* **2009**, *25*, 126–127. [CrossRef] [PubMed]
37. Nguyen, L.-T.; Schmidt, H.A.; von Haeseler, A.; Minh, B.Q. IQ-TREE: A fast and effective stochastic algorithm for estimating maximum-likelihood phylogenies. *Mol. Biol. Evol.* **2015**, *32*, 268–274. [CrossRef] [PubMed]
38. Guindon, S.; Dufayard, J.-F.; Lefort, V.; Anisimova, M.; Hordijk, W.; Gascuel, O. New algorithms and methods to estimate maximum-likelihood phylogenies: Assessing the performance of PhyML 3.0. *Syst. Biol.* **2010**, *59*, 307–321. [CrossRef] [PubMed]
39. Stamatakis, A. RAxML version 8: A tool for phylogenetic analysis and post-analysis of large phylogenies. *Bioinforma. Oxf. Engl.* **2014**, *30*, 1312–1313. [CrossRef] [PubMed]
40. Minh, B.Q.; Nguyen, M.A.T.; von Haeseler, A. Ultrafast approximation for phylogenetic bootstrap. *Mol. Biol. Evol.* **2013**, *30*, 1188–1195. [CrossRef] [PubMed]
41. Letunic, I.; Bork, P. Interactive Tree Of Life (iTOL): An online tool for phylogenetic tree display and annotation. *Bioinforma. Oxf. Engl.* **2007**, *23*, 127–128. [CrossRef] [PubMed]
42. Berezin, C.; Glaser, F.; Rosenberg, J.; Paz, I.; Pupko, T.; Fariselli, P.; Casadio, R.; Ben-Tal, N. ConSeq: The identification of functionally and structurally important residues in protein sequences. *Bioinform. Oxf. Engl.* **2004**, *20*, 1322–1324. [CrossRef] [PubMed]
43. Ashkenazy, H.; Erez, E.; Martz, E.; Pupko, T.; Ben-Tal, N. ConSurf 2010: Calculating evolutionary conservation in sequence and structure of proteins and nucleic acids. *Nucleic Acids Res.* **2010**, *38*, W529–W533. [CrossRef] [PubMed]
44. Lo, A.; Cheng, C.-W.; Chiu, Y.-Y.; Sung, T.-Y.; Hsu, W.-L. TMPad: An integrated structural database for helix-packing folds in transmembrane proteins. *Nucleic Acids Res.* **2011**, *39*, D347–D355. [CrossRef] [PubMed]
45. Zhou, Y.; Cierpicki, T.; Jimenez, R.H.F.; Lukasik, S.M.; Ellena, J.F.; Cafiso, D.S.; Kadokura, H.; Beckwith, J.; Bushweller, J.H. NMR solution structure of the integral membrane enzyme DsbB: Functional insights into DsbB-catalyzed disulfide bond formation. *Mol. Cell* **2008**, *31*, 896–908. [CrossRef] [PubMed]
46. Sali, A.; Blundell, T.L. Comparative protein modelling by satisfaction of spatial restraints. *J. Mol. Biol.* **1993**, *234*, 779–815. [CrossRef] [PubMed]
47. Emsley, P.; Cowtan, K. Coot: Model-building tools for molecular graphics. *Acta Crystallogr. D Biol. Crystallogr.* **2004**, *60*, 2126–2132. [CrossRef] [PubMed]
48. Zhang, Y. I-TASSER server for protein 3D structure prediction. *BMC Bioinform.* **2008**, *9*, 40. [CrossRef] [PubMed]
49. Davis, I.W.; Leaver-Fay, A.; Chen, V.B.; Block, J.N.; Kapral, G.J.; Wang, X.; Murray, L.W.; Arendall, W.B.; Snoeyink, J.; Richardson, J.S.; *et al.* MolProbity: All-atom contacts and structure validation for proteins and nucleic acids. *Nucleic Acids Res.* **2007**, *35*, W375–W383. [CrossRef] [PubMed]
50. Senes, A.; Gerstein, M.; Engelman, D.M. Statistical analysis of amino acid patterns in transmembrane helices: The GxxxG motif occurs frequently and in association with beta-branched residues at neighboring positions. *J. Mol. Biol.* **2000**, *296*, 921–936. [CrossRef] [PubMed]
51. Stevens, T.J.; Arkin, I.T. Substitution rates in alpha-helical transmembrane proteins. *Protein Sci. Publ. Protein Soc.* **2001**, *10*, 2507–2517. [CrossRef]

52. Raczko, A.M.; Bujnicki, J.M.; Pawlowski, M.; Godlewska, R.; Lewandowska, M.; Jagusztyn-Krynicka, E.K. Characterization of new DsbB-like thiol-oxidoreductases of Campylobacter jejuni and Helicobacter pylori and classification of the DsbB family based on phylogenomic, structural and functional criteria. *Microbiol. Read. Engl.* **2005**, *151*, 219–231. [CrossRef] [PubMed]
53. Rishavy, M.A.; Usubalieva, A.; Hallgren, K.W.; Berkner, K.L. Novel insight into the mechanism of the vitamin K oxidoreductase (VKOR): Electron relay through Cys43 and Cys51 reduces VKOR to allow vitamin K reduction and facilitation of vitamin K-dependent protein carboxylation. *J. Biol. Chem.* **2011**, *286*, 7267–7278. [CrossRef] [PubMed]
54. Doolittle, W.F. Phylogenetic classification and the universal tree. *Science* **1999**, *284*, 2124–2128. [CrossRef] [PubMed]
55. Schaap, P. Guanylyl cyclases across the tree of life. *Fron. Biosci.* **2005**, *10*, 1485–1498. [CrossRef]
56. Lake, J.A.; Skophammer, R.G.; Herbold, C.W.; Servin, J.A. Genome beginnings: Rooting the tree of life. *Philos. Trans. R. Soc. Lond B. Biol. Sci.* **2009**, *364*, 2177–2185. [CrossRef] [PubMed]
57. Gribaldo, S.; Brochier, C. Phylogeny of prokaryotes: Does it exist and why should we care? *Res. Microbiol.* **2009**, *23*, 23. [CrossRef] [PubMed]
58. Nakayama, T.; Archibald, J.M. Evolving a photosynthetic organelle. *BMC Biol.* **2012**, *10*, 35. [CrossRef] [PubMed]
59. Nowack, E.C.M.; Melkonian, M.; Glöckner, G. Chromatophore genome sequence of Paulinella sheds light on acquisition of photosynthesis by eukaryotes. *Curr. Biol. CB* **2008**, *18*, 410–418. [CrossRef] [PubMed]
60. Marin, B.; Nowack, E.C.M.; Melkonian, M. A plastid in the making: Evidence for a second primary endosymbiosis. *Protist* **2005**, *156*, 425–432. [CrossRef] [PubMed]
61. Singh, A.K.; Bhattacharyya-Pakrasi, M.; Pakrasi, H.B. Identification of an atypical membrane protein involved in the formation of protein disulfide bonds in oxygenic photosynthetic organisms. *J. Biol. Chem.* **2008**, *283*, 15762–15770. [CrossRef] [PubMed]
62. Matagrin, B.; Hodroge, A.; Montagut-Romans, A.; Andru, J.; Fourel, I.; Besse, S.; Benoit, E.; Lattard, V. New insights into the catalytic mechanism of vitamin K epoxide reductase (VKORC1)—The catalytic properties of the major mutations of rVKORC1 explain the biological cost associated to mutations. *FEBS Open Bio.* **2013**, *3*, 144–150. [CrossRef] [PubMed]
63. Fasco, M.J.; Preusch, P.C.; Hildebrandt, E.; Suttie, J.W. Formation of hydroxyvitamin K by vitamin K epoxide reductase of warfarin-resistant rats. *J. Biol. Chem.* **1983**, *258*, 4372–4380. [PubMed]
64. Rost, S.; Pelz, H.-J.; Menzel, S.; MacNicoll, A.D.; León, V.; Song, K.-J.; Jäkel, T.; Oldenburg, J.; Müller, C.R. Novel mutations in the VKORC1 gene of wild rats and mice—A response to 50 years of selection pressure by warfarin? *BMC Genet.* **2009**, *10*, 4. [CrossRef] [PubMed]
65. Kapadia, M.; Rolston, K.V.I.; Han, X.Y. Invasive streptomyces infections: Six cases and literature review. *Am. J. Clin. Pathol.* **2007**, *127*, 619–624. [CrossRef] [PubMed]
66. Berkner, K.L. Vitamin K-dependent carboxylation. *Vitam. Horm.* **2008**, *78*, 131–156. [PubMed]
67. Note 1: Readers interested in viewing features summarized in Figure 5 for the all-atoms molecular models of hVKORC1 and hVKORC1L1 can download these from the Protein Model DataBase (https://bioinformatics.cineca.it/PMDB/main.php, PMDB identifiers PM0075969, PM007). The NMR structure for DsbB (PDB entry 2K74, model 1) can be downloaded from the RCSB Protein Data Bank (http://www.rcsb.org/pdb/home/home.do).
68. White, S.H. Biophysical dissection of membrane proteins. *Nature* **2009**, *459*, 344–346. [CrossRef] [PubMed]
69. Wallin, E.; von Heijne, G. Genome-wide analysis of integral membrane proteins from eubacterial, archaean, and eukaryotic organisms. *Protein Sci.* **1998**, *7*, 1029–1038. [CrossRef] [PubMed]
70. Lundstrom, K. Structural genomics and drug discovery. *J. Cell Mol. Med.* **2007**, *11*, 224–238. [CrossRef] [PubMed]
71. Oberai, A.; Ihm, Y.; Kim, S.; Bowie, J.U. A limited universe of membrane protein families and folds. *Protein Sci.* **2006**, *15*, 1723–1734. [CrossRef] [PubMed]
72. Vitkup, D.; Melamud, E.; Moult, J.; Sander, C. Completeness in structural genomics. *Nat. Struct. Biol.* **2001**, *8*, 559–566. [CrossRef] [PubMed]
73. Zhang, Y. Protein structure prediction: When is it useful? *Curr. Opin. Struct. Biol.* **2009**, *19*, 1–11. [CrossRef] [PubMed]

74. Schwede, T.; Sali, A.; Honig, B.; Levitt, M.; Berman, H.M.; Jones, D.; Brenner, S.E.; Burley, S.K.; Das, R.; Dokholyan, N.V.; *et al.* Outcome of a workshop on applications of protein models in biomedical research. *Structure* **2009**, *17*, 151–159. [CrossRef] [PubMed]
75. Adams, P.D.; Afonine, P.V.; Grosse-Kunstleve, R.W.; Read, R.J.; Richardson, J.S.; Richardson, D.C.; Terwilliger, T.C. Recent developments in phasing and structure refinement for macromolecular crystallography. *Curr. Opin. Struct. Biol.* **2009**, *21*, 21. [CrossRef] [PubMed]
76. Barbar, E.; Lehoux, J.G.; Lavigne, P. Toward the NMR structure of StAR. *Mol. Cell Endocrinol.* **2009**, *300*, 89–93. [CrossRef] [PubMed]
77. Bax, A. Weak alignment offers new NMR opportunities to study protein structure and dynamics. *Protein Sci.* **2003**, *12*, 1–16. [CrossRef] [PubMed]
78. Rost, B. Twilight zone of protein sequence alignments. *Protein Eng.* **1999**, *12*, 85–94. [CrossRef] [PubMed]
79. Forrest, L.R.; Tang, C.L.; Honig, B. On the accuracy of homology modeling and sequence alignment methods applied to membrane proteins. *Biophys. J.* **2006**, *91*, 508–517. [CrossRef] [PubMed]
80. Malojcić, G.; Owen, R.L.; Grimshaw, J.P.A.; Glockshuber, R. Preparation and structure of the charge-transfer intermediate of the transmembrane redox catalyst DsbB. *FEBS Lett.* **2008**, *582*, 3301–3307. [CrossRef] [PubMed]
81. Inaba, K.; Murakami, S.; Nakagawa, A.; Iida, H.; Kinjo, M.; Ito, K.; Suzuki, M. Dynamic nature of disulphide bond formation catalysts revealed by crystal structures of DsbB. *Embo J.* **2009**, *28*, 779–791. [CrossRef] [PubMed]
82. Vogel, C.; Morea, V. Duplication, divergence and formation of novel protein topologies. *Bioessays* **2006**, *28*, 973–978. [CrossRef] [PubMed]
83. Grishin, N.V. Fold change in evolution of protein structures. *J. Struct. Biol.* **2001**, *134*, 167–185. [CrossRef] [PubMed]

14

Vitamin E as a Treatment for Nonalcoholic Fatty Liver Disease: Reality or Myth?

Hamza El Hadi, Roberto Vettor and Marco Rossato *

Internal Medicine 3, Department of Medicine—DIMED, University of Padova, Via Giustiniani 2, 35128 Padova, Italy; dr.hamza.elhadi@gmail.com (H.E.H.); roberto.vettor@unipd.it (R.V.)

* Correspondence: marco.rossato@unipd.it

Abstract: Obesity is one of the major epidemics of this millennium, and its incidence is growing worldwide. Following the epidemics of obesity, nonalcoholic fatty liver disease (NAFLD) has become a disease of increasing prevalence and a leading cause of morbidity and mortality closely related to cardiovascular disease, malignancies, and cirrhosis. It is believed that oxidative stress is a main player in the development and progression of NAFLD. Currently, a pharmacological approach has become necessary in NAFLD because of a failure to modify lifestyle and dietary habits in most patients. Vitamin E is a potent antioxidant that has been shown to reduce oxidative stress in NAFLD. This review summarizes the biological activities of vitamin E, with a primary focus on its therapeutic efficacy in NAFLD.

Keywords: vitamin E; nonalcoholic fatty liver disease; obesity; oxidative stress

1. Introduction

Nonalcoholic fatty liver disease (NAFLD) is defined as the accumulation of excessive fat in the liver, as demonstrated by imaging or by histology, in the setting of no significant alcohol consumptionand the absence of any secondary cause [1].

NAFLD encompasses a broad pathological spectrum of phenotypes ranging from isolated hepatic steatosis (IHS) to nonalcoholic steatohepatitis (NASH)—the progressive form of fatty liver disease associated with inflammation and cellular injury, which can lead to NASH-related cirrhosis and hepatocellular carcinoma [2]. This pathology is now regarded as a leading cause of chronic liver diseases and liver transplantation in most countries [3]. In addition, NAFLD has been also linked to extra-hepatic morbidity, including systemic metabolic complications, chronic kidney and cardiovascular disease, and malignancies, which all contribute to a higher mortality observed in NASH patients [4].

NAFLD is strongly associated with obesity and related metabolic disorders such as insulin resistance and dyslipidemia. In the last decades, adult and childhood obesity has reached epidemic levels, and as a consequence the global prevalence of NAFLD has increased significantly. According to a recent report, prevalence estimates in the general population of Europe and the Middle East are 20–30%, with higher prevalence in Western countries' populations with obesity or diabetes (75%) and with morbid obesity (90–95%) [5].

It is acknowledged that vitamin E is the major lipid-soluble chain-breaking antioxidant found in the human body. In addition to its anti-oxidative properties, molecules of the vitamin E family exertanti-atherogenicand anti-inflammatory activities [6]. Although the pathogenesis of NAFLD and its progression to fibrosis needs to be fully clarified, it is believed that oxidative stress plays a crucial role in producing the lethal hepatocyte injury associated with NAFLD.

Therefore, by targeting oxidative stress components, vitamin E appears as a promising therapeutic approach in NASH patients.

The present review briefly discusses the biological activities of vitamin E, focusing on its potential as a treatment for NAFLD/NASH. To this aim, we also highlight the role of oxidative stress in the pathogenesis of NAFLD.

2. Vitamin E: Brief Overview of Structure, Metabolism and Function

2.1. Structural Perspectives

The discovery of vitamin E dates back to 1922 due to the observations of Herbert Evans and his associate Bishop who isolated an as-yet uncharacterized fat-soluble compound from green leafy vegetables which is required for reproduction in rats [7]. Upon isolating this dietary compound, it was termed as tocopherol (Greek: tocos—child birth; pheros—to bear; ol—alcohol). Today the term "vitamin E" encompasses a group of eight lipophilic molecules that are synthesized by plants starting from homogentisic acid. It includes four tocopherols and four tocotrienols. Tocopherols and tocotrienols are subdivided into alpha (α), beta (β), gamma (γ), and delta (δ) forms based on the methyl and hydroxyl substitution in their phenolic rings [8] (Figure 1). The tocopherols are saturated forms of vitamin E, whereas the tocotrienols are unsaturated and possess an isoprenoid side chain [8]. α-Tocopherol is considered the most abundant form in nature, and is consequently the most widely studied. Common food oils including corn, peanut, and soybean oil contain largely α-tocopherol. In contrast, tocotrienols are relatively rarer in food sources and prevail in rice bran, barley, oats, and palm oil [9].

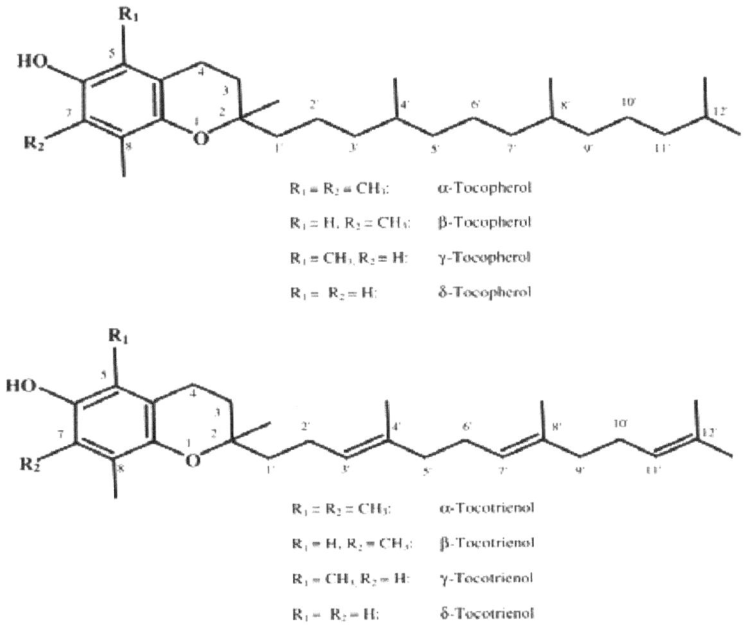

Figure 1. Structure of tocopherols and tocotrienols (with permission from reference [8]).

Currently, synthetic forms of vitamin E consist mainly of α-tocopherol, whichwas first synthesized in 1938 [10]. Unlike naturally-occurring d-RRR-α-tocopherol, synthesized α-tocopherol consists of a racemic mixture of eight stereoisomers named the all-racemic or (2RS, 4′RS, 8′RS) product [11].

2.2. Insight into Metabolism

Like other fat-soluble vitamins, the bioavailability of vitamin E depends on pancreatic function, biliary secretion, micellar formation, and penetration across intestinal membranes. After being cleaved by the enzyme esterase located in the stomach lining and partly processed enzymatically in the stomach by gastric lipase, vitamin E isoforms reach the basolateral side of enterocytes [12,13]. In the intestinal lumen, dietary tocopherols and tocotrienols appear to be similarly absorbed along with dietary fat, and are secreted in chylomicron particles together with triacylglycerol, phospholipids, and cholesterol [12,13]. The chylomicron-bound vitamin E isoforms are then transferred to peripheral tissues such as adipose tissues, bones, brain, lung, muscle, and skin via the lymphatic system. During their transport, chylomicrons are catabolized in the circulation by the endothelial-bound enzyme, which hydrolyzes triglycerides, releasing free fatty acids (FFAs) [12,13]. The resulting chylomicron remnants containing absorbed vitamin E are subsequently taken up by the liver, probably by a receptor-mediated process, and then preferentially incorporated within very low density lipoprotein (VLDL) and high-density lipoprotein (HDL) into the bloodstream [12]. After hepatic uptake, the α-tocopherol form of vitamin E is preferentially re-excreted into the circulation. α-Tocopherol transfer protein (α-TTP), a small cytoplasmic hepatic protein with differential affinity for various vitamin E forms, is responsible for the biodiscriminating process underlying the selective resecretion of α-tocopherol from the liver into plasma [14].

While α-TTP has a high affinity for α-tocopherol (100%), it has a lower affinity for other vitamin E isoforms: approximately 50% for β-tocopherol, 10–30% for γ-tocopherol, and 1% for δ-tocopherol [12]. In the liver, isoforms not bound to α-TTP will be susceptible to catabolization via cytochrome P450 (CYP4F2)-initiated ω-hydroxylation and oxidation by ω-hydroxylase, and thus vitamin E isoforms are metabolized to carboxychromanols, hydroxycarboxychromanol, and carboxyethylhydroxychroman derivatives [15]. Besides catabolism, it was estimated that metabolized vitamin E isoforms are also discarded via biliary excretion [16].

2.3. *Biological Activity of Vitamin E*

2.3.1. Antioxidant Activity

Oxidative stress is defined as the imbalance between the generation of reactive species and antioxidant defense, and leads to the damage of DNA and disturbances in cellular biology [17]. Vitamin E is widely accepted as one of the most potent antioxidants in nature [18]. The antioxidant property is attributed to the hydroxyl group from the aromatic ring of tocochromanols, which donates hydrogen to neutralize free radicals or reactive oxygen species (ROS). The antioxidant activity of α-, β-, γ-isoforms of tocotrienols and tocopherols is similar, but the γ-isoform showed weaker activity when tested in pyrogallolsulfonphthalein and 2,7-dichlorodihydrofluorescein diacetate methods [18,19].

In the same context, the antioxidant efficacy of vitamin E on reactive nitrogen species (RNS) has been gaining more attention recently. RNS include nitric oxide (NO), nitrogen dioxide (NO_2), and peroxynitrite ($ONOO^-$) [20–22].

On the other hand, in vitro studies have shown that vitamin E can alternatively switch to a pro-oxidant action under certain circumstances, such as a constant low-level flux of initiator free radicals and the absence of co-antioxidants as such as vitamin C [23]. In addition, current evidence from in vivo studies showed that vitamin E may produce pro-oxidant effects at high doses [24] or in cigarette smokers consuming a high polyunsaturated fat diet [25].

2.3.2. Beyond Vitamin E Antioxidant Activity

Vitamin E biological activity is not limited to antioxidant properties. In fact, vitamin E forms are involved in the regulation of inflammatory response, gene expression, membrane-bound enzymes, modulation of cellular signaling, and cell proliferation.

Over the last two decades, vitamin E has been shown to have direct and indirect effects on several enzymes involved in signal transduction, such as protein kinase C (PKC), protein phosphatase 2A (PP2A), protein tyrosine phosphatase (PTP), protein tyrosine kinase (PTK), diacylglycerol kinase (DAGK), 5-, 12- and 15-lipoxygenases (5-, 12-, and 15-LOX), phospholipase A2 (PLA2), cyclooxygenase-2 (COX-2), and the mitogen activated protein kinase (MAPK) signal transduction pathway [26,27].

The first evidence that vitamin E can modulate enzymes involved in signal transduction came from studies with PKC when α-tocopherol exerted an inhibitory effect unrelated to antioxidant action [28]. PKC inhibition by α-tocopherol is mainly correlated with the reduction of cell proliferation in many different cell types, including vascular smooth muscle cells, monocytes/macrophages, neutrophils, fibroblasts, mesangial cells, as well as various cancer cell lines [29]. In addition to interference with cell proliferation, the inhibition of PKC by α-tocopherol inhibited NADPH-oxidase assembly in monocytes, leading to lower superoxide production [30]. Additionally, PKC inhibition mediated by α-tocopherol and not by β-tocopherol suppressed endothelin secretion in endothelial cells [31].

Another evidence of a non-antioxidant function of α-tocopherol is related to its role in regulating the expression of specific genes not only coupled to oxidative stress but also involved in cholesterol homeostasis, inflammatory pathways, and cellular trafficking [32,33]. These genes include those encoding for proteins involved in inflammation and cell adhesion (such as E-selectin, intercellular adhesion molecule-1, vascular cell adhesion molecule [VCAM]-1, integrin, interleukin [IL]-1b, IL-2, IL-4, and transforming growth factor [TGF]-β), extracellular matrix formation and degradation (tropomyosin, glycoprotein IIb, collagen A1, matrix metalloproteinase [MMP]-1, MMP-19 and connective tissue growth factor), cell cycle regulation (cyclin D1, cyclin E1, and p27), transcriptional control lipoprotein (peroxisome proliferator-activated receptor [PPAR]-γ), receptors (CD36, scavenger receptor class B type 1, low density lipoprotein receptor), and metabolism (Cytochrome P450 3A4 [CYP3A4] and HMG-CoA reductase) [32,33].

3. Vitamin E and NAFLD

3.1. NAFLD/NASH Pathogenesis

NAFLD is a complex disease trait where inter-patient genetic and epigenetic variations and environmental factors are combined to define development and disease progression [34] (Figure 2).

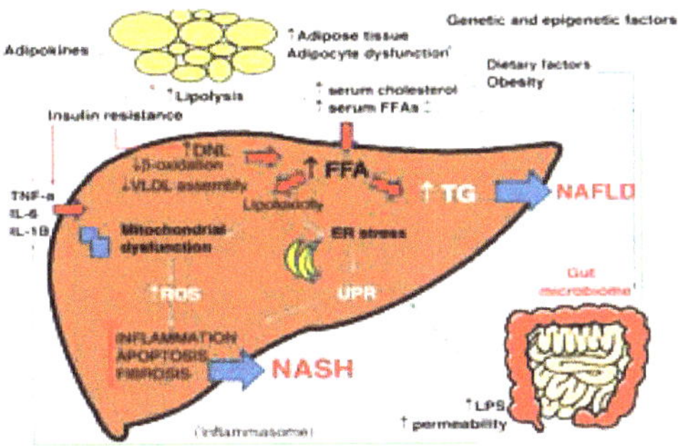

Figure 2. Multiple parallel-hit hypothesis of nonalcoholic fatty liver disease (NAFLD). Obesity together with dietary habits and environmental factors can lead to raised serum levels of free fatty acids (FFAs) and cholesterol, development of insulin resistance, adipocyte proliferation, and dysfunction in the intestinal microbiome. Insulin resistance acts on adipose tissue, worsening adipocyte dysfunction, induces hepatic de novo lipogenesis (DNL) and release of proinflammatory adipokines such as interleukin (IL)-6, IL-1β, and tumor necrosis factor (TNF)-α, which also exacerbates the insulin resistance state. The increased hepatic FFAs flux which derives from the above processes and from an altered activity of the gut microbiome leads to accumulation of triglycerides (TGs) and "toxic"levels of FFAs, free cholesterol, and other lipid metabolites which cause mitochondrial dysfunction, oxidative stress with the production of reactive oxygen species (ROS), and endoplasmic reticulum (ER) stress with the activation of the unfolded protein response (UPR), all leading to hepatic inflammation and fibrogenesis (nonalcoholic steatohepatitis, NASH). Increased intestinal permeability of gut-derived microbial products such as lipopolysaccharides (LPS) contributes to the activation of the inflammasome, ER stress, and activation of inflammatory cascades. Epigenetic factors are also involved in progression to NASH or persistence in a stable stage of disease (with permission from [34]). VLDL: very low density lipoprotein.

The generally accepted dogma in the pathogenesis of NAFLD is that insulin resistance—commonly associated with obesity—leads to the hepatic accumulation of triglycerides, a process that usually results from increased FFAs flux from adipose tissue to the liver, dietary fat via chylomicron metabolism, and increased de novo lipogenesis [35–37]. Obesity generates a state of low-grade inflammation characterized by the accumulation of immune cells in adipose tissue (particularly macrophages), and the production of proinflammatory cytokines by adipocytes contributes to the development of systemic and hepatic insulin resistance [35–37]. However, multiple pathways (multiple hits) are involved in the development of NASH and fibrosis. "Hits" that may contribute include oxidative stress, endotoxins, changes in the gut–liver axis, and mitochondrial dysfunction [34].

Oxidative stress and mitochondrial dysfunction were proposed as main triggers for the progression of steatosis to steatohepatitis [38]. FFAs catabolism in the liver takes place mainly via mitochondrial β-oxidation—a process that can lead to the generation of ROS, including superoxide, hydrogen peroxide, and hydroxyl radicals, in the case of increased FFAs delivery [38].

In the same context, impaired mitochondrial activity in NASH patients due to reduced enzymatic activities of mitochondrial electron transport chain and excessive in FA oxidation results in hepatic ATP depletion and may cause structural mitochondrial abnormalities consisting of enlargement (megamitochondria), paracrystalline inclusions, and loss of cristae [39,40].

In NAFLD, enhanced cytochrome P450 2E1 (CYP2E1) expression and activity seem to be an important source of ROS which trigger oxidative stress and perpetuate the hepatic mitochondrial dysfunction [41]. Moreover, it has been reported that upregulated microsomal CYP4A enzymes ω-hydroxylate fatty acids into dicarboxylic acids that are then preferentially oxidized by peroxisomes, thus promoting ROS production in NAFLD [42]. The ablation of a homolog of human CYP4A gene (CYP4A14) in animal models of steatohepatitis has shown to attenuate hepatic inflammation and fibrosis [43]. The abundant production of ROS induces the peroxidation of hepatic triglycerides with the release of reactive aldehydes such as 4-hydroxynonenal (4-HNE) and malondialdehyde (MDA) which can damage mitochondrial components [44].

Accumulating data have implicated the disruption of endoplasmic reticulum (ER) homeostasis (i.e., ER stress) in the development of NASH [45]. Factors that disturb ER folding capacity (e.g., excessive protein synthesis, mitochondrial dysfunction, oxidative stress) will lead to the activation of a physiologic mechanism called the "unfolded protein response" (UPR) in hepatocytes. This adaptive mechanism aims to increase the folding capacity of the ER, thus bringing the organelle and the cell into a state of equilibrium. When the activation of the UPR fails to promote cell survival, the cell is taken down the pro-apoptotic ER stress response pathway, which can ultimately lead to apoptotic cell death, inflammation, and/or fat accumulation [45].

Several studies have suggested a role of gut microbiome in NASH pathogenesis [46]. Intestinal barrier alterations cause increased intestinal permeability of bacteria, viruses, or microbial products such as lipopolysaccharide (LPS). These pathogens are recognized through specialized recognition receptors that include toll-like receptors (TLRs) and inflammasomes, inducing a signaling cascade leading to the production of inflammatory cytokines [46].

3.2. Vitamin E and NAFLD: Experimental Studies

The methionine and choline deficient (MCD) diet is a widely employed diet in NASH animal studies. The MCD diet is high in sucrose and fat (40% sucrose, 10% fat), and is deficient in methionine and choline, which are essential for hepatic beta-oxidation and the production of VLDL [47].

A trial carried out with rats fed with an MCD-diet showed that vitamin E significantly reduces the oxidative stress. In the control group, the authors observed a depletion in the liver glutathione stores and a notable increase in hepatic fibrosis, whereas vitamin E supplementation repleted hepatic glutathione, reduced steatosis, inflammation, hepatic stellate cell activation, and collagen mRNA expression, and ameliorated fibrosis [48].

In another animal NASH model, the combination of MCD diet and vitamin E significantly lowered serum transaminase levels and ameliorated hepatic steatosis and necroinflammation. These effects were associated with suppressed expression of the fibrotic genes TGF-β and MMP-2, inflammatory factor COX-2, and pro-apoptotic genes (Bax). In addition, vitamin E enhanced the activity of hepatic superoxide dismutase (SOD) and inhibited that of nuclear factor kappa B (NFkB) [49].

Similar effects were reported in arecent mouse model for NAFLD in which vitamin E therapy after partial hepatectomy significantly reduced the oxidative stress level and attenuated the progression of NAFLD [50].

In an obese (ob/ob) mouse model, α- or γ-tocopherol exerted a hepatoprotective role in alipopolysaccharide-induced NASH, as shown by suppressing hepatic malondialdehyde (MDA), tumor necrosis factor-α, and serum alanine aminotransferase levels [51].

Moreover, chickens fed ahigh-oxidant diet with the supplementation of vitamin E were able to normalize elevated hepatic transaminase levels [52]. In addition to the role of being an antioxidant, some studies have also proposed that vitamin E improves the liver integrity by down-regulating hepatic cluster of differentiation 36 protein (CD36)—a membrane transporter responsible for the uptake of fatty acids into the liver [53].

3.3. *Vitamin E and NAFLD: Human Studies*

Vitamin E has been used in monotherapy or with other agents in multiple clinical trials to treat NAFLD or NASH, with reported improvement in liver biochemistries and histology [54–68]. These trials varied in duration (24 weeks to >2 years) and dose (100–1200 IU/day) of vitamin E used. Long-term studies ($\geq$2 years) are summarized in Table 1.

Treatment with vitamin E combined with vitamin C and atorvastatin was demonstrated to be effective in reducing the odds of having hepatic steatosis in individuals with computed tomography (CT)-diagnosed NAFLD after 4 years of active therapy [63].

The combination of ursodeoxycholic acid (UDCA) with vitamin E has been evaluated in a small sample size compared with UDCA alone or placebo. Improvement in steatosis and transaminases level were observed only in the group who received combination therapy with UDCA and vitamin E [64]. By evaluating the long-term (>2 years) efficacy of a similar combination (UDCA with vitamin E) in patients with NASH, Piettu et al.demonstrated an improvement in histological lesions in the majority of patients [62].

Nobili et al.studied 90 children with NAFLD who were given calorie-restricted diet and exercise. Patients were randomized to treatment with vitamin E (600 IU/day) in combination with ascorbic acid (500 mg/daily; n = 45) or placebo (n = 45) [65]. At the end of 24 months, both groups had significant improvement in steatosis, lobular inflammation, hepatocyte ballooning. However, the addition of α-tocopherol and ascorbic acid was not associated with a greater histological or biochemical improvement as compared to placebo [65,66].

Clinical trials with vitamin E supplementation in NASH patients yielded promising results. In the PIVENS (Pioglitazone, Vitamin E or Placebo for Nonalcoholic Steatohepatitis) trial, vitamin E was evaluated as a treatment for NASH. The rate of achievement of the primary outcome was higher in patients treated with high-dose vitamin E (800 IU/day) for 96 weeks compared to placebo (43% vs. 19%, $p = 0.001$), while pioglitazone did not reach statistical significance. The histological analysis showed a reduction in hepatocyte ballooning (50% vs. 29%, $p = 0.005$) and lobular inflammation (54% vs. 35%, $p = 0.02$), thus reflecting its expected effect as an antioxidant leading to a decrease of oxidative stress-mediated injury. Interestingly, it significantly reduced liver steatosis and alanine aminotransferase (ALT), but had no significant changes on fibrosis [60].

Table 1. Effects of Vitamin E administration in patients with NAFLD.

Author	Study Design	Duration	Vitamin E Dosage	Effect of Vitamin E on NAFLD/NASH Histology and Biochemistry Compared to Placebo				
				ALT	Steatosis	Inflammation	Hepatocytes Ballooning	Fibrosis
Dufour et al., 2006 [64]	48 NASH patients randomized to vitamin E plus UDCA, UDCA versus placebo	2 years	400 IU twice daily	↓	↓	ns	NA	ns
Nobili et al., 2008 [66]	53 NAFLD patients randomized to vitamin E plus ascorbic and life style intervention versus placebo	2 years	600 IU/day	ns	ns	ns	ns	ns
Sanyal et al., 2010 [60]	247 NASH patients randomized to vitamin E, pioglitazone versus placebo	96 weeks	800 IU daily	↓		↓	↓	ns
Foster et al., 2011 [63]	1005 randomized to vitamin E combined with ascorbic acid and atorvastatin versus placebo. At baseline 80 had CT-diagnosed NAFLD	4 years	1000 IU daily	ns	↓ (Based on abdominal CT scan)	NA	NA	NA
Lavine et al., 2011 [61]	173 NAFLD patients randomized to vitamin E, metformin versus placebo	96 weeks	400 IU twice daily	ns	ns	ns	↓	ns
Pietu et al., 2012 [62]	101 patients treated with a combination of vitamin E with UDCA. 10 patients had a second liver biopsy during follow-up	4 years	500 IU daily	↓	↓3/10 ↑1/10 patients	↓3/10 ↑2/10 patients	↓3/10 ↑1/10patients	↓4/10 ↑1/10 patients

ALT: alanine aminotransferase; CT: computed tomography; NAFLD: nonalcoholic fatty liver disease; NASH: nonalcoholic steatohepatitis; ns: no significant statistical difference versus placebo; NA: not available; UDCA: ursodeoxycholic acid; ↑: worsening; ↓: improvement.

Following those studies, Lavine et al. conducted a multicenter, double-blind, double-placebo, randomized clinical trial in pediatric patients. The TONIC (Treatment of NAFLD in Children) trial involved 173 children and adolescents witha mean age of 13 years that received metformin (500 mg twice daily), vitamin E (400 IU twice daily), or placebo twice daily for 96 weeks. The primary outcome was sustained reduction in ALT level (defined as $\leq$50% baseline or $\leq$40 U/L from 48 weeks to 96 weeks of treatment). The only histologic feature of NASH that improved after treatment with both medications was the hepatocellular ballooning. Disappointingly, neither vitamin E nor metformin were superior to placebo in achieving sustained ALT reduction or in improving steatosis, lobular inflammation, or fibrosis scores [61].

In the light of these observations, today the European Association for the Study of the Liver (EASL) and the American Association for the Study of Liver Diseases (AASLD) (Alexandria, VA, USA) guidelines consider vitamin E as a potential short-term treatment for non-diabetic adults with biopsy-proven NASH [69]. Until further data supporting its effectiveness is available, vitamin E is not recommended to treat NASH in diabetic patients, NAFLD without liver biopsy, NASH cirrhosis, or cryptogenic cirrhosis [1,69].

3.4. Vitamin E: Safety Concerns

Long-term safety should be carefully discussed with NASH patients before starting therapy with vitamin E.A meta-analysis has suggested that high-dosage ($\geq$400 IU/day) vitamin E supplements may increase all-cause mortality [70]. However, this meta-analysis has been criticized because several studies with low mortality were excluded and concomitant vitamin A and the administration of other drugs as well as common factors such as smoking were not considered. Another meta-analysis where new clinical trials and updated results of mortality were included suggested that the higher mortality can be explained by a higher proportion of male patients that were included in these trials and not due to the higher dose of vitamin E supplementation [71]. On the other hand, large meta-analysis that included 57 trials showed that vitamin E supplementation appears to have no effect on all-cause mortality at doses up to 5500 IU/day [72].

Finally, a meta-analysis investigating the effect of vitamin E on the incidence of stroke reported an increase in the relative risk of hemorrhagic stroke by 22%, while the risk of ischemic stroke was reduced by 10% [73]. Another concern about vitamin E use is related to its association with a modest increase in the risk of prostate cancer [74].

Thus, patients chosen for treatment with vitamin E should be aware of these risks or be considered for alternative treatments.

4. Conclusions

Despite its high prevalence and the intensive research in the field, the treatment of NAFLD remains an unmet medical need. To date, no definite pharmacological treatment has been approved for NAFLD, and patients are often advised to engage in physical activity and lose weight, which is difficult to achieve and more difficult to maintain. However, policies to promote physical activity and the management of associated comorbidities (i.e., obesity and metabolic syndrome components) are expected to decrease both hepatic and cardiovascular-related morbidity and mortality in NASH patients.

Clinical trials for NAFLD or NASH showed a modest improvement in liver biochemistries and histology induced by vitamin E administration. However, some limitations of these trials should be noted. The duration of therapy may be not long enough to detect long-term histological change complications. Moreover, the number of randomized trials included was limited, and the number of participants in the trials was low. An additional reason for the lack of efficacy of vitamin E could be related to the use of oral preparations of varied dosage, which may not always guarantee an adequate bioavailability in patients with liver disease.

In this context, further monotherapy clinical trials and pharmacological evaluations are still needed to elucidate the underlying molecular mechanisms of prevention or therapy and possible adverse outcomes. This may also help to identify the optimal daily intake of vitamin E in both pediatric and adult patients.

In addition, more research is needed to seek novel biological activities of vitamin Emetabolites in the liver of NAFLD patients that may differ from those of parent compounds.

Finally, a better understanding of the pathophysiology of NAFLD/NASH will provide the opportunity to create trials of combination therapies that achieve high rates of therapeutic responses.

Author Contributions: Hamza El Hadi, Roberto Vettor and Marco Rossato designed the concept and wrote the manuscript.

References

1. Chalasani, N.; Younoss, Z.; Lavine, J.E.; Diehl, A.M.; Brunt, E.M.; Cusi, K.; Charlton, M.; Sanyal, A.J. The diagnosis and management of non-alcoholic fatty liver disease: Practice Guideline by the American Association for the Study of Liver Diseases, American College of Gastroenterology, and the American Gastroenterological Association. *Hepatology* **2012**, *55*, 2005–2023. [CrossRef] [PubMed]
2. Polyzos, S.A.; Kountouras, J.; Zavos, C. Nonalcoholic fatty liver disease: The pathogenetic roles of insulin resistance and adipocytokines. *Curr. Mol. Med.* **2009**, *72*, 299–314. [CrossRef]
3. Khan, R.S.; Newsome, P.N. Non-alcoholic fatty liver disease and liver transplantation. *Metabolism* **2016**, *65*, 1208–1223. [CrossRef] [PubMed]
4. Rinella, M.E. Nonalcoholic fatty liver disease: A systematic review. *JAMA* **2015**, *313*, 2263–2273. [CrossRef] [PubMed]
5. Review, T.; LaBrecque, D.R.; Abbas, Z.; Anania, F.; Ferenci, P.; Khan, A.G.; Goh, K.L.; Hamid, S.S.; Isakov, V.; Lizarzabal, M.; et al. World Gastroenterology Organisation global guidelines: Nonalcoholic fatty liver disease and nonalcoholic steatohepatitis. *J. Clin. Gastroenterol.* **2014**, *48*, 467–473.
6. El Hadi, H.; Vettor, R.; Rossato, M. Congenital Vitamin E deficiency. In *Handbook of Famine, Starvation, and Nutrient Deprivation*; Preedy, V.R., Patel, V.B., Eds.; Springer International Publishing AG: Basel, Switzerland, 2018; pp. 1–18, ISBN 978-3-319-40007-5.
7. Evans, H.M.; Bishop, K.S. On the existence of a hitherto unrecognized dietary factor essential for reproduction. *Science* **1922**, *56*, 650–651. [CrossRef] [PubMed]
8. Gee, P.T. Unleashing the untold and misunderstood observations on vitamin E. *Genes Nutr.* **2011**, *6*, 5–16. [CrossRef] [PubMed]
9. Sheppard, A.J.; Pennington, J.A.T.; Weihrauch, J.L. Analysis and distribution of vitamin E in vegetable oils and foods. In *Vitamin E in Health and Disease*; Packer, L., Fuchs, J., Eds.; Marcel Dekker Inc.: New York, NY, USA, 1993; pp. 9–31.
10. Karrer, P.; Fritzsche, H.; Ringier, B.; Salomon, H. Synthesis of alpha-tocopherol (vitamin E). *Nature* **1938**, *141*, 1057. [CrossRef]
11. Jensen, S.K.; Lauridsen, C. Alpha-tocopherol stereoisomers. *Vitam. Horm.* **2007**, *76*, 281–308. [PubMed]
12. Traber, M.G. Vitamin E regulatory mechanisms. *Annu. Rev. Nutr.* **2007**, *27*, 347–362. [CrossRef] [PubMed]
13. Kayden, H.J.; Traber, M.G. Absorption, lipoprotein transport, and regulation of plasma concentrations of vitamin E in humans. *J. Lipid Res.* **1993**, *34*, 343–358. [PubMed]
14. Kaempf-Rotzoll, D.E.; Traber, M.G.; Arai, H. Vitamin E and transfer proteins. *Curr. Opin. Lipidol.* **2003**, *14*, 249–254. [CrossRef] [PubMed]
15. Jiang, Q. Natural forms of vitamin E: Metabolism, antioxidant, and anti-inflammatory activities and their role in disease prevention and therapy. *Free Radic. Biol. Med.* **2014**, *72*, 76–90. [CrossRef] [PubMed]
16. Bardowell, S.A.; Duan, F.; Manor, D.; Swanson, J.E.; Parker, R.S. Disruption of mouse cytochrome p4504f14 (Cyp4f14 gene) causes severe perturbations in vitamin E metabolism. *J. Biol. Chem.* **2012**, *287*, 26077–26086. [CrossRef] [PubMed]
17. Birben, E.; Sahiner, U.M.; Sackesen, C.; Erzurum, S.; Kalayci, O. Oxidative stress and antioxidant defense. *World Allergy Organ J.* **2012**, *5*, 9–19. [CrossRef] [PubMed]

18. Peh, H.Y.; Tan, W.S.; Liao, W.; Wong, W.S. Vitamin E therapy beyond cancer: Tocopherol versus tocotrienol. *Pharmacol. Ther.* **2016**, *162*, 152–169. [CrossRef] [PubMed]
19. Yoshida, Y.; Saito, Y.; Jones, L.S.; Shigeri, Y. Chemical reactivities and physical effects in comparison between tocopherols and tocotrienols: Physiological significance and prospects as antioxidants. *J. Biosci. Bioeng.* **2007**, *104*, 439–445. [CrossRef] [PubMed]
20. Cooney, R.V.; Harwood, P.J.; Franke, A.A.; Narala, K.; Sundström, A.K.; Berggren, P.O.; Mordan, L.J. Products of gamma-tocopherol reaction with NO_2 and their formation in rat insulinoma (RINm5F) cells. *Free Radic. Biol. Med.* **1995**, *19*, 259–269. [CrossRef]
21. Christen, S.; Jiang, Q.; Shigenaga, M.K.; Ames, B.N. Analysis of plasma tocopherols α, γ, and 5-nitro-γ in rats with inflammation by HPLC coulometric detection. *J. Lipid Res.* **2002**, *43*, 1978–1985. [CrossRef] [PubMed]
22. Berbée, M.; Fu, Q.; Boerma, M.; Wang, J.; Kumar, K.S.; Hauer-Jensen, M. gamma-Tocotrienol ameliorates intestinal radiation injury and reduces vascular oxidative stress after total-body irradiation by an HMG-CoA reductase-dependent mechanism. *Radiat. Res.* **2009**, *171*, 596–605. [CrossRef] [PubMed]
23. Upston, J.M.; Terentis, A.C.; Stocker, R. Tocopherol-mediated peroxidation of lipoproteins: Implications for vitamin E as a potential antiatherogenic supplement. *FASEB J.* **1999**, *13*, 977–994. [PubMed]
24. Pearson, P.; Lewis, S.A.; Britton, J.; Young, I.S.; Fogarty, A. The pro-oxidant activity of high-dose vitamin E supplements in vivo. *BioDrugs* **2006**, *20*, 271–273. [CrossRef] [PubMed]
25. Weinberg, R.B.; VanderWerken, B.S.; Anderson, R.A.; Stegner, J.E.; Thomas, M.J. Pro-oxidant effect of vitamin E in cigarette smokers consuming a high polyunsaturated fat diet. *Arterioscler. Thromb. Vasc. Biol.* **2001**, *21*, 1029–1033. [CrossRef] [PubMed]
26. Zingg, J.M.; Azzi, A. Non-antioxidant activities of vitamin E. *Curr. Med. Chem.* **2004**, *11*, 1113–1133. [CrossRef] [PubMed]
27. Rimbach, G.; Minihane, A.M.; Majewicz, J.; Fischer, A.; Pallauf, J.; Virgli, F.; Weinberg, P.D. Regulation of cell signalling by vitamin E. *Proc. Nutr. Soc.* **2002**, *61*, 415–425. [CrossRef] [PubMed]
28. Boscoboinik, D.; Szewczyk, A.; Hensey, C.; Azzi, A. Inhibition of cell proliferation by alpha-tocopherol. Role of protein kinase C. *J. Biol. Chem.* **1991**, *266*, 6188–6194. [PubMed]
29. Cook-Mills, J.M. Isoforms of Vitamin E Differentially Regulate PKC α and Inflammation: A Review. *J. Clin. Cell. Immunol.* **2013**, *4*, 1000137. [CrossRef] [PubMed]
30. Venugopal, S.K.; Devaraj, S.; Yang, T.; Jialal, I. Alpha-tocopherol decreases superoxide anion release in human monocytes under hyperglycemic conditions via inhibition of protein kinase C-alpha. *Diabetes* **2002**, *51*, 3049–3054. [CrossRef] [PubMed]
31. Martin-Nizard, F.; Boullier, A.; Fruchart, J.C.; Duriez, P. Alpha-tocopherol but not beta-tocopherol inhibits thrombin-induced PKC activation and endothelin secretion in endothelial cells. *J. Cardiovasc. Risk* **1998**, *5*, 339–345. [CrossRef] [PubMed]
32. Rimbach, G.; Moehring, J.; Huebbe, P.; Lodge, J.K. Gene-regulatory activity of alpha-tocopherol. *Molecules* **2010**, *15*, 1746–1761. [CrossRef] [PubMed]
33. Ahsan, H.; Ahad, A.; Iqbal, J.; Siddiqui, W.A. Pharmacological potential of tocotrienols: A review. *Nutr. Metab.* **2014**, *11*, 52. [CrossRef] [PubMed]
34. Buzzetti, E.; Pinzani, M.; Tsochatzis, E.A. The multiple-hit pathogenesis of non-alcoholic fatty liver disease (NAFLD). *Metabolism* **2016**, *65*, 1038–1048. [CrossRef] [PubMed]
35. Hassan, K.; Bhalla, V.; El Regal, M.E.; A-Kader, H.H. Nonalcoholic fatty liver disease: A comprehensive review of a growing epidemic. *World J. Gastroenterol.* **2014**, *20*, 12082–12101. [CrossRef] [PubMed]
36. Fabbrini, E.; Mohammed, B.S.; Magkos, F.; Korenblat, K.M.; Patterson, B.W.; Klein, S. Alterations in adipose tissue and hepatic lipid kinetics in obese men and women with nonalcoholic fatty liver disease. *Gastroenterology* **2008**, *134*, 424–431. [CrossRef] [PubMed]
37. Sanyal, A.J.; Campbell-Sargent, C.; Mirshahi, F.; Rizzo, W.B.; Contos, M.J.; Sterling, R.K.; Luketic, V.A.; Shiffman, M.L.; Clore, J.N. Nonalcoholic steatohepatitis: Association of insulin resistance and mitochondrial abnormalities. *Gastroenterology* **2001**, *120*, 1183–1192. [CrossRef] [PubMed]
38. Hardwick, R.N.; Fisher, C.D.; Canet, M.J.; Lake, A.D.; Cherrington, N.J. Diversity in antioxidant response enzymes in progressive stages of human nonalcoholic fatty liver disease. *Drug Metab. Dispos.* **2010**, *38*, 2293–2301. [CrossRef] [PubMed]
39. Day, C.P. Pathogenesis of steatohepatitis. *Best Prac. Res. Clin. Gastroenterol.* **2002**, *16*, 663–678. [CrossRef]
40. Caldwell, S.H.; Chang, C.Y.; Nakamoto, R.K.; Krugner-Higby, L. Mitochondria in nonalcoholic fatty liver disease. *Clin. Liver Dis.* **2004**, *8*, 595–617. [CrossRef] [PubMed]

41. Aubert, J.; Begriche, K.; Knockaert, L.; Robin, M.A.; Fromenty, B. Increased expression of cytochrome P450 2E1 in nonalcoholic fatty liver disease: Mechanisms and pathophysiological role. *Clin. Res. Hepatol. Gastroenterol.* **2011**, *35*, 630–637. [CrossRef] [PubMed]
42. Leclercq, I.A.; Farrell, G.C.; Field, J.; Bell, D.R.; Gonzalez, F.J.; Robertson, G.R. CYP2E1 and CYP4A as microsomal catalysts of lipid peroxides in murine nonalcoholic steatohepatitis. *J. Clin. Investig.* **2000**, *105*, 1067–1075. [CrossRef] [PubMed]
43. Zhang, X.; Li, S.; Zhou, Y.; Su, W.; Ruan, X.; Wang, B.; Zheng, F.; Warner, M.; Gustafsson, J.Å.; Guan, Y. Ablation of cytochrome P450 omega-hydroxylase 4A14 gene attenuates hepatic steatosis and fibrosis. *Proc. Natl. Acad. Sci. USA* **2017**, *114*, 3181–3185. [CrossRef] [PubMed]
44. Demeilliers, C.; Maisonneuve, C.; Grodet, A.; Mansouri, A.; Nguyen, R.; Tinel, M.; Lettéron, P.; Degott, C.; Feldmann, G.; Pessayre, D.; et al. Impaired adaptive resynthesis and prolonged depletion of hepatic mitochondrial DNA after repeated alcohol binges in mice. *Gastroenterology* **2002**, *123*, 1278–1290. [CrossRef] [PubMed]
45. Dara, L.; Ji, C.; Kaplowitz, N. The contribution of endoplasmic reticulum stress to liver diseases. *Hepatology* **2011**, *53*, 1752–1763. [CrossRef] [PubMed]
46. Marra, F.; Svegliati-Baroni, G. Lipotoxicity and the gut-liver axis in NASH pathogenesis. *J. Hepatol.* **2017**. [CrossRef] [PubMed]
47. Larter, C.Z.; Yeh, M.M.; Williams, J.; Bell-Anderson, K.S.; Farrell, G.C. MCD-induced steatohepatitis is associated with hepatic adiponectin resistance and adipogenic transformation of hepatocytes. *J. Hepatol.* **2008**, *49*, 407–416. [CrossRef] [PubMed]
48. Phung, N.; Pera, N.; Farrell, G.; Leclercq, I.; Hou, J.Y.; George, J. Pro-oxidant-mediated hepatic fibrosis and effects of antioxidant intervention in murine dietary steatohepatitis. *Int. J. Mol. Med.* **2009**, *24*, 171–180. [PubMed]
49. Nan, Y.M.; Wu, W.J.; Fu, N.; Liang, B.L.; Wang, R.Q.; Li, L.X.; Zhao, S.X.; Zhao, J.M.; Yu, J. Antioxidants vitamin E and 1-aminobenzotriazole prevent experimental non-alcoholic steatohepatitis in mice. *Scand. J. Gastroenterol.* **2009**, *44*, 1121–1131. [CrossRef] [PubMed]
50. Karimian, G.; Kirschbaum, M.; Veldhuis, Z.J.; Bomfati, F.; Porte, R.J.; Lisman, T. Vitamin E Attenuates the Progression of Non-Alcoholic Fatty Liver Disease Caused by Partial Hepatectomy in Mice. *PLoS ONE* **2015**, *10*, e0143121. [CrossRef] [PubMed]
51. Chung, M.Y.; Yeung, S.F.; Park, H.J.; Volek, J.S.; Bruno, R.S. Dietary α- and γ-tocopherol supplementation attenuates lipopolysaccharide-induced oxidative stress and inflammatory-related responses in an obese mouse model of nonalcoholic steatohepatitis. *J. Nutr. Biochem.* **2010**, *21*, 1200–1206. [CrossRef] [PubMed]
52. Lu, T.; Harper, A.F.; Zhao, J.; Corl, B.A.; LeRoith, T.; Dalloul, R.A. Effects of a dietary antioxidant blend and vitamin E on fatty acid profile, liver function, and inflammatory response in broiler chickens fed a diet high in oxidants. *Poult. Sci.* **2014**, *93*, 1658–1666. [CrossRef] [PubMed]
53. Podszun, M.C.; Grebenstein, N.; Spruss, A.; Schlueter, T.; Kremoser, C.; Bergheim, I.; Frank, J. Dietary alpha-tocopherol and atorvastatin reduce high-fat-induced lipid accumulation and down-regulate CD36 protein in the liver of guinea pigs. *J. Nutr. Biochem.* **2014**, *25*, 573–579. [CrossRef] [PubMed]
54. Lavine, J.E. Vitamin E treatment of nonalcoholic steatohepatitis in children: A pilot study. *J. Pediatr.* **2000**, *136*, 734–738. [CrossRef]
55. Hasegawa, T.; Yoneda, M.; Nakamura, K.; Makino, I.; Terano, A. Plasma transforming growth factor-beta1 level and efficacy of alpha-tocopherol in patients with non-alcoholic steatohepatitis: A pilot study. *Aliment. Pharmacol. Ther.* **2001**, *15*, 1667–1672. [CrossRef] [PubMed]
56. Kugelmas, M.; Hill, D.B.; Vivian, B.; Marsano, L.; McClain, C.J. Cytokines and NASH: A pilot study of the effects of lifestyle modification and vitamin E. *Hepatology* **2003**, *38*, 413–419. [CrossRef] [PubMed]
57. Yakaryilmaz, F.; Guliter, S.; Savas, B.; Erdem, O.; Ersoy, R.; Erden, E.; Akyol, G.; Bozkaya, H.; Ozenirler, S. Effects of vitamin E treatment on peroxisome proliferator-activated receptor-alpha expression and insulin resistance in patients with non-alcoholic steatohepatitis: Results of a pilot study. *Intern. Med. J.* **2007**, *37*, 229–235. [CrossRef] [PubMed]
58. Bugianesi, E.; Gentilcore, E.; Manini, R.; Natale, S.; Vanni, E.; Villanova, N.; David, E.; Rizzetto, M.; Marchesini, G. A randomized controlled trial of metformin versus vitamin E or prescriptive diet in nonalcoholic fatty liver disease. *Am. J. Gastroenterol.* **2005**, *100*, 1082–1090. [CrossRef] [PubMed]

59. Vajro, P.; Mandato, C.; Franzese, A.; Ciccimarra, E.; Lucariello, S.; Savoia, M.; Capuano, G.; Migliaro, F. Vitamin E treatment in pediatric obesity-related liver disease: A randomized study. *J. Pediatr. Gastroenterol. Nutr.* **2004**, *38*, 48–55. [CrossRef] [PubMed]
60. Sanyal, A.J.; Chalasani, N.; Kowdley, K.V.; McCullough, A.; Diehl, A.M.; Bass, N.M.; Neuschwander-Tetri, B.A.; Lavine, J.E.; Tonascia, J.; Unalp, A.; et al. Pioglitazone, vitamin E, or placebo for nonalcoholic steatohepatitis. *N. Engl. J. Med.* **2010**, *362*, 1675–1685. [CrossRef] [PubMed]
61. Lavine, J.E.; Schwimmer, J.B.; Van Natta, M.L.; Molleston, J.P.; Murray, K.F.; Rosenthal, P.; Abrams, S.H.; Scheimann, A.O.; Sanyal, A.J.; Chalasani, N.; et al. Effect of vitamin E or metformin for treatment of nonalcoholic fatty liver disease in children and adolescents: The TONIC randomized controlled trial. *JAMA* **2011**, *305*, 1659–1668. [CrossRef] [PubMed]
62. Pietu, F.; Guillaud, O.; Walter, T.; Vallin, M.; Hervieu, V.; Scoazec, J.Y.; Dumortier, J. Ursodeoxycholic acid with vitamin E in patients with nonalcoholic steatohepatitis: Long-term results. *Clin. Res. Hepatol. Gastroenterol.* **2012**, *36*, 146–155. [CrossRef] [PubMed]
63. Foster, T.; Budoff, M.J.; Saab, S.; Ahmadi, N.; Gordon, C.; Guerci, A.D. Atorvastatin and antioxidants for the treatment of nonalcoholic fatty liver disease: The St Francis Heart Study randomized clinical trial. *Am. J. Gastroenterol.* **2011**, *106*, 71–77. [CrossRef] [PubMed]
64. Dufour, J.F.; Oneta, C.M.; Gonvers, J.J.; Bihl, F.; Cerny, A.; Cereda, J.M.; Zala, J.F.; Helbling, B.; Steuerwald, M.; Zimmermann, A. Swiss Association for the Study of the Liver. Randomized placebo-controlled trial of ursodeoxycholic acid with vitamin E in nonalcoholic steatohepatitis. *Clin. Gastroenterol. Hepatol.* **2006**, *4*, 1537–1543. [CrossRef] [PubMed]
65. Nobili, V.; Manco, M.; Devito, R.; Ciampalini, P.; Piemonte, F.; Marcellini, M. Effect of vitamin E on aminotransferase levels and insulin resistance in children with non-alcoholic fatty liver disease. *Aliment. Pharmacol. Ther.* **2006**, *24*, 1553–1561. [CrossRef] [PubMed]
66. Nobili, V.; Manco, M.; Devito, R.; Di Ciommo, V.; Comparcola, D.; Sartorelli, M.R.; Piemonte, F.; Marcellini, M.; Angulo, P. Lifestyle intervention and antioxidant therapy in children with nonalcoholic fatty liver disease: A randomized, controlled trial. *Hepatology* **2008**, *48*, 119–128. [CrossRef] [PubMed]
67. Sanyal, A.J.; Mofrad, P.S.; Contos, M.J.; Sargeant, C.; Luketic, V.A.; Sterling, R.K.; Stravitz, R.T.; Shiffman, M.L.; Clore, J.; Mills, A.S. A pilot study of vitamin E versus vitamin E and pioglitazone for the treatment of nonalcoholic steatohepatitis. *Clin. Gastroenterol. Hepatol.* **2004**, *2*, 1107–1115. [CrossRef]
68. Harrison, S.A.; Torgerson, S.; Hayashi, P.; Ward, J.; Schenker, S. Vitamin E and vitamin C treatment improves fibrosis in patients with nonalcoholic steatohepatitis. *Am. J. Gastroenterol.* **2003**, *98*, 2485–2490. [CrossRef] [PubMed]
69. European Association for the Study of the Liver (EASL); European Association for the Study of Diabetes (EASD); European Association for the Study of Obesity (EASO). EASL-EASD-EASO Clinical Practice Guidelines for the management of non-alcoholic fatty liver disease. *J. Hepatol.* **2016**, *64*, 1388–1402.
70. Miller, E.R.; Pastor-Barriuso, R.; Dalal, D.; Riemersma, R.A.; Appel, L.J.; Guallar, E. Meta-analysis: High-dosage vitamin E supplementation may increase all-cause mortality. *Ann. Intern. Med.* **2005**, *142*, 37–46. [CrossRef] [PubMed]
71. Gerss, J.; Köpcke, W. The questionable association of vitamin E supplementation and mortality–inconsistent results of different meta-analytic approaches. *Cell. Mol. Biol.* **2009**, *55* (Suppl. OL), 1111–1120.
72. Abner, E.L.; Schmitt, F.A.; Mendiondo, M.S.; Marcum, J.L.; Kryscio, R.J. Vitamin E and all-cause mortality: A meta-analysis. *Curr. Aging Sci.* **2011**, *4*, 158–170. [CrossRef] [PubMed]
73. Schurks, M.; Glynn, R.J.; Rist, P.M.; Tzourio, C.; Kurth, T. Effects of vitamin E on stroke subtypes: Meta-analysis of randomised controlled trials. *BMJ* **2010**, *341*, c5702. [CrossRef] [PubMed]
74. Klein, E.A.; Thompson, I.M.; Tangen, C.M.; Crowley, J.J.; Lucia, M.S.; Goodman, P.J.; Minasian, L.M.; Ford, L.G.; Parnes, H.L.; Gaziano, J.M.; et al. Vitamin E and the risk of prostate cancer: The Selenium and Vitamin E Cancer Prevention Trial (SELECT). *JAMA* **2011**, *306*, 1549–1556. [CrossRef] [PubMed]

15

Tocotrienols: A Family of Molecules with Specific Biological Activities

Raffaella Comitato, Roberto Ambra and Fabio Virgili *

Council for Agricultural Research and Economics, Research Centre for Food and Nutrition (CREA-AN) via Ardeatina 546, 00178 Rome, Italy; raffaella.comitato@crea.gov.it (R.C.); roberto.ambra@crea.gov.it (R.A.)

* Correspondence: fabio.virgili@crea.gov.it

Abstract: Vitamin E is a generic term frequently used to group together eight different molecules, namely: α-, β-, γ- and δ-tocopherol and the corresponding tocotrienols. The term tocopherol and eventually Vitamin E and its related activity was originally based on the capacity of countering foetal re-absorption in deficient rodents or the development of encephalomalacia in chickens. In humans, Vitamin E activity is generally considered to be solely related to the antioxidant properties of the tocolic chemical structure. In recent years, several reports have shown that specific activities exist for each different tocotrienol form. In this short review, tocotrienol ability to inhibit cancer cell growth and induce apoptosis thanks to specific mechanisms, not shared by tocopherols, such as the binding to Estrogen Receptor-β (ERβ) and the triggering of endoplasmic reticulum (EndoR) stress will be described. The neuroprotective activity will also be presented and discussed. We propose that available studies strongly indicate that specific forms of tocotrienols have a distinct mechanism and biological activity, significantly different from tocopherol and more specifically from α-tocopherol. We therefore suggest not pooling them together within the broad term "Vitamin E" on solely the basis of their putative antioxidant properties. This option implies obvious consequences in the assessment of dietary Vitamin E adequacy and, probably more importantly, on the possibility of evaluating a separate biological variable, determinant in the relationship between diet and health.

Keywords: tocopherols; tocotrienols; estrogen receptors; endoplasmic reticulum stress; neuroprotection

---

1. Introduction

The term "natural Vitamin E" is commonly used to group together eight different molecules, namely α-, β-, γ- and δ-tocopherol and the corresponding tocotrienols. The original description of Vitamin E is: "a fat soluble vitamin that inhibits oxidative destruction of biological membranes and is necessary for fertility and to prevent hemolysis in rats and muscle dystrophy in poultry" [1]. If we held that this definition is biologically true and descriptive of the vitamin functions, we must face the evidence that, with the exception of a "generic" putative antioxidant activity in protecting biological membranes from peroxidation, in comparison to α-tocopherol, β-, γ- and δ-tocopherol and all tocotrienols have very low (if any) biological activity in the fetal re-absorption test. Their relative efficiency, in fact, ranges from zero to about 40% for β-tocopherol, which is the only alternative form significantly active in this test [1]. Accordingly, the units definition provided by the United States Pharmacopoeia of the different Vitamin E analogues is standardized on the efficiency of α-tocopherol, whereas β-, γ- and δ-tocopherol and the tocotrienols are much less active (either inactive) in this assay [2].

If we agree in considering that the only biological function of Vitamin E is acting as an "antioxidant", the inclusion of tocotrienols in the Vitamin E family should not be questioned but, accordingly, we should include in the "Vitamin E family" several other molecules displaying a "lipid peroxidation chain breaking activity" within biological membranes. Conversely, if we accept that the biological role of α-tocopherol is more complex and goes beyond its activity as a membrane antioxidant, we must accept that this role is not shared by other tocols, and solely assign the term Vitamin E to α-tocopherol.

In fact, it is possible to describe similarities and differences between the members of the Vitamin E family. Dietary α-tocopherol, non-α-tocopherols and tocotrienols are all absorbed by intestinal cells by passive diffusion; and receptor-mediated transport and delivered to the lymph and then to the liver via chylomicron [3]. However, the efficiency of absorption is not the same, being apparently higher for tocotrienols than for α-tocopherol. This latter has been reported to significantly inhibit the cellular uptake of δ-tocotrienol (and probably of other tocotrienols), at least in endothelial cells by a still unknown mechanism [4].

Once in the liver, α-tocopherol is immediately transferred to the α-tocopherol transfer protein (α-TTP) (see below) and further disposed to the peripheral tissues after the incorporation into VLDL/LDL/HDL [3]. If not delivered to peripheral tissues, α-tocopherol, non-α-tocopherols and tocotrienols are metabolized by phase I and II enzymes and excreted as glucuronide or sulfate [3], but tocotrienols have been reported to be degraded to a larger extent than their counterparts with saturated side chains. The significant quantitative differences in the metabolism between each tocopherol and between tocotrienols and tocopherols that have been reported in vitro, suggest that similar differences may exist also in vivo [5].

Very importantly, the biological activity of Vitamin E is highly dependent upon regulatory mechanisms exerted by the intracellular α-TTP that enrich the plasma with α-tocopherol while non-α-tocopherols molecules are directed to metabolism. α-TTP specifically recognizes α-tocopherol by the three methyl groups on the chromanol ring, by the hydroxyl group on the chromanol ring and the structure and orientation of the phytyl side chain. Thanks to these multiple "recognition mechanisms", α-TPP preferably and efficiently only binds α-tocopherol while all the other Vitamin E forms display a very low or null binding activity [6,7]. As the result of this specificity, only α-tocopherol, once taken up from the liver from dietary derived chilomicrons, can be released to peripheral extrahepatic tissues via lipoprotein VLDL trafficking, while the other tocopherols and the tocotrienols are rapidly metabolized by phase I and phase II enzymes and finally excreted in the bile, feces or urine [3]. Interestingly, a linear relationship between the relative affinity and the known biological activity obtained from the rat resorption-gestation assay exists, clearly indicating that the ability to bind to α-TTP is critical to determine the biological activity. However, it has been demonstrated that long oral supplementation of tocotrienol to mice and rats results in the delivery to vital organs including the brain, liver, heart, skin, lungs, adipose tissue, and whole blood independently of α-TTP expression [8,9]. These findings strongly demonstrate the existence of TTP-independent, still partially unknown, mechanisms of transport for oral tocotrienol. Moreover, the presence of α-tocopherol leads to decreased binding and to an acceleration of metabolism of non-α-tocopherols and tocotrienols [9].

Significant differences also exist in plasma concentration of α-tocopherol and tocotrienols. The administration of high doses (750 mg and 1000 mg) of a tocotrienol mixture from Annatto (*Bixa orellana*), results in a maximum plasma concentration levels at 3–4 h for all isomers, while α-tocopherol is reported to peak at 6 h, suggesting a different distribution mechanism [10]. Even though γ- and δ-tocotrienols have been probably studied more in the detail, α-tocotrienol has been found as the most abundant form circulating in plasma, chilomicrons, LDL, and HDL after the dietary supplementation with a mixture from palm (*Elaeis guineensis)* oil, also containing α-tocopherol. According to the study mentioned above [10], concentrations are in the order of μM and peak at less than 5 h for γ- and δ-tocotrienol and at 6 h for α-tocotrienol [11].

Overall, in conclusion, it is quite surprising that α-, β-, γ- and δ-tocotrienol are still pooled together with tocopherols in spite of a significantly different steric hindrance due to the unsaturated phytyl tail, and of several evidences indicating that they have a distinct metabolism and different routes of tissue delivery and storage [12]. All these evidences suggest that tocotrienol should be a candidate to play a different biological role than α-tocopherol [13]. A "side-to side" visualization of D-α-tocopherol and D-α-tocotrienols (Figure 1) highlights the evident differences between these two molecules at the tridimensional level that are frequently ignored in a two-dimensional, planar visualization. A dynamic view of these two molecules would further underline their different spatial seizures, due to the presence of two *trans* double bonds in the phytyl tail of tocotrienols limiting the rotational freedom of carbon-carbon bonds.

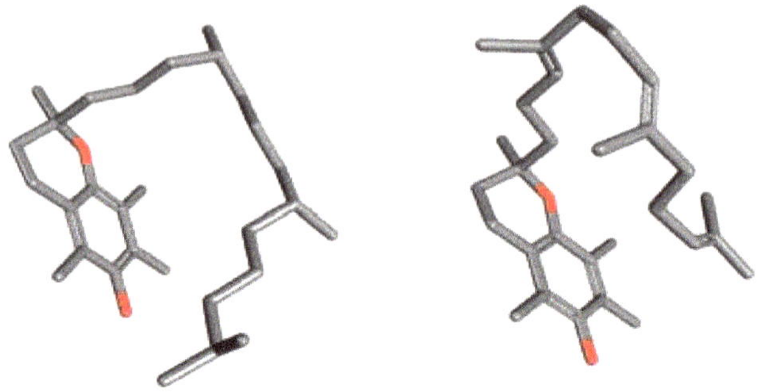

D-α-tocopherol D-α-tocotrienol

Figure 1. Structural differences between α-tocotrienol and α-tocopherol (from https://pubchem.ncbi.nlm.nih.gov/).

A plethora of papers, also published by high impact factor journals (including those by the authors) encourage a kind of confusion. In fact, the term Vitamin E is frequently introduced as (e.g.,): " ... *Tocotrienols and tocopherols are natural forms of the Vitamin E family* ... ", even though it is always admitted that (e.g.,) " ... *Vitamin E deficiency syndromes cannot be prevented by supplying non-α-tocopherols or tocotrienols* ... " and that (e.g.,) "*Although all natural forms of Vitamin E display potent antioxidant activity, the activity of tocotrienols is mediated independently of their antioxidant activity..*" and also: " ... *current studies of the biological functions of Vitamin E indicate that members in the Vitamin E family possess unique biological functions often not shared by other family members*".

Starting from the "contradictions" described above, this review focuses on some of the most evident specific activities reported for tocotrienols, not shared by α-tocopherol or by other tocopherols, namely the estrogen receptor-β (ERβ) binding activity and endoplasmic reticulum (EndoR) response activation both leading to a pro-apoptotic cellular response by γ- and δ-tocotrienol. The specificity of α-tocotrienol in protecting neuronal cells after ischemia will also be presented and discussed together with other tocotrienol-specific mechanisms on cell functions and survival.

2. Tocotrienols as Ligands of ERβ

Interestingly, one of the first studies reporting the antiproliferative/pro-apoptotic effects of tocotrienols, excluded the possibility of a mechanism related to the binding to estrogen receptors [14]. This early paper reported a study that was conducted somehow before the discovery and characterization of the β form of ERs [15]. The experimental design was in fact based on the assumption that the human breast cancer cell line estrogen-independent (MDA-MB-231) was void of any ER form and utilized to compare the effects of tocotrienols on the estrogen responsive breast cancer cell line, MCF7. Conversely, MDA cells have been eventually demonstrated to express a functional β form, while MCF7 express both α- and β-ER. In this study, authors observed that a tocotrienol-rich fraction (TRF) of palm (*Elaeis guineensis*) oil, containing α-tocopherol and α-, γ- and δ-tocotrienol, inhibited MCF7 cells growth in both the presence and absence of estradiol with a nonlinear dose-response. MDA-MB-231 cells were also inhibited by TRF but with a linear dose-response. In the same study, the authors reported, after fractionation of TRF, γ- and δ-tocotrienols containing fractions were the most inhibitory ones. On the other hand, and according to the matter of the present paper, α-tocopherol had no effect on the growth rate of both cell lines. The authors ruled out the contribution of ER activity on the basis that TRF (and therefore tocotrienols) did not affect the expression of a gene, the breast cancer estrogen inducible sequence-trefoil factor 1 (pS2-TFF1), known to be driven by estradiol due to the presence of an ERα responsive elements in its promoter. The original conclusion has been reconsidered under the light of an "*omic*" approach utilized in subsequent studies performed by our laboratory. In a first study [16], utilizing cultured cells as an experimental model, we performed a cDNA array analysis of cancer-related gene expression in estrogen-dependent (MCF-7) and estrogen-independent (MDA-MB-231) human breast cancer cells. In this study, we utilized the best transcriptomic platform available at that time (1200 gene) that allowed us to conclude that the supplementation tocotrienol rich fraction form palm oil (TRF) was associated to the modulation of a number of genes encoding for proteins involved in cell cycle and therefore to inhibitory effects on cell growth and differentiation of the tumor cell lines. Previous studies had already demonstrated that α-tocopherol, the only tocopherol form present in TRF, had no effect on the induction of apoptosis in both cell lines, the only one having some pro-apoptotic activity being δ-tocopherol [17].

In a second study, based on a more sophisticated in vivo model [18], MCF-7 breast cancer cells were injected into athymic nude mice also fed with TRF. At the end of 20 wk dietary treatment there was a significant delay in the onset, incidence, and size of the tumors in nude mice supplemented with TRF compared with the controls. In addition, a cDNA array technique providing the differential expression of 1200 genes was performed on excised tumor tissues and, in agreement with the study performed on cultured cells, a significant number of genes was affected by TRF treatment. According to a "gene-ontology" analysis we identified a set of genes involved in the regulation of immune response and in the functional class of intracellular transducers/effectors/modulators. Data obtained in the course of these studies, further interrogated in silico provided a consistent hypothesis for a direct interaction of tocotrienols with estrogen pathway. In silico docking analysis, and in vitro binding-displacement test to purified ER protein demonstrated a high affinity of tocotrienols for ERβ but not for ERα. We also demonstrated that in ERβ-containing MDA-MB-231 breast cancer cells, tocotrienols, but not α-tocopherol, increase ERβ translocation into the nucleus and the expression of a spectrum of pro-apoptotic estrogen-responsive genes such as the Macrophage-inhibiting Cytokine-1 (MIC-1), the Early Growth Response-1 (EGR-1) and Cathepsin-D and accompanied by typically apoptotic-like alterations of cell morphology, DNA fragmentation, and caspase-3 activation [19]. These results have been corroborated and completed by a second study conducted on MCF-7 breast cancer cell, expressing both ERα and ERβ [20]. Furthermore, in this cell line, treatment with TRF and in particular with γ-tocotrienol, but not α-tocopherol, was associated with ERβ nuclear translocation and ER-dependent genes expression (MIC-1, EGR-1 and Cathepsin-D). At same time, the treatment induced a very evident inhibition of ERα activity finally leading to DNA fragmentation and apoptosis [20]. cDNA-array data obtained within this study also suggested the presence of an alternative pathway activated by γ- and δ-tocotrienols that will be presented below.

It is well known that ERβ activation can produce different cellular outcomes according to the balance between the "non genomic" signaling triggered by ERα and ERβ and other specific characteristics of cellular and tissue environment [21,22]. Accordingly, Nakaso and coworkers have more recently reported a cytoprotective, rather than pro-apoptotic effect of γ- and δ-tocotrienol in SH-SY5Y neuroblastoma cells, a cellular model addressing the pathogenesis of human Parkinson's disease [23]. In agreement with our original studies, this study confirmed that purified γ- and δ-tocotrienol bind to ERβ in vitro and that γ- and δ-tocotrienol were cytoprotective against Parkinson's disease-related toxicities such as 1-methyl-4-phenylpyridinium ion (MPP^+) thanks to a marked activation of the phosphoinositide-3-kinase/serine/threonine kinase-1 (PI3K/Akt) signaling pathway downstream to ERβ binding. The pivotal and functional role of γ- and δ-tocotrienol binding to ERβ was confirmed by ERβ silencing that was associated to the abrogation of cytoprotection and Akt phosphorylation [23].

The same authors also reported that the silencing of caveolin-1 and/or caveolin-2, candidates for the early events of signal transduction, prevented the cytoprotective effects of γ- and δ-tocotrienol, but not Akt phosphorylation. In agreement with us, the authors conclude that tocotrienols, in particular γ- and δ-tocotrienol, have distinct biological activities, unrelated to their putative antioxidant capacity, and that they can exert a specific neuro-protective activity mediated by ERβ binding and PI3K/Akt signaling activation [23].

Remarkably, one early study reported that tocotrienols induce apoptosis and a significant delay in cell growth in normal mammary cells obtained from midpregnant BALB/c mice [24]. However, neither the same authors, nor other research groups, have eventually confirmed these observations. Conversely, the same authors more recently, reported that γ-tocotrienol has a potent antiproliferative and cytotoxic effects by autophagy in MCF-7 and MDA-MD-231 cancer cell [25]. In contrast to the reports of Nakaso and coworkers mentioned above [23], γ-tocotrienol is reported to induce a reduction in PI3K/Akt/ mechanistic target of rapamycin kinase (mTOR) signaling and a corresponding increase in the Bax/Bcl-2 ratio, cleaved caspase-3, and cleaved poly (ADP-ribose) polymerase (PARP) levels in these cancer cell lines. These events suggest that γ-tocotrienol-induced autophagy may be involved in the initiation of apoptosis. In contrast, the same treatment was not found to increase autophagy marker expression in immortalized mouse (CL-S1) and human (MCF-10 A) normal mammary epithelial cell lines [25].

It seems therefore possible to speculate that γ-tocotrienol induces opposite effects in cancer and normal (or pseudo-normal) cells in agreement with the established perturbation of PI3K/Akt/mTOR signaling pathway in cancer cells [26]. Similarly, a specific effect of tocotrienols on Bax/Bcl2 mediated apoptosis has been also reported in prostate tumorigenesis in the transgenic adenocarcinoma mouse prostate (TRAMP) mouse model. In this study, a dietary supplementation with of a tocotrienol mixture induced a decrease in the levels of high-grade neoplastic lesions associated with an increased expression of proapoptotic proteins BAD a Bcl2 antagonist of cell death and cleaved caspase-3 and cell cycle regulatory proteins cyclin dependent kinase inhibitors p21 and p27 [27].

3. Tocotrienols as Inducers of Apoptosis via Endoplasmic Reticulum (EndoR) Stress

The first report of an EndoR stress mediated apoptosis by tocotrienols dates back about 10 years. Wali and coworkers [28] tested the effect of γ-tocotrienol in highly metastatic +SA rodent mammary epithelial cells. This study identified that 15–40 μM γ-tocotrienol induces a dose dependent apoptotic response paralleled by an increase of poly (ADP-ribose) polymerase (PARP)-cleavage and activation of a pathway distinctive of EndoR stress response, the protein kinase-like endoplasmic reticulum kinase/eukaryotic translational initiation factor/activating transcription factor 4 (PERK/eIF2α/ATF-4). γ-tocotrienol treatment also caused a large increase of key components of EndoR stress mediated apoptosis, tribbles 3 (TRB3) and C/emopamil binding protein (EBP) homologous protein (CHOP). The silencing of this latter gene significantly quenched γ-tocotrienol-induced PARP-cleavage and TRB3 expression. The same study [28] also reports that γ-tocotrienol treatment was associated to a decrease of full-length caspase-12 levels, indicating an activation of caspase-12 cleavage.

Park and collaborators have later confirmed these observations in a syngeneic mouse mammary tumor model and in cultured human breast cancer cells [29]. In the animal study, after the subcutaneous implantation of 66cl-4-GFP murine mammary tumor cells, female BALB/c mice were fed a diet enriched with purified α- and γ-tocotrienol to approximately provide 0.625 mg of each tocotrienol/mouse/day. The authors excluded a possible interference from Vitamin E supplementation, by adjusting Vitamin E in the diet with 30 IU/kg diet of DL-α-tocopheryl acetate to fully meet the animal's requirement. Dietary γ-tocotrienol suppressed tumor growth by inhibiting cell proliferation and inducing apoptosis. In fact, tumors excised from the γ-tocotrienol fed animals had significant more TUNEL (terminal deoxynucleotidyl transferase mediated nick end labeling assay) and less Ki-67 (a biomarker for cell division) positive cells (386% and 55%, respectively) compared to the animal fed the basal diet group. The same study reports no effects on tumor vascularization, and that the feeding with α-tocotrienol supplementation was not associated to comparable activities potential, at the tested dose. When utilizing cultured cells (MDA-MB-231 and MCF-7 human breast cancer cells and 66cl-4-GFP murine mammary tumor cells) the authors could confirm that α-, γ- and δ-tocotrienols induce apoptosis, independently of cell estrogen receptors' expression profile [29]. γ-tocotrienol was the most active form and was studied in deeper detail. The authors observed a significant activation of c-Jun NH(2)-terminal kinase (JNK) and p38-mitogen activated kinase-like protein (MAPK) accompanied by the upregulation of the expression death receptor 5 (DR5) and C/EBP homologous protein (CHOP), an endoplasmic reticulum (EndoR) stress marker, these events finally leading to the PARP, caspase-8, -9, and -3 cleavage. The silencing of JNK or p38 MAPK was associated to a reduced increase of DR5 and CHOP and partially inhibiting apoptosis. α-tocotrienol did not reduce tumor burden in vivo, but had inhibitory effects on colony formation in all three cell lines at relatively high concentrations in comparison to γ- and δ-tocotrienols, corroborating the evidence that the observed effects are strongly specific.

A further indication for the involvement of EndoR stress in tocotrienol-induced apoptosis was provided by Patacsil and coworkers [30] in MDA-MB 231 and MCF-7 breast cancer cells. This study demonstrates that 40 μM γ-tocotrienol induces PARP cleavage and caspase-7 activation in MCF-7 cells, accompanied by alterations in the expression of genes involved in cell growth and proliferation, cell death, cell cycle, cellular development, cellular movement and gene regulation. Among the categories studied by means of in silico Pathway Analysis the paper reports the modulation of signal transduction mediated by NRF-2-mediated "hormetic" oxidative stress response, transforming Growth Factor-β (TGF-β) signaling and EndoR stress response. Moreover, in agreement with other studies conducted on the same cellular models [31], the same study reports that MCF-7 and MDA-MB 231 cells respond to γ-tocotrienol by inducing the activation of PERK and pIRE1α pathways. The strong up-regulation of the Activating transcription factor 3 (ATF3) (16.8-fold) associated to EndoR stress and the abrogation of the apoptotic response after ATF3 silencing suggests this protein as a potential molecular target for γ-tocotrienol in breast cancer cells.

The specific activity of γ-tocotrienol on CHOP expression and EndoR stress has been also reported in several human malignant mesothelioma H2052 (sarcomatoid), H28 (epithelioid), H2452 (bi-phasic), and MSTO-211H (biphasic). In these cells, statins (atorvastatin and simvastatin) and 20 μM γ-tocotrienol have been observed to have synergistic effect on cell growth inhibition and acting through the inhibition of mevalonate pathway [32]. The authors report that, in H2052 and MSTO-211H cells, the treatment with γ-tocotrienol alone was sufficient to induce a significant increase of the expression of the endoplasmic reticulum stress markers CHOP and glucose regulated protein-78 (GRP-78). Conversely, the intrinsic apoptotic marker, caspase 3 activation, was induced only in the presence of statins. It is well known that the Bcl-2 family plays a pivotal role in apoptosis, either as an activator (through Bax and Bak) or as an inhibitor (Bcl-2 and Bcl-xL), Bcl-2 to Bax ratio is recognized as a key factor in the regulation of the apoptotic process or cell death [33]. According to this notion, this study also considered the possibility that γ-tocotrienol could affect Bax to Bcl2 ratio. Consistently with a previous report indicating that γ-tocotrienol induced a mitochondrial disruption pathway without affecting Bax/Bcl-2 expression in human breast cancer MDA-MB-231 cells [34], the Bax/Bcl2 ratio was not affected by any of the treatments.

We have also studied the involvement of EndoR stress on the effects of δ-tocotrienol on the growth of two different lines of human melanoma cells, BLM and A375 [35]. In agreement to observations obtained utilizing different tumor lines, the treatment with 5–20 μM δ-tocotrienol had a significant proapoptotic effect on both cell lines, involving the intrinsic apoptosis pathway. Very importantly, we observed no effect on the viability of normal human melanocytes. δ-tocotrienol effects were associated to the activation of the PERK/p-eIF2α/ATF4/CHOP, Inositol-requiring enzyme-1α (IRE1α) and caspase-4 strongly suggesting the involvement of EndoR stress upstream to the apoptotic response. We confirmed this hypothesis observing the quenching of the apoptotic response after a treatment with Salubrinal, an inhibitor of the EndoR stress. In the same study, in disagreement with observations reported by others [32,34], but in agreement with the observations by Barve and coworkers [27], we observed cytochrome c release from mitochondria, indicating a disruption of the mitochondrial outer membrane potential, associated to a significant increase of Bax/Bcl2 ratio. In vivo experiments performed in nude mice bearing A375 cells xenografts confirmed that a supplementation with dietary δ-tocotrienol (100 mg/kg daily, 5 days/week) up to 35 days, results in a reduced tumor volume and tumor mass and in significant delay of tumor progression [35].

A final confirmation of the ability of specific tocotrienol forms to activate EndoR stress is reported in a very recent study from our laboratory [31]. We reported a series of experiments based on the analysis of transcriptomic data obtained within our previous studies [18,19]. These data, interrogated by different bio-informatics tools, suggested the existence of an alternative pathway, activated by specific tocotrienols forms and leading to apoptosis, also in tumor cells not expressing ERs. This hypothesis was, in fact, confirmed utilizing HeLa cells, a line of human cervical cancer cells void of any canonical ER form. Once synchronized and treated either with the tocotrienol-rich fraction (α, γ and δ form) from palm oil (10–20 μg/mL) or with purified α-, γ- and δ-tocotrienol (5–20 μg/mL), HeLa cells underwent apoptosis which was accompanied by a significant expression of caspase 8, caspase 10 and caspase 12. Following the interrogation of additional data obtained from transcriptomic platforms, we considered the hypothesis that the administration of γ- and δ-tocotrienol could induce a release of Ca^{2+} from the EndoR. Accordingly, in living cells, we observed a significant activation of Ca-dependent signals. This event was followed by the expression and activation of IRE-1α and by the splicing and activation of X-box binding protein 1 (XBP-1), another molecule involved in the unfolded protein response, the core pathway coping with EndoR stress in eukaryotic cells, finally leading to apoptosis. Very importantly, and not very commonly indeed, our study considered α-tocopherol as a negative control, confirming that only γ- and δ-tocotrienol, not the proper Vitamin E D-α-tocopherol, are responsible for the observed effects. In the same paper [31], addressing the molecular mechanism underlying tocotrienols' activity, we wanted to speculate about the possible presence of a putative (orphan) receptor, possibly located at the level of the cellular membrane and able to accept tocotrienols and other estrogen mimetics as selective ligands. We based this speculation on the observation that the treatment with the specific ER inhibitor ICI-182,780 weakens the effects of tocotrienols on the upregulation of pro-apoptotic genes and the apoptotic response in cells lacking ERs. According to the chemo-physical characteristics of tocotrienols, the candidate downstream target(s) of the activity of this receptor could reasonably be located at the level of EndoR. The activation of this hypothetical (orphan) receptor would sequentially trigger EndoR stress, IRE-1 activation and XBP-1 splicing, finally inducing apoptosis.

The ability of γ-tocotrienol to induce apoptosis through activation of both the intrinsic and extrinsic pathway has been also confirmed in Jurkat cells, a human T-cell lymphoma [36]. In this study, γ-tocotrienol but not α-tocotrienol inhibited proliferation and induced apoptosis in this cell line in a dose dependent manner. The administration of 10–50 μM γ-tocotrienol resulted in elevated mitochondrial ROS production, JNK activation and suppression of extracellular regulated MAP kinase (ERK) and p38-MAPK. In agreement with our observations [31], γ-tocotrienol induced intracellular calcium release and, in agreement with others [27] a loss of mitochondrial membrane potential and cytochrome c release. These changes were found to be associated with an increase Bax/Bcl-xL expression rate and to an increased expression of Fas and FasL. Similarly to other studies [24,25,35], γ-tocotrienol had no effects on normal human peripheral blood mononuclear cells suggesting a specific cytotoxicity towards transformed lymphoma cells [36].

γ-Tocotrienol has also been demonstrated to induce paraptosis, a type of caspase independent programmed cell death, morphologically distinct from apoptosis, in that it displays cytoplasmic vacuolation and lacks of the typical apoptotic morphology. Zhang and collaborators [37] focused on the effects of δ-tocotrienol on human colon cancer SW620 cells and observed that δ-tocotrienol inhibits proliferation in a dose-dependent manner, correlated with cytoplasmic vacuolation possibly resulting from welling and fusion of mitochondria and/or EndoR. No changes in caspase 3 activation and other morphological (blebbing) or molecular markers of apoptosis were observed. The authors also report that δ-tocotrienol treatment (10 to 40 μM) was associated to a reduced β-catenin and wnt-1 expression and to lower cyclin D1, c-jun and matrix metallopeptidase 7 (MMP-7) protein levels, indicating the triggering of paraptosis-like cell death, with the suppression of the Wnt signaling pathway. The same authors have more recently reported similar results after the treatment with γ-tocotrienol both in SW620 and HCT-8 cells, another type of human ileocecal colorectal adenocarcinoma also associated to the suppression of Wnt signaling pathway [38].

4. Neuroprotection and Lipoxygenase Inhibition by α-Tocotrienol

While γ- and δ-tocotrienol have been demonstrated to induce specific responses in cancer cells with little or no effects on normal cells, α-tocotrienol has been frequently reported to play a protective activity on normal neuronal cells and, in general, on central nervous system. A study by Fukui and collaborators [39] utilized neuro2a cells, a line obtained from a spontaneous neuroblastoma in an albino strain A mouse frequently utilized as a model to study neurite outgrowth, neurotoxicity, Alzheimer disease and in general for neuronal tumourigenicity studies. This study, even appearing somehow an oversimplification in comparison with other studies based on a more complex experimental design, demonstrated that 5 μM α-tocotrienol counters the effects of the water-soluble free radical generator 2,2′-azobis(2-methylpropionamide) dihydrochloride (AAPH) on neurite degeneration and dynamics.

More specific research, directly targeting the protective effects of α-tocotrienol against neurodegeneration, has been conducted by the group of Sen and collaborators [40]. These authors originally reported the ability of nanomolar concentrations of α-tocotrienol, but not α-tocopherol to block glutamate-induced cell death. Glutamate is one of the most important neurotransmitters but, at high concentrations, it induces a rise of intracellular Ca^{2+} and mitochondrial dysfunction followed by cell death [41]. α-tocotrienol inhibits cell death by suppressing the activation of c-Src kinase and ERK phosphorylation in HT4, an embryonal carcinoma from metastatic lung with neural characteristics and expressing Simian vacuolating polyoma virus 40 (SV40) [42]. Very interestingly, the concentrations utilized in this study were 4–10-fold lower than levels detected in plasma of supplemented humans, indicating that α-tocotrienol regulates a specific signal transduction pathway insensitive to comparable concentrations of tocopherol, clearly suggesting that this activity is completely independent of its antioxidant capacity.

In a following study [43], the same group demonstrated that, in the same tumor cell line (HT4) and in immature primary cortical neurons, glutamate toxicity is mediated by the activation of neuronal 12-lipoxygenase that precede the production of peroxides, increased influx of Ca^{2+} and cell death. At lower physiologically achievable concentrations (nanomolar), α-tocotrienol displayed potent neuroprotective properties in both cell lines challenged by glutamate apparently interacting with 12-lipoxygenase, suppressing arachidonic acid metabolism. This observation was confirmed in vitro, by testing the activity of a purified enzyme in the presence of α-tocotrienol and by an in silico docking study suggesting that α-tocotrienol hampers the access of lipoxygenase substrate, to the enzyme catalytic site [43]. Even though a 12-lipoxygenase inhibiting activity has been reported also for α-tocopherol [44], the IC50 was in the order of μM, which is an order of magnitude higher than that reported for α-tocotrienol and, therefore, possibly due to a different mechanism.

The same group has further investigated the neuroprotective activity of α-tocotrienol in a sophisticated model based on single neuron microinjection technique on HT4 cells. The same study also reports the effects of dietary supplementation of α-tocotrienol in 12-lipoxigenase deficient mice undergoing surgically induced stroke and in spontaneously hypertensive rats [45]. The authors observed that very low quantities (sub-attomole) of α-tocotrienol, but not of α-tocopherol, protected isolated neurons from glutamate challenge. In agreement with the observations of a rapid 12-lipoxygenase tyrosine phosphorylation catalyzed by c-Src, lipoxygenase-deficient mice were more resistant to stroke-induced brain injury than their wild-type controls. Oral supplementation of α-tocotrienol to spontaneously hypertensive rats was associated to increased levels in the brain and to a protection against stroke-induced injury, associated with lower c-Src activation and 12-lipoxygenase phosphorylation at the stroke site.

In a study that followed [46], the same group addressed the comparison between the antioxidant-independent and -dependent neuroprotective properties of α-tocotrienol in HT4 cells cytotoxicity elicited by homocysteic acid and linoleic acid, respectively. Homocysteic acid administration was associated to a significant neurodegeneration presenting features similar to those previously observed in glutamate-induced neurotoxicity, in particular, the activation of c-Src and 12-lipoxygenase phosphorylation as early events. The administration of both homocysteic and linoleic acid was associated to an increased ratio of oxidized to reduced glutathione and to the triggering of an EndoR stress, as indicated by raised intracellular Ca^{2+} concentration and altered mitochondrial membrane potential eventually followed by cell death [46]. As the oxidative stress is considered a late event in apoptosis induced by homocysteic acid, the antioxidant component of α-tocotrienol protection was verified by inducing oxidative stress and cell death by linoleic acid. In all cases, the presence of nanomolar concentrations of α-tocotrienol, but not of α-tocopherol, was significantly protective. The authors concluded that α-tocotrienol protection against neurotoxicity is attributable to a combination of an antioxidant-independent and to antioxidant-dependent mechanisms.

The neuroprotective activity tocotrienols and, in particular, of α-tocotrienol has been confirmed by Osakada and coworkers [47]. In their study, the authors observed that a tocotrienol mixture from palm oil, further purified in order to eliminate α-tocopherol, purified α-, γ- and δ-tocotrienol (0.1–10 μM) significantly protects primary neuronal cells from rat striatum challenged by different pro-oxidants. Namely, hydrogen peroxide, a superoxide generating molecule (paraquat), nitric oxide donors (*S*-nitrosocysteine and 3-morpholinosydnonimine) and an inhibitor of glutathione synthesis L-buthionine-[*S*,*R*]-sulfoximine were utilized. In the same paper, only α-tocotrienol, but not γ- and δ-tocotrienol prevented the apoptosis induced by a protein kinase inhibitor, staurosporine, suggesting a specific mechanism underlying α-tocotrienol activity, totally independent of its putative antioxidant capacity. Conversely, α-tocopherol was ineffective in all cases, corroborating the evidence of a specific tocotrienol activity unrelated to their nucleophilic, antioxidant, properties.

It is worth noting that Wang and coworkers have elegantly demonstrated that the arylating oxidative product of γ-tocopherol, γ-tocopherol quinone, but not the non-arylating α-tocopherol quinone, induces EndoR stress affecting activation of PERK/CHOP proteins in N2A neuroblastoma cells [48]. As mentioned above, γ- and δ-tocotrienol have been also reported to affect this pathway in melanoma [35], mesothelioma H2052 and MSTO-211H cells [32], while our recent study indicated that EndoR stress induced by tocotrienols was mediated by IRE1 activation and not by PERK, suggesting a separate mechanism of action [31]. However, the paper by Wang and collaborators [48] clearly identifies the arylating activity of γ-tocopherol quinone as the mechanism underlying the activation of EndoR stress, while other investigations and in particular our study [31], did not take this event into consideration, on the basis of the indications of a receptor-mediated mechanism.

Finally, it is possible that the relative intracellular concentration and the specific localization of α-tocopherol and γ- and δ-tocotrienol can affect the cell response, eventually determining the final outcome. At present, very few studies [45] addressed this important issue and more investigation is surely warranted.

5. Other Tocotrienol-Triggered Cellular Responses

Besides ERβ activation and EndoR stress mediated apoptosis, γ-tocotrienol has also recently been observed to significantly alter sphingolipids composition in various types of cancer cells such as Human colon HCT-116, pancreatic PANC-1 and breast MCF-7 [49]. In particular, the authors observed a rapid elevation of dihydrosphingosine and dihydroceramides associated with increased cellular stress, phosphorylation of the mitogen-activated protein kinase, JNK and apoptosis. The inhibition of the de novo synthesis of sphingolipids was associated to a parallel inhibition of γ-tocotrienol-induced apoptosis and autophagy. γ-tocotrienol was demonstrated to inhibit dihydroceramide desaturase

(DEGS) activity but not its protein expression or de novo synthesis of sphingolipids. The increase of dihydroceramides paralleled by a relative decrease of ceramides coincides with the induction of apoptosis and autophagy. Overall, the authors conclude that γ-tocotrienol inhibits ceramide desaturase activity inducing an early elevation of dihydro-sphingolipids and late increase of saturated ceramide suggesting a role of these sphingolipid in tocotrienol-induced cell stress and death [49].

According to the evidence that several chemopreventive agents negatively affect cell growth by targeting p53 pathway, Agarwal and coworkers [50], utilized the human colon carcinoma RKO cell line, to investigate the effects of a TRF on the components of p53 signaling network. The authors report that the treatment with TRF results in a dose- and time- dependent inhibition of growth and colony formation associated to the induction of cyclin dependent kinase inhibitor 1A (WAF1)/p21, independent of cell cycle regulation and is transcriptionally upregulated in p53 dependent fashion.

In agreement with observations from our group and by others [27,35], but in disagreement with other reports [32,34], Agarwal and collaborators [50] reported that TRF induces the release of cytochrome c and induction of apoptotic protease-activating factor-1 upon a significant alteration of Bax/Bcl2 ratio. The altered ratio between the members of the Bax family triggered in turn by the activation of initiator caspase-9 followed by activation of effector caspase-3 finally lead to apoptosis characterized by chromatin condensation, DNA fragmentation and shrinkage of cell membrane.

Other biological activities have been reported specifically for γ- and δ-tocotrienol. A recent paper by Wong and coworkers [51] reports that the supplementation with 85 mg/kg/day γ- and δ-tocotrienol, but not with α-tocotrienol and α-tocopherol, improves cardiovascular functions in rats fed for 16 weeks a diet high in simple carbohydrates (fructose) and fats (beef tallow), in comparison to a corn starch based diet. In the same study [51], only δ-tocotrienol was associated with improved glucose tolerance, insulin sensitivity, lipid profile and abdominal adiposity. In the liver, these interventions reduced lipid accumulation, inflammatory infiltrates and plasma liver enzyme activities. In agreement with previous investigations [8,9], despite low or no detection of tocotrienols in plasma, the authors found detectable levels in heart, liver and adipose tissue confirming that chronic oral administration is associated to tocotrienols delivery and accumulation to these organs [51].

6. Conclusions

We have provided some references that strongly indicate that specific tocotrienols forms, and in particular α-, γ- and δ-, have biological activities distinct from that of tocopherols and in particular of D-α-tocopherol, the only molecule that, in our opinion should be considered as "Vitamin E".

In this review, we focused our interest on the ability of γ- and δ-tocotrienol to induce cell growth arrest and apoptosis in different tumor cell types, by specific mechanisms apparently not shared by tocopherols. Even though other specific effects have been reported, the ability to act as "productive" ligands of ERβ and to trigger Ca^{2+} release from EndoR, seem the most evident features of δ- and γ-tocotrienol, eventually associated with the expression of pro-apoptotic genes, finally leading to apoptosis or paraptosis. Interestingly, the pathway associated to cell death depends, at least in part, on the tumor type and pro-apoptotic effects have not been reported in non-tumor cells.

These observations not only suggest that specific forms of tocotrienols (in this case, δ- and γ-tocotrienol) have a specific capacity in inducing programmed death in tumor cells, but also that their specific activity occurs through diverse specific mechanisms, according to the cell type. Under this perspective, specific forms of tocotrienols and, in particular, δ-tocotrienol could be proposed as an expedient, potentially effective option for novel chemopreventive/therapeutic strategies in different types of solid tumors. On the other hand, α-tocotrienol displays a specific neuroprotective capacity due to its ability to inhibit 12-lipoxygenase, a key enzyme in the execution of cellular death induced by glutamate and by homocysteic acid. Taken together, current findings strongly indicate that tocotrienols may have a significant role in different specific pathological conditions, which are not necessarily affected by Vitamin E (α-tocopherol). Figure 2 shows the different molecular targets of tocotrienols in the representative cell types we have considered in this review, namely cancer cells expressing

ER, cancer cells not expressing ER and normal neuronal cells submitted to specific stressors such as glutamate or homocysteic acid.

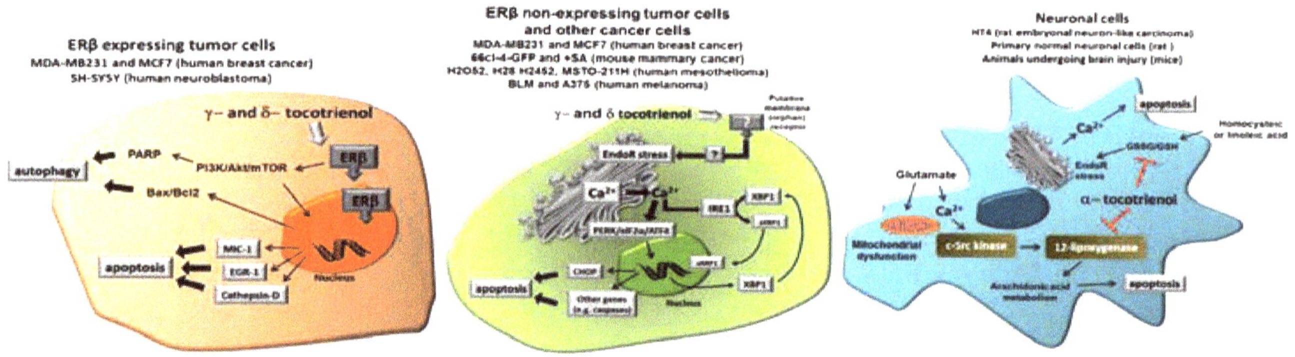

Figure 2. Different molecular targets of tocotrienols in the representative cell types we have considered in this review, namely cancer cells expressing Estrogen Receptor (ER), cancer cells not expressing ER and normal neuronal cells submitted to specific stressors such as glutamate or homocysteic acid. See text for more details. (Modified from [31]).

In spite of the relative abundance of studies dealing with the effects associated to the administration of tocotrienols, either in cultured cells or in experimental animals, very few studies considered the mechanism of action. In fact, very often, the terms "mechanism" and "effects" are utilized interchangeably, when they should refer to different concepts. In our opinion, the term mechanism should be solely utilized to describe the molecular events leading to the observed effects, such as (e.g.,) in the case of the tocotrienol binding to ERβ (mechanism) leading to the transcriptional activation of gene expression (effects). To our knowledge, our laboratory and few others [20,43] are the only ones that addressed this issue by the combination of in silico *docking* analysis, to build up the hypothesis of ER (either other nuclear receptors) binding or the inhibition of 12-lipoxygenase, respectively, eventually confirmed in vitro, in cultured cells and in animals. Further studies, dealing with the understanding of the molecular (mechanistic) basis underlying the observed effects of specific tocotrienol forms are surely warranted, in order to define the real limits of these molecules as a possible alternative for cancer treatment or co-adjuvant in cancer treatment.

Besides this, a major problem in the correct interpretation of some of studies reported herein is, in general, the absence of a treatment, either in cultured cells or in animals, with α-tocopherol. In fact, for instance, studies utilizing mixtures administered to cultured cells or to animals contained significant amounts of α-tocopherol. This experimental weakness make it unclear if the observed effects can be totally ascribed to tocotrienols or also to α-tocopherol, as several authors tend to claim. However, studies correctly performing this specific "negative" control published by our laboratory [19,20,31] and by others [29,40,42,43,45–47] provide indirect but solid indications about the differential ability of α-, γ- and δ-tocotrienol, but not α-tocopherols to trigger specific cellular response in different cell types.

7. Practical Consequences at Nutritional Level

If we accept that each tocotrienol form has a distinct, specific biological activity, different cellular targets and molecular mechanisms of action, significantly different from tocopherol and more specifically from α-tocopherol, we must necessarily stop pooling them together on solely the basis of their putative antioxidant properties. Consequently, tocotrienols should be excluded from the "Vitamin E family". This option would probably imply some consequences in the assessment of dietary Vitamin E adequacy even though more studies are surely needed to investigate their relative body distribution and plasma levels in normal dietary conditions. More importantly, the distinction between Vitamin E (α-tocopherol) and specific non-α-tocopherol molecules will allow for investigations aiming to evaluate a separate biological variable determinant in the relationship between diet and health.

Finally, a system biology approach, accompanied by high throughput methodologies, appears an indispensable tool for a better understanding of the role of molecules of nutritional interest in human health and disease. Classical "hypothesis driven studies", even when very well conducted and designed, may risk consolidating original weaknesses, possibly leading to a *"narrowing of perspective and from there false expectation"*.

References

1. Machlin, L.J. *Vitamin E*, 2nd ed.; Marcel Dekker, Inc.: New York, NY, USA, 1991.
2. Board, F.A.N.; Medicine, I.O. *Dietary Reference Intakes for Vitamin C, Vitamin E, Selenium, and Carotenoids*; The National Academies Press: Washington, DC, USA, 2000.
3. Schmölz, L.; Birringer, M.; Lorkowski, S.; Wallert, M. Complexity of vitamin E metabolism. *World J. Biol. Chem.* **2016**, *7*, 14–43. [CrossRef] [PubMed]
4. Shibata, A.; Nakagawa, K.; Tsuduki, T.; Miyazawa, T. Alpha-Tocopherol suppresses antiangiogenic effect of delta-tocotrienol in human umbilical vein endothelial cells. *J. Nutr. Biochem.* **2015**, *26*, 345–350. [CrossRef] [PubMed]
5. Jiang, Q. Natural forms of vitamin E: Metabolism, antioxidant, and anti-inflammatory activities and their role in disease prevention and therapy. *Free Radic. Biol. Med.* **2014**, *72*, 76–90. [CrossRef] [PubMed]
6. Hosomi, A.; Arita, M.; Sato, Y.; Kiyose, C.; Ueda, T.; Igarashi, O.; Arai, H.; Inoue, K. Affinity for alpha-tocopherol transfer protein as a determinant of the biological activities of vitamin E analogs. *FEBS Lett.* **1997**, *409*, 105–108. [CrossRef]
7. Manor, D.; Morley, S. The alpha-tocopherol transfer protein. *Vitam. Horm.* **2007**, *76*, 45–65. [PubMed]
8. Patel, V.; Khanna, S.; Roy, S.; Ezziddin, O.; Sen, C.K. Natural vitamin E alpha-tocotrienol: Retention in vital organs in response to long-term oral supplementation and withdrawal. *Free Radic. Res.* **2006**, *40*, 763–771. [CrossRef] [PubMed]
9. Khanna, S.; Patel, V.; Rink, C.; Roy, S.; Sen, C.K. Delivery of orally supplemented alpha-tocotrienol to vital organs of rats and tocopherol-transport protein deficient mice. *Free Radic. Biol. Med.* **2005**, *39*, 1310–1319. [CrossRef] [PubMed]
10. Qureshi, A.A.; Khan, D.A.; Silswal, N.; Saleem, S.; Qureshi, N. Evaluation of Pharmacokinetics, and Bioavailability of Higher Doses of Tocotrienols in Healthy Fed Humans. *J. Clin. Exp. Cardiol.* **2016**, *7*, 434. [CrossRef] [PubMed]
11. Fairus, S.; Nor, R.M.; Cheng, H.M.; Sundram, K. Alpha-tocotrienol is the most abundant tocotrienol isomer circulated in plasma and lipoproteins after postprandial tocotrienol-rich vitamin E supplementation. *Nutr. J.* **2012**, *11*, 5. [CrossRef] [PubMed]
12. Patel, V.; Rink, C.; Gordillo, G.M.; Khanna, S.; Gnyawali, U.; Roy, S.; Shneker, B.; Ganesh, K.; Phillips, G.; More, J.L.; et al. Oral tocotrienols are transported to human tissues and delay the progression of the model for end-stage liver disease score in patients. *J. Nutr.* **2012**, *142*, 513–519. [CrossRef] [PubMed]
13. Peh, H.Y.; Tan, W.S.; Liao, W.; Wong, W.S. Vitamin E therapy beyond cancer: Tocopherol versus tocotrienol. *Pharmacol. Ther.* **2016**, *162*, 152–169. [CrossRef] [PubMed]
14. Nesaretnam, K.; Stephen, R.; Dils, R.; Darbre, P. Tocotrienols inhibit the growth of human breast cancer cells irrespective of estrogen receptor status. *Lipids* **1998**, *33*, 461–469. [CrossRef] [PubMed]
15. Mosselman, S.; Polman, J.; Dijkema, R. ER beta: Identification and characterization of a novel human estrogen receptor. *FEBS Lett.* **1996**, *392*, 49–53. [CrossRef]
16. Nesaretnam, K.; Ambra, R.; Selvaduray, K.R.; Radhakrishnan, A.; Reimann, K.; Razak, G.; Virgili, F. Tocotrienol-rich fraction from palm oil affects gene expression in tumors resulting from MCF-7 cell inoculation in athymic mice. *Lipids* **2004**, *39*, 459–467. [CrossRef] [PubMed]
17. Yu, W.; Simmons-Menchaca, M.; Gapor, A.; Sanders, B.G.; Kline, K. Induction of apoptosis in human breast cancer cells by tocopherols and tocotrienols. *Nutr. Cancer* **1999**, *33*, 26–32. [CrossRef] [PubMed]
18. Nesaretnam, K.; Ambra, R.; Selvaduray, K.R.; Radhakrishnan, A.; Canali, R.; Virgili, F. Tocotrienol-rich fraction from palm oil and gene expression in human breast cancer cells. *Ann. N. Y. Acad. Sci.* **2004**, *1031*, 143–157. [CrossRef] [PubMed]
19. Comitato, R.; Nesaretnam, K.; Leoni, G.; Ambra, R.; Canali, R.; Bolli, A.; Marino, M.; Virgili, F. A novel mechanism of natural vitamin E tocotrienol activity: Involvement of ERbeta signal transduction. *Am. J. Physiol. Endocrinol. Metab.* **2009**, *297*, E427–E437. [CrossRef] [PubMed]

20. Comitato, R.; Leoni, G.; Canali, R.; Ambra, R.; Nesaretnam, K.; Virgili, F. Tocotrienols activity in MCF-7 breast cancer cells: Involvement of ERbeta signal transduction. *Mol. Nutr. Food Res.* **2010**, *54*, 669–678. [CrossRef] [PubMed]
21. Acconcia, F.; Totta, P.; Ogawa, S.; Cardillo, I.; Inoue, S.; Leone, S.; Trentalance, A.; Muramatsu, M.; Marino, M. Survival versus apoptotic 17beta-estradiol effect: Role of ER alpha and ER beta activated non-genomic signaling. *J. Cell. Physiol.* **2005**, *203*, 193–201. [CrossRef] [PubMed]
22. Lewis-Wambi, J.S.; Jordan, V.C. Estrogen regulation of apoptosis: How can one hormone stimulate and inhibit? *Breast Cancer Res.* **2009**, *11*, 206. [CrossRef] [PubMed]
23. Nakaso, K.; Tajima, N.; Horikoshi, Y.; Nakasone, M.; Hanaki, T.; Kamizaki, K.; Matsura, T. The estrogen receptor beta-PI3K/Akt pathway mediates the cytoprotective effects of tocotrienol in a cellular Parkinson's disease model. *Biochim. Biophys. Acta* **2014**, *1842*, 1303–1312. [CrossRef] [PubMed]
24. McIntyre, B.S.; Briski, K.P.; Tirmenstein, M.A.; Fariss, M.W.; Gapor, A.; Sylvester, P.W. Antiproliferative and apoptotic effects of tocopherols and tocotrienols on normal mouse mammary epithelial cells. *Lipids* **2000**, *35*, 171–180. [CrossRef] [PubMed]
25. Tiwari, R.V.; Parajuli, P.; Sylvester, P.W. Gamma-Tocotrienol-induced autophagy in malignant mammary cancer cells. *Exp. Biol. Med.* **2014**, *239*, 33–44. [CrossRef] [PubMed]
26. Porta, C.; Paglino, C.; Mosca, A. Targeting PI3K/Akt/mTOR Signaling in Cancer. *Front. Oncol.* **2014**, *4*, 64. [CrossRef] [PubMed]
27. Barve, A.; Khor, T.O.; Reuhl, K.; Reddy, B.; Newmark, H.; Kong, A.N. Mixed tocotrienols inhibit prostate carcinogenesis in TRAMP mice. *Nutr. Cancer* **2010**, *62*, 789–794. [CrossRef] [PubMed]
28. Wali, V.B.; Bachawal, S.V.; Sylvester, P.W. Endoplasmic reticulum stress mediates gamma-tocotrienol-induced apoptosis in mammary tumor cells. *Apoptosis* **2009**, *14*, 1366–1377. [CrossRef] [PubMed]
29. Park, S.K.; Sanders, B.G.; Kline, K. Tocotrienols induce apoptosis in breast cancer cell lines via an endoplasmic reticulum stress-dependent increase in extrinsic death receptor signaling. *Breast Cancer Res. Treat.* **2010**, *124*, 361–375. [CrossRef] [PubMed]
30. Patacsil, D.; Tran, A.T.; Cho, Y.S.; Suy, S.; Saenz, F.; Malyukova, I.; Ressom, H.; Collins, S.P.; Clarke, R.; Kumar, D. Gamma-tocotrienol induced apoptosis is associated with unfolded protein response in human breast cancer cells. *J. Nutr. Biochem.* **2012**, *23*, 93–100. [CrossRef] [PubMed]
31. Comitato, R.; Guantario, B.; Leoni, G.; Nesaretnam, K.; Ronci, M.B.; Canali, R.; Virgili, F. Tocotrienols induce endoplasmic reticulum stress and apoptosis in cervical cancer cells. *Genes Nutr.* **2016**, *11*, 32. [CrossRef] [PubMed]
32. Tuerdi, G.; Ichinomiya, S.; Sato, H.; Siddig, S.; Suwa, E.; Iwata, H.; Yano, T.; Ueno, K. Synergistic effect of combined treatment with gamma-tocotrienol and statin on human malignant mesothelioma cells. *Cancer Lett.* **2013**, *339*, 116–127. [CrossRef] [PubMed]
33. Lindqvist, L.M.; Vaux, D.L. BCL2 and related prosurvival proteins require BAK1 and BAX to affect autophagy. *Autophagy* **2014**, *10*, 1474–1475. [CrossRef] [PubMed]
34. Takahashi, K.; Loo, G. Disruption of mitochondria during tocotrienol-induced apoptosis in MDA-MB-231 human breast cancer cells. *Biochem. Pharmacol.* **2004**, *67*, 315–324. [CrossRef] [PubMed]
35. Montagnani Marelli, M.; Marzagalli, M.; Moretti, R.M.; Beretta, G.; Casati, L.; Comitato, R.; Gravina, G.L.; Festuccia, C.; Limonta, P. Vitamin E delta-tocotrienol triggers endoplasmic reticulum stress-mediated apoptosis in human melanoma cells. *Sci. Rep.* **2016**, *6*, 30502. [CrossRef] [PubMed]
36. Wilankar, C.; Khan, N.M.; Checker, R.; Sharma, D.; Patwardhan, R.; Gota, V.; Sandur, S.K.; Devasagayam, T.P. γ-Tocotrienol induces apoptosis in human T cell lymphoma through activation of both intrinsic and extrinsic pathways. *Curr. Pharm. Des.* **2011**, *17*, 2176–2189. [CrossRef] [PubMed]
37. Zhang, J.S.; Li, D.M.; He, N.; Liu, Y.H.; Wang, C.H.; Jiang, S.Q.; Chen, B.Q.; Liu, J.R. A paraptosis-like cell death induced by delta-tocotrienol in human colon carcinoma SW620 cells is associated with the suppression of the Wnt signaling pathway. *Toxicology* **2011**, *285*, 8–17. [CrossRef] [PubMed]
38. Zhang, J.S.; Li, D.M.; Ma, Y.; He, N.; Gu, Q.; Wang, F.S.; Jiang, S.Q.; Chen, B.Q.; Liu, J.R. Gamma-Tocotrienol induces paraptosis-like cell death in human colon carcinoma SW620 cells. *PLoS ONE* **2013**, *8*, e57779.
39. Fukui, K.; Sekiguchi, H.; Takatsu, H.; Koike, T.; Urano, S. Tocotrienol prevents AAPH-induced neurite degeneration in neuro2a cells. *Redox Rep.* **2013**, *18*, 238–244. [CrossRef] [PubMed]
40. Sen, C.K.; Khanna, S.; Roy, S. Tocotrienol: The natural vitamin E to defend the nervous system? *Ann. N. Y. Acad. Sci.* **2004**, *1031*, 127–142. [CrossRef] [PubMed]

41. Kritis, A.A.; Stamoula, E.G.; Paniskaki, K.A.; Vavilis, T.D. Researching glutamate—Induced cytotoxicity in different cell lines: A comparative/collective analysis/study. *Front. Cell. Neurosci.* **2015**, *9*, 91. [CrossRef] [PubMed]
42. Sen, C.K.; Khanna, S.; Roy, S.; Packer, L. Molecular basis of vitamin E action. Tocotrienol potently inhibits glutamate-induced pp60(c-Src) kinase activation and death of HT4 neuronal cells. *J. Biol. Chem.* **2000**, *275*, 13049–13055. [CrossRef] [PubMed]
43. Khanna, S.; Roy, S.; Ryu, H.; Bahadduri, P.; Swaan, P.W.; Ratan, R.R.; Sen, C.K. Molecular basis of vitamin E action: Tocotrienol modulates 12-lipoxygenase, a key mediator of glutamate-induced neurodegeneration. *J. Biol. Chem.* **2003**, *278*, 43508–43515. [CrossRef] [PubMed]
44. Reddanna, P.; Rao, M.K.; Reddy, C.C. Inhibition of 5-lipoxygenase by vitamin E. *FEBS Lett.* **1985**, *193*, 39–43. [CrossRef]
45. Khanna, S.; Roy, S.; Slivka, A.; Craft, T.K.; Chaki, S.; Rink, C.; Notestine, M.A.; DeVries, A.C.; Parinandi, N.L.; Sen, C.K. Neuroprotective properties of the natural vitamin E alpha-tocotrienol. *Stroke* **2005**, *36*, 2258–2264. [CrossRef] [PubMed]
46. Khanna, S.; Roy, S.; Parinandi, N.L.; Maurer, M.; Sen, C.K. Characterization of the potent neuroprotective properties of the natural vitamin E alpha-tocotrienol. *J. Neurochem.* **2006**, *98*, 1474–1486. [CrossRef] [PubMed]
47. Osakada, F.; Hashino, A.; Kume, T.; Katsuki, H.; Kaneko, S.; Akaike, A. Alpha-tocotrienol provides the most potent neuroprotection among vitamin E analogs on cultured striatal neurons. *Neuropharmacology* **2004**, *47*, 904–915. [CrossRef] [PubMed]
48. Wang, X.; Thomas, B.; Sachdeva, R.; Arterburn, L.; Frye, L.; Hatcher, P.G.; Cornwell, D.G.; Ma, J. Mechanism of arylating quinone toxicity involving Michael adduct formation and induction of endoplasmic reticulum stress. *Proc. Natl. Acad. Sci. USA* **2006**, *103*, 3604–3609. [CrossRef] [PubMed]
49. Jang, Y.; Rao, X.; Jiang, Q. Gamma-tocotrienol profoundly alters sphingolipids in cancer cells by inhibition of dihydroceramide desaturase and possibly activation of sphingolipid hydrolysis during prolonged treatment. *J. Nutr. Biochem.* **2017**, *46*, 49–56. [CrossRef] [PubMed]
50. Agarwal, M.K.; Agarwal, M.L.; Athar, M.; Gupta, S. Tocotrienol-rich fraction of palm oil activates p53, modulates Bax/Bcl2 ratio and induces apoptosis independent of cell cycle association. *Cell Cycle* **2004**, *3*, 205–211. [CrossRef] [PubMed]
51. Wong, W.Y.; Ward, L.C.; Fong, C.W.; Yap, W.N.; Brown, L. Anti-inflammatory gamma- and delta-tocotrienols improve cardiovascular, liver and metabolic function in diet-induced obese rats. *Eur. J. Nutr.* **2017**, *56*, 133–150. [CrossRef] [PubMed]

Permissions

All chapters in this book were first published by MDPI; hereby published with permission under the Creative Commons Attribution License or equivalent. Every chapter published in this book has been scrutinized by our experts. Their significance has been extensively debated. The topics covered herein carry significant findings which will fuel the growth of the discipline. They may even be implemented as practical applications or may be referred to as a beginning point for another development.

The contributors of this book come from diverse backgrounds, making this book a truly international effort. This book will bring forth new frontiers with its revolutionizing research information and detailed analysis of the nascent developments around the world.

We would like to thank all the contributing authors for lending their expertise to make the book truly unique. They have played a crucial role in the development of this book. Without their invaluable contributions this book wouldn't have been possible. They have made vital efforts to compile up to date information on the varied aspects of this subject to make this book a valuable addition to the collection of many professionals and students.

This book was conceptualized with the vision of imparting up-to-date information and advanced data in this field. To ensure the same, a matchless editorial board was set up. Every individual on the board went through rigorous rounds of assessment to prove their worth. After which they invested a large part of their time researching and compiling the most relevant data for our readers.

The editorial board has been involved in producing this book since its inception. They have spent rigorous hours researching and exploring the diverse topics which have resulted in the successful publishing of this book. They have passed on their knowledge of decades through this book. To expedite this challenging task, the publisher supported the team at every step. A small team of assistant editors was also appointed to further simplify the editing procedure and attain best results for the readers.

Apart from the editorial board, the designing team has also invested a significant amount of their time in understanding the subject and creating the most relevant covers. They scrutinized every image to scout for the most suitable representation of the subject and create an appropriate cover for the book.

The publishing team has been an ardent support to the editorial, designing and production team. Their endless efforts to recruit the best for this project, has resulted in the accomplishment of this book. They are a veteran in the field of academics and their pool of knowledge is as vast as their experience in printing. Their expertise and guidance has proved useful at every step. Their uncompromising quality standards have made this book an exceptional effort. Their encouragement from time to time has been an inspiration for everyone.

The publisher and the editorial board hope that this book will prove to be a valuable piece of knowledge for researchers, students, practitioners and scholars across the globe.

List of Contributors

Kotaro Azuma
Department of Systems Aging Science and Medicine, Tokyo Metropolitan Institute of Gerontology, 35-2 Sakae-cho, Itabashi-ku, Tokyo 173-0015, Japan

Satoshi Inoue
Department of Systems Aging Science and Medicine, Tokyo Metropolitan Institute of Gerontology, 35-2 Sakae-cho, Itabashi-ku, Tokyo 173-0015, Japan
Division of Gene Regulation and Signal Transduction, Research Center for Genomic Medicine, Saitama Medical University, 1397-1 Yamane, Hidaka-shi, Saitama 350-1241, Japan

Mario Cozzolino, Michela Mangano and Andrea Galassi
Renal Division, Department of Health Sciences, University of Milan, 20142 Milan, Italy

Paola Ciceri and Piergiorgio Messa
Renal Research Laboratory, Department of Nephrology, Dialysis and Renal Transplant, Fondazione IRCCS Ca' Granda, Ospedale Maggiore Policlinico & Fondazione D'Amico per la Ricerca sulle Malattie Renali, 20122 Milan, Italy

Sagar Nigwekar
Department of Medicine, Division of Nephrology, Massachusetts General Hospital, Boston, MA 02114, USA

Junshi Doi, Amika Moro, Masato Fujiki, Bijan Eghtesad, Cristiano Quintini, Koji Hashimoto and Kazunari Sasaki
Department of General Surgery, Digestive Disease & Surgery Institute, Cleveland Clinic, Cleveland, OH 44195, USA

K. V. Narayanan Menon
Department of Gastroenterology and Hepatology, Cleveland Clinic, Cleveland, OH 44195, USA

Irma Elisa Cupone, Eleonora Dellera, Fabio Marra and Andrea Maria Giori
IBSA Farmaceutici Italia, 26900 Lodi, Italy

Atsushi Shioi and Tetsuo Shoji
Department of Vascular Medicine and Vascular Science Center for Translational Research, Osaka City University Graduate School of Medicine, Osaka 545-8585, Japan

Tomoaki Morioka and Masanori Emoto
Department of Metabolism, Endocrinology, and Molecular Medicine, Osaka City University Graduate School of Medicine, Osaka 545-85858, Japan

Eliza Glowka, Joanna Stasiak and Janina Lulek
Department of Pharmaceutical Technology, Poznan University of Medical Sciences, 6 Grunwaldzka Street, 60-780 Poznan, Poland

Emmanuelle Reboul
Aix Marseille University, INRA, INSERM, C2VN, 13005 Marseille, France

Johannes Oldenburg
Institute of Experimental Haematology and Transfusion Medicine, University Clinic Bonn, Bonn 53105, Germany

Carville G. Bevans
Im Hermeshain 6, Frankfurt am Main 60388, Germany

Martin Schubert, Stefan Kluge, Lisa Schmölz and Stefan Lorkowski
Department of Biochemistry and Physiology of Nutrition, Friedrich-Schiller-University Jena, 07743 Jena, Germany
Competence Center for Nutrition and Cardiovascular Health (nutriCARD), Halle-Jena-Leipzig, 07743 Jena, Germany

Maria Wallert
Department of Biochemistry and Physiology of Nutrition, Friedrich-Schiller-University Jena, 07743 Jena, Germany
Baker IDI Heart and Diabetes Institute, Melbourne VIC 3004, Australia

Francesco Galli
Department of Pharmaceutical Sciences, Laboratory of Nutrition and Clinical Biochemistry, University of Perugia, 06123 Perugia, Italy

Marc Birringer
Department of Nutrition, Food and Consumer Sciences, University of Applied Sciences Fulda, 36037 Fulda, Germany

Katrin J. Czogalla
Institute of Experimental Hematology and Transfusion Medicine, University Clinic Bonn, Bonn 53105, Germany

Johannes Oldenburg
Institute of Experimental Hematology and Transfusion Medicine, University Clinic Bonn, Bonn 53105, Germany
Center for Rare Diseases Bonn (ZSEB), University Clinic Bonn, Bonn 53127, Germany

Siti Syairah Mohd Mutalip
Faculty of Pharmacy, Universiti Teknologi MARA (UiTM) Puncak Alam Campus, Selangor 42300, Malaysia

Sharaniza Ab-Rahim and Mohd Hamim Rajikin
Faculty of Medicine, Universiti Teknologi MARA (UiTM) Sg. Buloh Campus, Selangor 42300, Malaysia

Emily S. Mohn, Nirupa R. Matthan, Chung-Yen Oliver Chen and Elizabeth J. Johnson
Jean Mayer US Department of Agriculture Human Nutrition Research Center on Aging, Tufts University, Boston, MA 02111, USA

Matthew J. Kuchan
Discovery Research, Abbott Nutrition, Columbus, OH 43229, USA

John W. Erdman Jr.
Department of Food Science and Human Nutrition, University of Illinois at Urbana-Champaign, Urbana, IL 61802, USA

Martha Neuringer
Oregon National Primate Research Center, Oregon Health and Science University, Beaverton, OR 97006, USA

Christoph Krettler and Christoph Reinhart
Department of Molecular Membrane Biology, Max Planck Institute of Biophysics, 60388 Frankfurt am Main, Germany

Matthias Watzka and Johannes Oldenburg
Institute of Experimental Haematology and Transfusion Medicine, University Clinic Bonn, 53105 Bonn, Germany

Hamza El Hadi, Roberto Vettor and Marco Rossato
Internal Medicine 3, Department of Medicine—DIMED, University of Padova, Via Giustiniani 2, 35128 Padova, Italy

Raffaella Comitato, Roberto Ambra and Fabio Virgili
Council for Agricultural Research and Economics, Research Centre for Food and Nutrition (CREA-AN) via Ardeatina 546, 00178 Rome, Italy

Index